Carla Curtis covers extensive ground in her powerful in-depth coverage of modern-day and antiquated gender myths. Her thought-provoking book brings understanding to how the resurgence of inflexible stereotypical gender roles is causing less freedom, less acceptance, and more regression and harm to anyone who does not fit nicely in the conventional female or male box. A must-read.

—Erin Friday, Esq.
co-lead of Our Duty USA (www.OurDuty.group/usa) and
Protect Kids California (www. ProtectKidsCA.com),
support networks for parents who wish to protect their children from gender ideology

Parents deserve accurate information when making decisions for their children and unfortunately American medical institutions have not been honest with them about the harms of puberty blockers and cross sex hormones. I am incredibly thankful for all of the members of Gays Against Groomers standing in solidarity with Moms for Liberty as we work to protect all of our children. *The Gender Trap* brilliantly lays out the case as to why transitioning children is the greatest medical abuse scandal we have ever seen in our country. I believe that when parents have accurate information about the irreversible harms of these drugs and surgeries, we will see a drastic drop in the amount of parents agreeing to put their children through it.

—Tiffany Justice
award-winning journalist and
co-founder, Moms for Liberty (www.MomsForLiberty.org),
an organization that stands up for parental rights at all levels of government

Gender ideology is a regressive, homophobic cult, teaching vulnerable kids who defy stereotypes that they might have been born in the wrong body. It especially preys on children with autism, and those who would grow up to be gay. *The Gender Trap* beautifully lays out everything you need to know to protect your kids from the greatest child abuse scandal in modern history.

—Chris Elston (Billboard Chris),
activist and gender dysphoria critic (www.BillboardChris.com)

It's about time this book got written. A radical, destructive movement that targets our children and our society has taken over, and it has done so by hiding behind the good names of gays and lesbians around the world. This book is a clear explanation and a much-needed antidote to this wicked movement in our society.

—James Lindsay, Ph.D.
 author and social critic,
 founder of New Discourses,
 and co-author of Cynical Theories: How Activist Scholarship Made Everything About Race, Gender, and Identity—and Why This Harms Everybody

I'm old enough to remember how absolutely awful gay conversion therapy was—as though through therapy, someone could be somehow talked out of being gay. Jump to 2024, and there seems to be little to no discussion in the medical community or society at large about how much worse and evil are today's child surgical mutilations and chemical conversions called puberty blockers (repurposed castration drugs). Laying out the history and science debunking the most stereotypical nonsensical reasoning for these drastic life-altering procedures that were literally laughed at only a few short years ago—namely that only boys play with trucks and only girls play with dolls—Carla Curtis of Gays Against Groomers methodically breaks down the myths and cuts through the lies of medicine's biggest malpractice and crime since lobotomies.

—Rob Schneider
 American actor, comedian, screenwriter, and director

This book helps readers demystify gender ideology and its pervasive institutional capture of all aspects of American life.

—Andy Ngo
 Journalist and author

There aren't many groups braver than Gays Against Groomers. Imagine the threats they get and the abuse they take. Who'd sign up for something like that? Only someone who really meant it, and who understood the stakes. The rest of us ought to be grateful for what they've done—and for this book.

—Tucker Carlson
 American political commentator and author

The Gender Trap

**The Trans Agenda's
War Against Children**

© 2024 by Carla Curtis

Gays Against Groomers Publishing

The Gender Trap: The Trans Agenda's War Against Children
© 2024 by Carla Curtis

Published by:

Gays Against Groomers
333 W Brown Deer Road, Suite G4100
Bayside, Wisconsin 53217

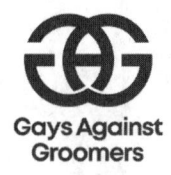

Cover and graphics: Jaimee Michell
Text formatting and layout: Carla Curtis
Text templates: Nicolas Blooms
Index: Carla Curtis
Editorial advice: Michael Costa

Attention vendors:

For wholesale and bulk orders, contact info@GaysAgainstGroomers.com

for more information:

www.GaysAgainstGroomers.com
www.TheGenderTrap.com

ISBN: 978-0-9668352-4-3

Any use of this intellectual property for text and data mining or computational analysis, including as training material for artificial intelligence systems, is strictly prohibited without express written consent.

This book is dedicated to all people
who have the courage to live and love
with the bodies they were dealt,
and who do not see themselves as victims,
but instead approach life
with grace, discernment,
and reverent respect.

Acknowledgements

It's not often that I, as a writer, feel that my words are inadequate. But to say that I appreciate the enthusiastic support of Gays Against Groomers is an understatement. My most heartfelt thanks go to a small but dynamic core group. Their excitement about this manuscript has given me inspiration and energy to expand, organize, and polish it in ways that I otherwise would not have. It has truly been a privilege getting to know some of these extraordinary people.

Robert Wallace, with his generous welcoming spirit, was my initial contact with Gays Against Groomers. His passion for saving children, spiritual development, and serving the general public through many different venues has led to his hosting The Dark Side of the Rainbow podcast. Robert was also featured in the must-see 2024 documentary, *Beneath Sheep's Clothing*.

Michael Costa, head of Gays Against Groomers Publishing, impressed me with his encyclopedic grasp of research and legislation. I greatly enjoyed our exhilarating talks, which reminded me of an earlier (and saner) era. Michael's encouragement, eloquence, and always candid editorial advice helped make this a better book. I also thank his team of volunteers who spent many hours proofreading.

Nicolas Blooms, wise beyond his years, lovingly and patiently held my hand while I navigated the typesetting program used for this manuscript. He offered not only assistance, but friendship. I will always treasure his luminous presence.

Sasha Leigh brought the same skill to the book's distribution that she devotes to Gays Against Groomers in her role of Executive Director and Treasurer. I am truly in awe of her organizational talent and am very grateful for her assistance.

Last but not least, I thank graphic artist Jaimee Michell, who not only designed the cover for this book, but is the inspired founder of Gays Against Groomers and created its spectacular logo. Since its inception in 2022, Gays Against Groomers has made a considerable impact on public awareness and convinced lawmakers to pass legislation that safeguards children from physical and psychological harm. I deeply appreciate Jaimee's tireless promotion and masterful outreach to ensure that *The Gender Trap* reaches a diverse and wide-ranging audience.

As appreciative as I am to Gays Against Groomers members for their support and material assistance, I am also indebted to them on a deeply personal level. Their insight, bravery, and unwavering commitment to the truth have given me hope for the future of humankind. Thank you for helping to save our children.

TABLE OF CONTENTS

FOREWORD   xi

INTRODUCTION   xiii

PART I. BIOLOGY

Chapter 1. Male and Female Development   3
Beyond Nature   3
Hormones, Body Structure, and Physiology   3
The Brain   7
    Neuroplasticity of the Brain   7
    The Corpus Callosum Conundrum   9
    Male and Female Brains: Fact or Fable?   11
    Some Neurotransmitters and Their Effects   21
Divergences of Sexual Development, Including Intersexuals   24
    Atypical Chromosomes and Hormonal Departures   24
    Some Common Variations   27
    Surgical "Corrections"   32
Categorizing Versus Assigning   38

PART II. CULTURE

Chapter 2. Sex Role Stereotypes   43
Clarifying Gender   43
Fraudulent Research   45
Masculinity and Femininity   48
Expectations of Stereotyped Gendered Behavior   51
    Epigenetics: Imprinting the Brain   51
    Girls and Boys in School   55
    The Math Myth   58
    Verbal Virtuosity and Spatial Skill   61
    Boys Aren't Good at Feelings   65
    Girls Aren't Good at Science   70
    The "Niceness" Syndrome   74
    Empathy Quotient, Motherhood, and Fatherhood   76
    Clothes Make the Man—and Woman   80
Sex Role Nonconformity: Homosexuals, Lesbians and Bisexuals   82

PART III. THE TRANS AGENDA

Chapter 3. Becoming Transgender   87
- Gender "Reassignment" Basics   87
  - Overview   87
  - What Should Happen   88
  - What Really Happens   89
  - Parents As Enemies   93
- Hormones that Give Males Some Features of Females   95
- Hormones that Give Females Some Features of Males   97
- Puberty Blockers for Children   98
- Surgeries for Males Who Want to Resemble Females (MtF)   105
- Surgeries for Females Who Want to Resemble Males (FtM)   107

Chapter 4. Gender Dysphoria and Mental Illness   109
- Fallout of the "Wrong Body" Myth   109
- Civil Rights and Violence   118
- The Suicide Threat   122
  - Falsified Data   122
  - Drug-Induced Death   125
- Drugs and Surgeries Versus Psychotherapy   128

Chapter 5. Why Someone Might Transition   131
- What Am I?   131
- Before the Trend   132
- Boys   133
- Girls   139
- Children Who Have Divergences of Sexual Development   144
- Men   145
- Women   148
- Adults Who Have Divergences of Sexual Development   153

Chapter 6. Trans Regret and Detransitioners   157
    Roadblocks to Detransitioning   157
    Detransitioner Accounts   162

Chapter 7. Who's Behind the Trans Agenda   175
    Transgendering is Expensive   175
    Bombardment from All Sides   177
    Politics in Our Pants   183
    Transhumanism, a Step Up   186

Chapter 8. Stifling Dissent   191
    The Adulteration of Language and Use of Reversals   191
        Language as Propaganda   191
        Being "Affirmed"   192
        What Member of the Alphabet Are You?   193
        "Cis" Terminology   194
        Words That Eliminate Women   196
    Punishing the Non-Believers   200
    The Cult(ure) of Victimhood   206
    Legal Battles   214

PART IV. HEALING

Chapter 9. Making Peace With Your Birth Body   221
    Emotional Awareness   221
        The Mind-Body Connection   221
        A Strong Foundation in Genuine Pleasure   231
    Confronting Trauma   235
    How to Help Children (and Adults) Considering Transition   238
    Beyond Stereotypes   242
        What Equality Really Means   242
        A Stereotype-Free World   246

Appendix A. Highlights of the Gender Wars 251
    First Wave Feminism 251
    Second Wave Feminism 254
    Third Wave Feminism 258
        Phony Feminists 258
        Toxic Masculinity 258
        Toxic Femininity 262
        Male Bashing 264
        The Aborting of Girls 264
        Rape 266
        The Enemy Within 274

Appendix B. Transgender Athletes in Sports 275
    Biology and Physiology of Male and Female Athletes 275
    Male-Born Transgenders (MtFs) Who Compete Against Women 279
        The First MtF Trans Athlete 279
        Same Privilege, New Package 280
        Men in Women's Spaces 285
        Injuries 288
    Female-Born Transgenders (FtMs) Who Compete Against Men 290
    Intersex Individuals Who Compete in Sports 292
    The Future of Sports 298
        Lawsuits 298
        Quitting 299
        Rules That Don't Apply to Everyone 300
        Where To Go From Here 303

Notes 305

Selected References 363

Index 379

About the Author and Gays Against Groomers 387

Resources 388

Foreword

When I founded Gays Against Groomers in 2022, I had no idea it would become the powerful force it is today. I began the organization because I could no longer stand idly by as a full-scale assault on children unfolded before my eyes, and I figured it was time to stand up and fight back. Our organization serves as a rallying cry from *within* the gay community. We needed a movement with *teeth*—one that loudly advocates not only for equality but also for the well-being of society as a whole. It is a call to action against a system hell-bent on sexualizing, indoctrinating, and mutilating children. Gays Against Groomers is on a mission, and we will not stop until the war on children is ended.

The heart of our advocacy lies in safeguarding children from irreversible harm. What masquerades as "gender-affirming care" is, in actuality, an attempt at conversion—and is a form of medical abuse. Subjecting children to procedures that rob them of their identity and sterilize their bodies is morally bankrupt. The ramifications last a lifetime. Through legislative action and grassroots efforts, we've done outreach, disseminated information, and helped pass laws to prohibit these barbaric practices. As of this writing, twenty-two states have passed legislation to ban the sexual mutilation of minors—rightfully so. And we are working to get legislation passed in every state of the U.S.

The so-called scientific research supporting this medical malpractice of transgendering is riddled with faulty statistics and ideological biases. These lies have become perceived as facts due to their propagation by non-governmental organizations (NGOs), which have created a framework that is not grounded in physical reality. In less than a decade, the medically abusive practices have already had disastrous consequences on the gay community and on an entire generation of children. This book provides a thoroughly cited compilation of data and studies on the topic, offering an accurate understanding of the current state of affairs.

When Carla Curtis approached us with her manuscript, she was concerned that its candid language might deter publishers. It was difficult for her to find a platform for her unapologetic narrative, and she sought a home for her work among those unafraid to confront uncomfortable truths. We embraced Carla's project wholeheartedly, driven by our dedication to showing people the truth, regardless of potential backlash or hurt feelings. In *The Gender Trap*, Carla Curtis delivers a brilliant biopsychosocial analysis of sex and gender, delving into the corrupt underpinnings of gender ideology while shedding light on the need to separate gay liberation from trans activism. Curtis exposes how the trans agenda is the most anti-gay movement of our time, utterly antithetical to the very essence of gay liberation. Carla Curtis's personal history, rooted in both women's rights and gay and bisexual activism, gives her a unique perspective on the societal onslaught of gender ideology. Drawing from decades of experience, she navigates the gender war with unwavering honesty, acknowledging that not every reader will agree with every point presented. Yet *The Gender Trap* still offers something unique and valuable for everyone—mothers, fathers, women, men, therapists, gays and lesbians, heterosexuals, detransitioners, and especially individuals who are questioning their identity. Throughout these pages, Curtis explains the incontrovertible facts of biology, leaving no questions unanswered. She reveals the fallacies perpetuated by the trans agenda and analyzes its insidious nature and dire consequences, particularly for children. She exposes the dark forces and financial interests driving the trans agenda. And she dismantles the ideological biases that have allowed the radical transgender movement to thrive.

The Gender Trap stands as a reminder that there is nothing hateful about speaking the truth, nor is there anything wrong with clarifying and defending biological reality. The timely and urgent publication of this book cannot be overstated. As gender ideology permeates and erodes the fabric of our institutions, wreaking havoc and silencing dissenting voices, *The Gender Trap* stands as a fearless reminder that tyranny cannot prevail, and gives readers the inspiration to speak out against the encroachment of the trans agenda—either through individual acts of courage, or with the support of groups like Gays Against Groomers. This book urges us to stand united in our commitment to a future grounded in rationality, where "equality" and "discovering one's identity" do not occur at the expense of society's most vulnerable.

The Gender Trap is a testament to the resilience of the gay community that, even in the face of adversity, is unwilling to make peace with a belief system that puts children in danger. The talented members of Gays Against Groomers who brought this project to life refuse to sugarcoat the horrors of the biggest medical scandal since the lobotomy, thus giving a voice to the millions of gay people who disagree with the human atrocities being pushed in their name. This is *our* side of the story—one grounded in facts, not propaganda. As the trans agenda crumbles under the weight of its own corruption, *The Gender Trap* stands as a beacon of hope for those who refuse to comply with or blindly follow a destructive path. Let this book serve as a *public record* of our refusal to surrender to tyranny. And let *The Gender Trap* be testimony to our resistance against an agenda that threatens to undermine the progress we have fought so hard to achieve. The time to speak out is now—and this written masterpiece provides the platform for those voices to finally be heard.

Jaimee Michell
Founder, President & CEO
Gays Against Groomers

Introduction

The second wave women's liberation movement, which began in the 1960s and gained momentum well into the 1980s, had many facets to it. "Equal rights for women" meant that women deserved the same pay as men for equivalent work. Women also demanded opportunities for professional advancement based on their skill and competence rather than their reproductive organs. Intimate connections were not exempt from scrutiny, either: Women wanted sexual relationships based on mutual caring and respect between peers, without coercion. Behind all these demands for change, the one unifying question—which we are still grappling with today—was what it meant to be male and what it meant to be female.

Back then, there was no aspect of living that sexual stereotypes didn't touch: work, play, education, entertainment, relationships. Both women and men grappled with society's expectations of what was supposed to be the correct behaviors and aspirations for each. As studies showed, women were assumed to be passive and men, assertive. Women were emotional and even hysterical, while men were rational and often stoic. Women could be nurses but it was not common for them to be doctors, and for men it was the opposite. It wasn't considered feminine for women to be corporate executives, just as it wasn't considered masculine for a man to be happy at home changing diapers while his wife was out working. It was widely assumed that males and females had different aptitudes. Males were perceived as better at science and math while females were understood to be more verbally skilled. These beliefs, which feminists called "sex role stereotypes," were so ingrained that they were accepted as immutable. A few innovative scholars pointed out that studies designed to detect differences in mental capacities between men and women contained inherent design flaws. Researchers selectively presented data from their experiments that confirmed only what they already believed. As it was eventually discovered, which I'll address in detail in Chapter 2, a great deal of scientific bias was indeed forcing both females and males into a box. Educational institutions, aligned with the bias of scientists, were eager to reinforce sex roles—to the detriment of everybody. Even the entertainment industry promoted stereotypes. In films and television, caricatures of women and men were almost constantly pitted against each other. The hostility between them, called "the battle of the sexes," was callously encouraged by the media as coy entertainment.

Adherence to sex role stereotypes played a huge role in society's intolerance of homosexuality. By definition, a romantic relationship consisted of polar opposites—someone who was masculine (a male) and someone who was feminine (a female). But if both partners in a couple were men or both partners were women, who was the male and who was the female? It was a confusing time indeed for those whose lives were based on faithfully adhering to culturally defined sex roles. Stereotypes informed everything that we were taught about how the world was supposed to operate. Although culturally assigned scripts often conflicted with who they actually were, both men and women felt obliged to follow them to be accepted—or at least achieve the appearance of respectability.

Second wave feminists worked as hard as they did to eliminate sex role stereotyping because they wanted to ensure greater freedom of choice in all areas of life, both professionally and personally. Increasing numbers of women became doctors rather than nurses, and corporate executives instead of secretaries. Men began to relax as the burden of earning a living for an entire family was shared by their spouses. As more men explored their emotional lives—realizing that they could retain their strength and self-respect while allowing themselves to be more emotionally vulnerable—they discovered the fulfillment that greater intimacy with their partners and friends could bring. Some women started feeling more comfortable with their choice not to have children at all. And an admittedly small handful of fathers stayed home with their sons and daughters while their wives worked outside the home. Men who supported the women's liberation movement understood that sex role stereotypes were unfair to everyone, not just women. We don't hear much today about the pro-feminist men's movement, but back then it had considerable visibility and was a powerful catalyst for the personal growth of men and boys.

Sadly, the progress that women and men made is not only at a standstill today, it's backsliding. Just when our culture was becoming more balanced, a sabotage of enormous magnitude began to occur. We no longer hear the phrases *sex role stereotypes* or *gender roles*, which had been used by feminists to mean the same thing. Instead, *gender* is now being used to designate someone who is either biologically male or female—a confusing and deceptive replacement for the uncomplicated and straightforward word *sex*. This linguistic shift allowed biological sex (someone is male or female, based on their reproductive organs) and sex roles (different behavior and aptitudes expected for males and females) to merge into the single word *gender*. This merging of two distinctly different concepts has not only caused enormous confusion for both the lay public and scientists, but it serves an insidious agenda. If people—young people especially, born post-1980 after the second wave feminist movement was dwindling down—conflate biological sex with sex roles, and their interests don't fit the conventional roles that they're taught belong to a specific set of reproductive organs, then surely they must be in the wrong body. Now the sabotage, for which the ground had been carefully cultivated, can be seen in stark relief. It's none other than the rapidly growing radical transgender movement, whose entire reason for existing is to convince the public—especially children, who grew up with the linguistic deception—that they need to change their bodies to fit their preferred roles.

The word *transgender* comes from the Latin *trans*, which means "across," "beyond," "through," "on the other side of," "to go beyond," and *gender*, which (depending on the source) refers either to the behavioral, cultural and psychological traits typically associated with one sex, or to one's biological sex itself.[1] People who consider themselves transgender say that they do not mentally or emotionally identify with their natal bodies, the biology they were born with. A man will insist that he is actually a woman, while a woman will declare that she is in fact a man. Very young children are especially vulnerable to falling prey to this mindset, as verified by a number of internet videos featuring boys who state with complete conviction that they are really girls. With their long hair, frilly dresses, and angelic pretty faces untouched by the onslaught of pubescent hormones, they certainly look the part. But transgenderism constitutes much more than dressing in clothing commonly ascribed to the opposite sex. In an effort to cosmetically transform their bodies, people are taking hormones in massively larger amounts than what their own bodies naturally produce and were innately designed to handle. Many are also receiving surgery. Women who want to be men are having their breasts removed, and men who want to be women are receiving breast implants. In addition, a small percentage of men and women are undergoing even more radical plastic surgery. Genitals are remodeled, reshaped, or removed. Some subjects are even having their faces sculpted. A surgeon might shave off part of a man's Adam's apple, chin and brow to create a softer look, or augment the chin line of a woman to create a more chiseled appearance.

Transgenders, who are regularly being spotlighted in the news today, haven't always been this visible. In the mid-1950s, a man who became known as Christine Jorgensen was the first well-known recipient of sexual "reassignment" surgery in the United States. The mid-1970s featured MtF (male-to-female) transgender, Renée Richards, who competed in women's professional tennis amid much controversy. In 1979, one of the first critiques of the practice of transgendering was published: Janice Raymond's *The Transsexual Empire: The Making of the She-Male*. The publication of Raymond's book reflected, as well as inflamed, the intense disagreements among feminists about allowing transsexuals (as transgenders were known at that time) in women-only spaces. Lesbian feminists especially opposed the presence, and even the concept, of trans "women." Nevertheless, in the 1980s and 1990s, organizations of gay men and women chose to form an alliance with people who identified as trans. All of the so-called sexually deviant minorities, as the majority culture saw them, were lumped together—even though sexual orientation (designating to whom one is sexually attracted) is not the same as actually perceiving oneself as the opposite sex. Appended to the acronym LGB, short for "lesbian, gay and bisexual," was T for "transgender." Still later "queer" was added, resulting in LGBTQ.

That string of letters keeps getting longer as more labels are deemed necessary, but it was the "T" in that political alphabet soup that began to turn back the clock at warp speed. Documentaries extolled boys, girls, men and women who came out as transgender. There was a proliferation of websites advising adults and even children how to manifest their true trans selves—in other words, take high-dose hormones and undergo surgery to alter genitals and perhaps other body parts.

Transgenderism was celebrated as a courageous act of liberation when in fact it was based on a slavish adherence to sex role stereotypes. These stereotypes, which for so long had so rigidly circumscribed men's and women's behaviors and goals—and from which people were finally starting to break free—returned with a vengeance.

In 2014, Sheila Jeffreys published her well-researched book *Gender Hurts: A feminist analysis of the politics of transgenderism*. Jeffreys focused chiefly on the psychological and social damage to straight and gay women that transgenderism causes. Not surprisingly, transgenders found her book highly controversial and tried to silence her. In 2020, Abigail Shrier's *Irreversible Damage: The Transgender Craze Seducing Our Daughters*, focused on how social media, peer pressure, and negative attitudes toward maturing encourage thousands of teenage girls to wish they were boys, and how the medical industry is happy to oblige. The author did not condemn transgenders per se; in fact, she pointed out that she became friends with several trans individuals. Her focus was strictly on impressionable teenage girls who are too young to understand the ramifications of receiving dangerous levels of hormones and life-altering surgery at a young age. Nevertheless, like the authors before her, Shrier was maligned by radical trans activists and unfairly branded as transphobic (the fear or hatred of transgenders). In 2023, psychiatrist Miriam Grossman published *Lost in Trans Nation: A Child Psychiatrist's Guide Out of the Madness*. Dr. Grossman emphasized the dangers of cross-sex hormones and genital surgeries to help parents and children understand what they're getting into should they decide to follow the transgender path. Critics of the trans activist agenda—medical professionals, psychotherapists, journalists, and even some transgenders themselves—are continuing to speak out against attempts to indoctrinate impressionable children. People who had started or completed the transgendering process and then decided that it was a mistake, are also coming forward.

Why has there been an explosion of transgenderism in the last decade? Who is ideologically and financially behind the trans movemen? What is the proper medical procedure for evaluating people in a gender "reassignment" clinic and what is actually occurring? What kinds of medical, psychological, and social problems plague people who believe that they're trans—and what problems existed before the individuals even began their trans journey? What are the negative effects and complications of cross-sex hormones and surgeries—complications that most medical professionals are reluctant to disclose? Most importantly, what makes children, teens, the gay community, and people with ambiguous genitalia especially vulnerable to the trans agenda? How are they being convinced they're the opposite sex, and how can we counteract that manipulation? Finally, what do we need to know in order to help people feel whole and accept themselves, so that hormones and surgeries are not considered necessary?

My search for answers led me to a wide range of disciplines: biology, physiology, medicine, psychology, sociology, politics, feminist history, and even economics. The answers are complex and multifaceted. But what consistently appears as the key to advancing the transgender scheme is sex role stereotypes, which some people simply call "gender."

We cannot understand or resist transgender ideology unless we have a grounding in basic science. Part I, "Biology," is devoted to the sexual development of males and females. The data I summarize describes differences between the sexes on chromosomal, hormonal, biological, anatomical, and physiological levels. There are psychological differences, too, but these are often exaggerated by environment and upbringing, and what those differences are depend on the culture in which one is raised. Scientific researchers, themselves products of stereotyped upbringing, almost always allow cultural bias to color their experiments—which means that conclusions about sex-linked differences are not necessarily correct. That is why I devote considerable space to discussing brain research, including the science of epigenetics that shows the enormous potential for mental flexibility. Vital to this section is a discussion of people whose genitals don't conform to rigid and arbitrary standards of appearance and as a result, have become casualties of gender stereotyping in palpably cruel ways.

Part II, "Culture," explores important differences between sex (biology) and gender (societal beliefs). Some studies that were intended to settle the "nature versus nurture" debate yielded unanticipated results, very different from what the experimenters had expected to find. Research on boys' and girls' aptitudes in math, science, spatial acumen, and verbal skills shows how the prejudices of parents and teachers reinforce boys' and girls' weaknesses as well as their strengths. There are many assumptions we make about the emotional lives of boys and girls and men and women, and this too is explored in depth. Also covered are biases against males and females in the professions, and how the clothing we wear defines us. Finally, I discuss sexual orientation and the connection (or lack of it) between transgenders and the gay community, whose members are dwindling as a result of the trans agenda.

Each of the many chapters in Part III, "The Trans Agenda," details an aspect of transgender life. In order to craft a body intended to resemble that of the opposite sex, immense medical manipulation is involved. Taking high doses of hormones and undergoing sexual "reassignment" surgery are not only dangerous, but they have complicated and far-reaching effects. Becoming a transgender, which can happen only slowly over time, requires immense effort, dedication, and financial resources. It also involves unimaginable physical pain, even under the most favorable circumstances when there are no complications from surgery. Mental illness, gender dysphoria and trans suicide are discussed, and some of the data may surprise you. The question "Why would someone want to transition?" is addressed as well. The reasons are complex. Because the reasons are different for boys, girls, men and women, I give each group its own section.

Part III also devotes a chapter to detransitioners—people who started to transition, and then decided they weren't transgender after all. The poignant personal accounts will move you. These accounts describe unhappy childhoods and sometimes sexual trauma, but what they all have in common is extreme psychological manipulation. Anyone who's considering making a radical change to their body will want to read what these detransitioners faced. Another chapter discusses some of the people and institutions behind the trans movement—among them, powerful and wealthy politicians (one of them a well-known transgender individual)—who fund hospitals, clinics, mainstream media, schools, universities, and other institutions. Finally, in Part III, I discuss ways in which those who object to the trans movement are being deliberately misrepresented, threatened, undermined, and silenced. Various forms of manipulation, rather than being random, have been systematically and steadily occurring for some time. Because language directly informs how we see the world, the trans strategy relies heavily on the manipulation of language. Some of the language has become so entrenched that the indoctrination has become invisible. The deconstruction of these linguistic mind games will help you resist the trans agenda. Close accomplices of this agenda, educational institutions, are also using such tactics. But they are also destabilizing students in other ways—ways that are so insidious, it can be hard to recognize them. After reading this section, you will understand the extent to which this agenda has taken hold, and will be able to take steps to diffuse the numerous attempts that are being made to cripple our nation's youth.

Solid research continues to show that most people who are drawn toward transgendering need counseling, not hormones and surgery. Part IV, "Healing," addresses in detail what happens to us—emotionally, physically, mentally, energetically, and spiritually—when we are not willing or able to face difficult experiences and traumas. The section on how to help those considering transition contains a list of carefully worded questions that parents can ask young children and teens and adults can ask themselves, with additional questions that can be introduced by experienced psychotherapists. These questions are designed to help people break free of stereotypes and access the root causes of why they might wish to escape their body. Prospective trans candidates who contemplate these issues will think hard about making decisions that are likely to impact them negatively for the rest of their lives.

There are two chapter-long appendices related to the main topic of this book. Appendix A is for readers who wonder how—from the time of the second wave feminist movement—we regressed from approaching a more egalitarian climate to the current backlash against both women and men. A half century ago, while some issues did elicit passionate debate, the dialogue was much more rational than it is today, where it's becoming increasingly common to malign a person simply for possessing a penis. I am of course, referring to the practice known as male bashing. In addition, I address not only toxic masculinity but also toxic femininity—because in our polarized world, neither can exist without its counterpart. The selective aborting of female fetuses is discussed in depth as well as rape, which unfortunately is now being widely perpetrated on both sexes. In today's climate, there are many institutionalized ways in which people mistreat each other irrespective of sex or gender roles.

Appendix B is devoted to the ramifications of transgenders infiltrating amateur and professional sports for both females and males. This includes biological men who claim to be transgender or "identify" as female, and compete against natal women. Intersexuals are included in this discussion—an even more complex and multifaceted issue that requires some novel analysis and out-of-the-box thinking.

During the writing of this book, I thought a great deal about my readers. People from all walks of life, of all ages, races and sexual orientations, and across the entire political spectrum, are recognizing the dangers of the trans agenda. But with such a diverse audience, it can be difficult to use language with which everyone agrees or feels comfortable. I have done my best to clearly define terms and concepts so there can be no mistake about my intentions. However, because in today's climate there can be so much misunderstanding, I want to make some additional points now.

The following remarks are directed to women, some of whom may consider themselves feminists. In the past, the biological, physiological, and psychological differences between women and men have been both exaggerated and minimized by women's rights advocates. These two extreme positions, while contradicting each other, have always shared the goal of helping women attain full social, professional, legal, and sexual equality. While it was incorrect to claim that sex-linked differences were essentially nonexistent, this was done because of the valid fear that differences (including reproductive functions) would be used to justify the subordination of women. I need to emphasize that whatever differences do exist do not indicate value judgments of better or worse. Nor do they justify mistreatment or the withholding of opportunities. It's important for women to remember this, even if some institutions and individuals still behave as though females are inferior and disposable.

My next comments are directed to men, especially those who have negative associations with feminism. When I participated in the second wave feminist movement, I was gratified and uplifted to see men work alongside women. Everyone recognized the common goal: to promote respect between the sexes and more freedom and opportunities for everyone. But those were very different times. As I will show in later chapters, the political machine that has financially supported radical trans activists has also infiltrated virtually every aspect of our lives, including the feminist movement. This same machine also owns mainstream media. That is why television programs, movies, and even advertisements have started to portray men in a disparaging manner. And it's why we are seeing an increase in the belittling and demonizing of males, especially white males. There is also a very small but vocal minority of women who are bashing males. They see all men through the most extreme stereotype and regard every problem in the world as exclusively the fault of men. These saboteurs are not feminists and they do not represent the majority of females. However, their visibility is sowing the seeds of distress and hatred. I am asking men to keep in mind that none of the divisive elements represent, or speak for, those of us who are trying to implement genuine positive change. If men can avoid being baited, they can utilize the power they still have in the world to help humanity through some very rough times.

The one question I keep asking throughout this book is why we must automatically accept gender roles as an inevitable and necessary part of life. To some readers, questioning sexual stereotypes—or disregarding them entirely—may feel like a defiance of the laws of nature. But as I will show in many ways, human beings have the capacity to express an almost unlimited range of behaviors. If some of our inclinations happen to correspond to those of a culturally typical male or a culturally typical female, there's nothing wrong with that. But let it be a choice, rather than the result of explicit or implicit cultural coercion. We have the right to our preferences, and to behave in ways that might or might not conform to an assigned role, as long as we are not physically inflicting harm or infringing on the rights of others.

The trend toward transgenderism, rather than representing freedom from the so-called binary system of gendered attitudes, is instead forcing us to be even more firmly entrenched in them—and in the most stereotypical ways possible. Yet despite the enormous harm caused by the radical trans movement, we can still extract a positive message from the rubble: *It's possible to live a life free of gender stereotypes*. At the very least, our freedom from stereotypes is something to which we should all aspire, as it can only lead to a richer life. We may lose the love and respect of some, but we'll gain it from others. Most importantly, we will have more love and respect for ourselves. Refusing to be limited by gender roles is the most effective way to resist the trans agenda. It's also the most effective way to protect our children. The world is at a crisis point. We urgently need to reevaluate our ideas about what it means to be male and female.

It is my earnest hope that this book will help bring about a new era of accepting who we truly are, inside and out.

Carla Curtis, Gays Against Groomers
United States, 2024

PART I

BIOLOGY

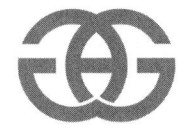

1

MALE AND FEMALE DEVELOPMENT

Beyond Nature

Young people today are facing a crisis that their parents are unlikely to have ever experienced: the notion that the bodies they were born with are not the bodies they were meant to have. All across the globe, and most certainly in the United States, people are going to great lengths to alter their physical appearance so they can resemble the opposite sex as much as possible. In order to advance the belief that people are born into the wrong body, radical transgender activists and their allies are challenging the reality of basic biology. We are being told that males can become females and females can become males. Simple biology has not only been vilified, but outright misrepresented and reversed.

Can men really transform into women, and can women really transform into men? To find out, we need to review some basic biology, physiology, and anatomy.

Hormones, Body Structure, and Physiology

In high school, older students used to be taught the basics of human reproduction and development. It starts when a male's sperm cell and a female's egg—each containing 23 chromosomes—fuse together to form a single cell consisting of 46 chromosomes (23 pairs). *Chromosomes* are strands of very tightly coiled DNA, containing various biochemicals, that are located inside the nucleus of almost every cell in the body. Inside the chromosomes are thousands of smaller units called *genes*. Males and females share about 99.8 percent of the same genes.

Except when rare deviations occur (discussed later in this chapter), most human males have XY chromosomes and most human females have XX chromosomes.

We all start out in life the same, at least genitally speaking. The embryo begins with primitive reproductive glands called *gonads* whose appearance is neither male nor female. At about the seventh week of gestation, if the embryo possesses the XX chromosomes of a female, the gonads will become ovaries. If the embryo possesses the XY chromosomes of a male, the gonads will become testes. About one week later, the testes of a male start to produce masculinizing hormones including testosterone. It's the presence or absence of testosterone that exerts the most significant impact on the gestating male fetus. In female fetuses, there is no outpouring of testosterone. Secretions from the ovaries are not required for female sex differentiation, so the baby continues to develop into a female.[1] Nevertheless, as University of Melbourne associate professor Cordelia Fine points out, "Female development is as active and complex a process as male development....*many* genes are involved in sex determination: *SRY* [sex-determining region Y gene] on the Y chromosome; a few on the X chromosome...[and] surprisingly, dozens of others located on other chromosomes."[2] If testosterone output halts, the system is again female.

As the fetus continues to develop, the appearance of its genitals becomes more defined. During this process of sexual differentiation, the hormones that are produced suffuse both body and brain. The amounts of hormones depend on the sex of the fetus. After testosterone is introduced to males, it remains at a high peak until week 24 of gestation. There will be a surge of testosterone soon after birth, peaking when the child is three to four months, and again during puberty.[3]

Boys grow more quickly than girls due to their higher metabolic rate. Lise Eliot, associate professor of neuroscience at the Chicago Medical School of Rosalind Franklin University of Medicine and Science, hypothesizes that the higher metabolic rate allows a male embryo to develop testes before the mother's estrogen—which progressively rises during early pregnancy—hinders the further maturation of the male sex organs. The faster growth of boys means that they are born larger and heavier than girls. Their greater weight and mass make it more difficult for the mother to deliver, and with males there's a slightly longer labor. More boys than girls are born via C-section.

Many hormones are involved in the development of a human being. *Steroid hormones*, or simply *steroids*—which the body manufactures from cholesterol (produced mostly in the liver)—are secreted by three types of glands: the testes in a male, which rest inside the scrotum that hangs outside the body (referred to in slang as "balls"); the small, almond-shaped ovaries in a female, located in the abdominal cavity on either side of the uterus (womb); and in both males and females, the cortex of the adrenal glands, which rest on top of either kidney.

The adrenals are unusual because in many ways they act like two separate glands. The medulla (center) secretes different substances than the thin cortex that surrounds it. Hormones produced by the medulla include adrenaline (also known as epinephrine) and noradrenaline (or norepinephrine). Both are involved in the fight-or-flight response, which I'll discuss in detail in the final chapter. For now, I want to focus on the adrenal cortex. It creates hormones that are anti-inflammatory and help maintain normal blood pressure and the balance of salt and water in the body. But its secretions are also directly involved in sexual development.

Androgens is a catch-all term for any steroid hormone that has masculinizing effects. These hormones are vital to a male's sexual development, bestowing the characteristics that we associate with typical maleness. *Testosterone* is the most well known androgen. It's produced by the testes in fairly large amounts, by the ovaries in much smaller amounts, and in the adrenal cortex of both sexes in small amounts. In women, the skin, fat cells and liver can convert androgens into testosterone. Testosterone is largely responsible for the development and maintenance of reproductive function in men, as well as the stimulation of secondary sex characteristics such as body hair on the male during puberty. The same androgen hormones that make boys grow faster *in utero* tend to suppress immune function, which is probably why boys are more susceptible to ear and other types of infections in early life. Testosterone is very familiar to sports fans. Until the practice became illegal, many athletes (especially males) would routinely inject themselves with testosterone and other steroid hormones to help build muscle mass, thereby augmenting strength, and to increase stamina. Some male athletes still take testosterone, hoping they won't get caught. Testosterone's role in sports will be discussed in depth in Appendix B.

Estrogens are vital to a female's sexual development. They give her the characteristics that we associate with typical femaleness. Of the three types of estrogen, the most potent is estradiol. It catalyzes and maintains mature reproductive function in women, and at the start of puberty, stimulates secondary sex characteristics such as the enlargement of breasts. Estradiol also increases the body's secretion and receptivity of the hormone oxytocin. *Oxytocin* stimulates milk production during pregnancy. It also arouses emotional closeness in both sexes under a variety of circumstances. Estrogens are produced by the ovaries in fairly large amounts, by the testes in much smaller amounts, and by specialized fat cells in women.

Progestins, the most important of which is progesterone, are also produced by the ovaries. They are responsible for maintaining a healthy pregnancy. If a woman's progesterone levels are too low, she may have irregular periods and trouble conceiving. She may also suffer mood changes and insomnia, among other symptoms. Men create progesterone as well, in their adrenal glands and testes. It helps them make testosterone and keeps estrogen in balance. If a man's progesterone levels are too low, his sleep will be impaired and he will be at a higher risk for developing arthritis, osteoporosis, and cancer.

By popular association, testosterone equals male and estrogen equals female—because most people believe that only males produce testosterone and only females produce estrogen. But males and females produce *all* of the same hormones, and require them all, though in different amounts. Testosterone is not only critical for males. It's such an integral part of female functioning that menopausal women are given minute amounts of it to supplement what their tired adrenals can no longer produce. This gives them extra energy, more intense and frequent orgasms, and an overall rise in libido. Likewise, estrogen—balanced in the appropriate ratio with testosterone—is vitally important to male sexual function. It helps regulate men's sex drive, the production of sperm, and the ability to have an erection. In fact, if the estrogen levels in a man are too low his libido will decrease, no matter how high his testosterone levels are. Sometimes, in both male and female bodies, testosterone is converted to a form of estrogen.

Testosterone and estrogen are typically regarded as sex hormones, but they do much more. They affect the brain, blood vessels, bones, intestine, liver and lungs, and regulate growth. The nonsexual roles of testosterone include better sleep, cholesterol control, improved insulin sensitivity, enhanced bone density, and improved function of the endothelial cells that line the blood and lymph vessels (which help normalize blood pressure). The nonsexual roles of estrogen include enhanced memory, mediating levels of the neurotransmitter serotonin, improved function of the fuel-burning mitochondria in the cells, blood flow regulation in the brain, protection against bone loss, and catalyzing the production of anti-inflammatory molecules. It's important to remember that *none of these hormones operate singly*. Their beneficial effects depend on the proper amounts and ratios of *all* the hormones.

For both sexes, the production of hormones intensifies at puberty, conferring those secondary sex characteristics that most adolescents agonize over. Males acquire hair in the underarm, pubic, and facial regions. Their voices become lower, the testes start to produce sperm cells, and the Adam's apple grows. (The so-called Adam's apple is a colloquial term for the thyroid cartilage that has a different angle in men's necks than in women's, which is why it protrudes more in men after they finish puberty.) Females acquire underarm and pubic hair. Their breasts enlarge, their hips widen, and the ovaries start releasing egg cells (the onset of the menstrual cycle). The primary sex organs—testes, scrotum and penis or ovaries, vulva, clitoris, vagina and uterus—and later the secondary sex characteristics, are all part of each sex's distinctive sexual development.[4] Another important sex-linked difference is body fat distribution. Women tend to store more body fat than men, possessing a much higher ratio of adipose (fat) tissue to lean muscle.[5]

Once puberty is in full swing, one of the most obvious differences between males and females is musculature. Testosterone gives men as much as 40 percent more muscle mass than women. Men's skeletal muscle fibers are also different than women's. They contract more quickly and produce more force.[6] About one in twenty women is as strong as the average man. Males and females also differ in skeleton shape and bone mass. The bone mass in men can be up to 50 percent higher than in women.[7] Each sex has a unique body shape, in part due to their bone structure. A man has wide shoulders and narrow hips. A woman has narrow shoulders and wide hips, designed to more easily allow a baby to have room to grow and be born. The waist of a man is below the navel and the waist of a woman is above the navel. Some of their bones are shaped differently, too. A male has a heavier ridge at the brow; hers is more muted. A male's forehead is sloped at an angle from the brow; a female's is more rounded. His jaw is more square; her jaw is generally rounder. In a man, the legs attach to the pelvis in a more parallel manner than that of a woman. Therefore, how men and women walk and stand are dissimilar—so different, in fact, that each has their own identifiable gait. In recognition of women's distinctive (non-male) physiology, sports coaches, physical therapists, and sports medicine doctors are finally instructing women and administering to their injuries appropriately according to their own unique structure, rather than treating them as though they were men.

Each sex has advantages. Men are physically stronger than women, but women have more resistance to disease and live longer. Many of the metabolic functions between the sexes vary so widely that the ways in which clinical drug trials are conducted are changing. The effects of medications used to be studied mostly on all-male groups—unless the drug was specifically meant for women, which means related to their reproductive function. It was assumed that females responded to pharmaceuticals as males did, which is not the case. Doctors are finally acknowledging that the effects of drugs are often very different for females than males, and are designing drug trials according to who the subjects are.

Sex-linked differences are embedded in sperm and egg cells before they ever make their voyage to the womb. So even if an adult takes high doses of hormones—in amounts equal to or greater than what's produced by the opposite sex—the original skeleton and musculature remain. Secondary opposite-sex characteristics might be introduced, such as a beard on women or more and redistributed fat on men; but the body you're born with is the one you'll have until you die. It can be very difficult to conceal the effects of the hormones secreted in the womb.

The Brain

Neuroplasticity of the Brain

It's the nature of human beings to learn through repetition. Neural circuits typically develop in the brain by traveling the path of least resistance, and they are reinforced when we continue doing the same thing over and over. A good analogy is a horse-drawn carriage traveling a dirt road. At first the road is completely even. But every day the horse steps in the same place, and the carriage wheels start to make a groove in the dirt. Pretty soon, even if the horse or driver want to swerve to the right or left, it becomes more difficult because the wheels are now fitting into the groove in the road. Soon, it's unthinkable that there might be any other way to travel.

So far the brain doesn't sound that remarkable, does it? But there are potentially unlimited exceptions to the above process. That's because the average brain contains one hundred billion nerve cells (neurons), and each neuron is connected to between 1,000 and 10,000 other neurons. There are sixty-three possible ways in which four nerve cells can be connected to other nerve cells, and one chance of no connection at all. Every time the brain grows new cells, the number of possible connections grows exponentially.[8] Returning to our analogy, these many connections and new brain cells allow us to introduce a different route. Say we deliberately steer the horse on an unfamiliar course. Even if that path doesn't feel natural or easy—because the carriage wheels keep bumping into ridges in the dirt that were created alongside the previous grooves—those wheels eventually start to make new indentations along the path. This is due to the brain's neuroplasticity.

Neuroplasticity is the synthetic-sounding name for an elegant natural process: the brain's ability to adapt and change due to input from our environment. More than a mere metaphor, neuroplasticity indicates actual changes in the structures of the brain and nervous system in response to being challenged. Our brains are never static. Cells grow and are replenished. They switch places with other cells. Neural pathways might disappear while others are made, thanks to continual feedback. The environment can be generated from within us or come from outside of ourselves—the experiences we've had and the conclusions we've drawn from those experiences, what others have told us about ourselves, what we tell ourselves about who we are, what we learn in school or on social media, and even the chemicals we're exposed to and the nutrients we receive from the foods we eat. Neuroplasticity encompasses motor function, muscle memory, cognition, recall, perception—everything. It resides in neurons, which transmit information, and in the specialized glia, which comprise half the cells in the central nervous system. Glial cells help maintain synaptic activity (communication) between neurons. They keep the overall nervous system running smoothly. And they alter neuron structure and function when necessary.

Even if you're unfamiliar with neuroplasticity, you may have heard of therapies based on the ability of the neuroplastic brain to adapt and evolve. For example, people who suffer strokes or brain injuries are given rehabilitation that stimulates brain cells to regenerate. Over time, they learn to talk. Or they might reclaim their motor function as intact, seemingly unrelated portions of their brain assume new duties. Sometimes new cells grow in or near the areas of injury while learning to assume the functions of the damaged tissue.

Neuroplasticity is also evident when a skilled psychotherapist treats clients for post-traumatic stress disorder. The practitioner eliminates symptoms by decreasing the reactivity of certain parts of the brain while introducing more positive, supportive stimuli into other neural pathways. Under most circumstances, more neural fibers can be created in the brain. And existing nerve cells can reorganize themselves and make more, or different, connections to other nerves.

World class athletes use our modern understanding of the brain to develop their skills. Even when they're not physically participating in their sport they're mentally active, practicing in a different way. Professional golfer Tiger Woods is known for contemplating various scenarios in his mind before he ever steps onto the green. His technique of reviewing his game first is used by athletes all over the world. Similarly, some musicians mentally rehearse the music even when they're not holding their instrument. They tap into their recollection of moving their fingers across a keyboard, or blowing into a mouthpiece, or pressing down on the valves or strings of their instrument. By doing this, they strengthen the neural circuitry in their brains and bodies involved with playing the instrument. Reinforcing muscle memory makes everyone better at what they do.

If neural imprinting and muscle memory are intensified by thinking and imagining, what about exposure to an idea or belief system—particularly if that exposure is repeated? And what if the concept involves ideas about the brain itself? Including the idea that there are male brains and female brains? Do such ideas influence neural imprinting, and hence the brain's structure and function? As it turns out, they do. Trained neuroscientists, well versed in neuroplasticity, are now pointing out the fallacies of believing that males and females have innately different brains leading to disparate character traits and mental abilities. One neuroscientist is Lise Eliot, author of *Pink Brain Blue Brain*. The brain also changes "when you figure out if you're a boy or a girl," she writes. "Learning and practice rewire the human brain, and considering the very different ways boys and girls spend their time while growing up, as well as the special potency of early experience in molding neuronal connections, it would be shocking if the two sexes' brains *didn't* work differently by the time they were adults."[9]

Closely related to neuroplasticity is *epigenetics*, the study of how behavior and environment can cause actual changes in our DNA. There are a great many variables that can switch a gene on or off, and cause it to express itself in unique ways. I will be discussing epigenetics in more detail in the next chapter. For now, let's look at how rumors become so established that they are believed to be science—when they are anything but that.

The Corpus Callosum Conundrum

Many researchers who believe that males and females have innately dissimilar aptitudes, preferences and behaviors, cite differences in the corpus callosum as the reason. The *corpus callosum* is a central, rope-like cable of white matter that connects the left and right hemispheres of the cerebrum, which is the largest and uppermost portion of the brain at the front of the skull. There's a widespread belief that a woman's corpus callosum is thicker than a man's, leading to more and faster connections between the left and right hemispheres. This means, the reasoning goes, that women have more coordinated activity between the two hemispheres, in contrast to men's greater brain activity within each separate hemisphere. All of this helps explain, it's further believed, women's ability to multitask and see the big picture while men excel in being hyper-focused on a single task without being distracted by other input. This theory sounds good—but is it true? As it turns out, only sometimes. The following account is a good example of how just one poorly executed study can create an ongoing myth. It also shows how someone in the public eye—even someone who's not a scientist—can perpetuate rumors that are then accepted as scientific reality.

As explained by biologist Anne Fausto-Sterling, the corpus callosum fiasco began with a short article that was first published in 1982 in the journal *Science*. Even though the authors studied only five female and nine male brains, they made a sweeping generalization that for visuospatial functions, men and women have different degrees of lateralization. *Lateralization* simply means that each hemisphere of the cerebrum is responsible for different functions. Translated, males and females were believed to use their brain hemispheres differently for visuospatial tasks because certain regions of the corpus callosum were thought to be larger in females than in males.[10] This insignificant paper skyrocketed to fame when the talk show host Phil Donahue, in a book loaded with biased and outright falsified research, inaccurately credited the authors with describing, in female brains, "an extra bundle of neurons that was missing in male brains."[11] This, he concluded, accounted for women's intuition. After *Time* and *Newsweek* repeated this inaccuracy—so much for fact checking!—it took only a short while for this hypothesis to become cemented as scientific fact by both the public and scientists. The general public, which as a rule doesn't read medical literature, might be forgiven; but when scientists repeat and promote speculation without proper follow-up research, this is sloppy science and there's no excuse for it.

Fausto-Sterling describes the structure of the corpus callosum in detail, which may point to more problems with that ill-fated study. Dead tissue is not like living tissue, and thus requires a different imaging system. For dead samples of the corpus callosum—which always shrink, due to loss of fluids—most researchers measure a 2D slice. For living tissue inside a person, researchers measure the entire 3D structure using MRI (magnetic resonance imaging). Thus we have two dissimilar tissue types, with inherently different thicknesses and spatial resolution, each requiring very different tools to measure them. Neither the samples nor the measuring methods are interchangeable across different experiments. Another problem is, the boundaries between the corpus callosum and adjacent structures are difficult to define. If the samples themselves are not clear, how can experimental results be correctly interpreted? Lise Eliot drew similar conclusions, reminding readers that the news media failed to mention several studies that reported *no* statistically significant sex differences in the corpus callosums of men and women, boys and girls, or male and female fetuses.

To add more perspective, originally the corpus callosum was studied to determine presumed differences between people with dark and light skin. In 1906, a paper was published called "Some racial peculiarities of the Negro brain."[12] "The methods used to measure the size and shape of the corpus callosum in cadavers has not changed...since the [paper's] publication," observes Fausto-Sterling. "Once freed from the body and domesticated for laboratory observation, the CC [corpus callosum] can serve different masters. In a period of preoccupation with racial difference, the CC, for a time, was thought to hold the key to racial difference. Now, the very same structure serves at...[the] beck and call" of biological sex.[13]

While animal studies can give us a starting point of inquiry, we cannot assume that the data automatically pertains to human beings. It's also unscientific to allow personal bias to influence an experiment. Eliot writes:

> If you've read anything about boy-girl differences, you're probably... convinced that scientists have discovered all kinds of disparities in brain structure, function, and neurochemistry—that girls' brains are wired for communication and boys' for aggression; that they have different amounts of serotonin and oxytocin circulating in their heads; that boys do math using the hippocampus while girls use the cerebral cortex; that girls are left-brain dominant while boys are right-brain dominant.
>
> These claims have spread like wildfire, but there are problems with every one. Some are blatantly false, plucked out of thin air because they sound about right. Others are cherry-picked from single studies or extrapolated from rodent research without any effort to critically evaluate all the data, account for conflicting studies, or even state that the results have never been confirmed in humans. And yet such claims are nearly always presented to parents, with great authority, as well-proven and dramatic facts about boys' and girls' brains, with seemingly dire implications.[14]

Theories abound as to why sex-linked differences occur and why there are exceptions to these differences. According to "Prenatal and postnatal hormone effects on the human brain and cognition," the effects of hormones depend not only on the dose, but also when they're secreted—and the deciding period is during prenatal development. Later in life, additional hormonal output merely fine tunes the early organization of the brain. Thus one's sexual identity is set in the womb; and any decision made later in life that one "is actually the opposite sex" is not supported by the biology of either the body or brain.[15] However, other researchers contradict these findings, stating that postnatal periods of hormone secretion are more powerful than prenatal surges.[16] So how do we know what's true? Let's try and sift through a morass of complicated data.

Male and Female Brains: Fact or Fable?

This section was very difficult to write. The entire chapter was intended to be devoted solely to biology, but cultural expectations—discussed in great detail in the next chapter on sex role stereotypes—began to intrude. It's not surprising that this would occur, because in any discussion of sex differences, biology (nature) always interacts with environment (nurture). An almost obsessive analysis of possible biases is required because the assumptions we grow up with are so ingrained that they become invisible, appearing as immutable truths when they are not.

The "nature versus nurture" debate has been raging for decades. On one side are scientists and academics who claim that being either male or female has nothing to do with biology and everything to do with culture. Purveyors of this viewpoint seem to forget (or fail to acknowledge) that if hormones are powerful enough to alter the shape and function of the body, they must also exert at least some influence on the brain. The other side of this debate features scientists and academics who claim that there exist naturally-occurring traits labeled "masculine" and "feminine"—and that their basis in biology overrides any and all cultural influences. Purveyors of *this* argument don't understand that biology can change depending on the environment, and the human brain, especially of a young child, is extremely malleable.[17]

The "biology is fixed" position always tries to bolster its argument with that seemingly magical hormone, testosterone. So before I analyze specific behaviors and discuss what they actually indicate, I need to delve a bit into how testosterone—which is (still) associated with all things male—operates in the body and affects the brain. It's not as simple or direct as you might think.

I already described how testosterone levels surge at critical junctures during a male's physical development. What about in the brain? There are many ways in which testosterone affects it. The hormone can influence already-existing neural pathways within minutes, or over a period of weeks. It can increase or decrease the sensitivity of brain cells. For a rapid, short-term effect, testosterone attaches to a nerve cell membrane and alters chemical pathways to change how easily that cell will fire. The hormone may bind to an androgen receptor. Once testosterone enters the nucleus of a neuron, it switches on certain genes by altering the cell's production of proteins and peptides. Assisted by the biochemical catalyst aromatase, testosterone may convert into estrogen and bind to an estrogen receptor—although this doesn't always occur because the brains of both males and females already manufacture estrogen. What happens in the brain depends on how much estrogen it's producing; the sensitivity of brain receptors to estrogen, testosterone and other hormones; the location of the estrogen receptor sites; how well testosterone is converted to estrogen; how much aromatase is available for the conversion; and other factors. As you can see, testosterone's activity isn't simple. With so much going on in the brain, using blood or saliva testosterone levels as a measure of how much testosterone a person possesses is simplistic and misleading.[18]

It's also simplistic and misleading to think that behavior can be inferred or predicted based *solely* on testosterone levels, regardless of where the hormone is stationed. "Sex effects in the brain don't always serve to create different behavior," Cordelia Fine explains. "Sometimes instead, one sex effect counteracts or compensates for another, *enabling similarity of behavior, despite dissimilarity of biology*....One researcher, for instance, suggests that male exposure to the testosterone surge *in utero* somehow *desensitizes* the brain to testosterone's effects later in life. This would be a smart way, maybe achieved through sex differences in neural sensitivity, of *enabling males to tolerate the higher levels of testosterone their bodies need to develop and maintain male secondary sexual characteristics, without having an excessively large effect on behavior.*" [emphasis added][19]

One thing we do know is that male and female brains can reach the same goal via different means. Take the African forest weaver, a type of songbird. In most species of birds, it's the males who sing. But both male and female African forest weaver birds sing (in unison, which is remarkable when you think about it). The male's brain region devoted to singing is larger than the corresponding brain region in females. However, in the female bird's brain, Fine reports, "the genes involved in song production areas 'express' (produce brain-altering proteins) at a much higher rate than in males, compensating for their smaller neural real estate."[20] She proposes that because "males and females need to be able to potentially behave in similar ways to get by in day-to-day life, evolution has to work out a way for this to be achieved in [their] somewhat different bodies...[W]e can't assume that neurobiological sex differences always act to *create* differences in behavior. Sometimes, they may in fact serve to iron them out."[21]

Nevertheless, myths die hard, and some people still believe that testosterone can create a distinctly "male" brain. To find out, authors of "Sex beyond the genitalia: The human brain mosaic" analyzed MRIs of more than 1,400 live human brains. After examining gray matter, white matter, and neural connections, they found that fewer than one percent of the subjects had solely stereotypical "masculine" or "feminine" characteristics. All other brains had a "mosaic" of features—"some more common in females compared with males, some more common in males compared with females, and some common in both females and males....These findings are corroborated by a similar analysis of personality traits, attitudes, interests, and behaviors of more than 5,500 individuals....Our study demonstrates that, although there are sex/gender differences in the brain, human brains do not belong to one of two distinct categories."[22] Three years later, in 2018, a similar study was conducted by some of the same researchers. "Unsupervised clustering algorithms [a simple way researchers generally use to classify data] revealed that common brain 'types' are similarly common in females and in males and that a male and a female are almost as likely to have the same brain 'type' as two females or two males....[S]ex category (i.e., whether one is female or male), is not a major predictor of the variability of human brain structure. Rather, the brain types typical of females are also typical of males, and vice versa...[except] in some rare brain types."[23]

If a man can have a "feminine" brain and a women can have a "masculine" one, does it make sense to label a brain according to sex? "Which of the many combinations of characteristics that males display should be considered male nature?" Fine asks. "Is it a profile of pure masculinity that appears to barely exist in reality? What does it mean to say that 'boys will be boys,' or to ask why a woman can't be more like a man? *Which* boy? Which woman, and which man?"[24]

Another problem arises with this type of labeling, Fine explains. "Although we're used to thinking of certain kinds of behavior as 'testosterone fueled,' in many cases it would make more sense to instead think of actions and situations as being 'testosterone fueling.' Social context modulates T [testosterone] levels (up or down), which influences behavior (presumably via changes in perception, motivation, and cognition), which influences social outcome, which influences T levels...and so on....[T]he effects of the social world have even been seen at the genetic level, with social interactions changing androgen and estrogen receptor expression in the brain."[25] Simply put, *context is everything*. Our experiences cause certain neural pathways to deepen, others to disappear, and still others to be formed (and sometimes, nothing changes). Plus, the simple act of living causes hormones to interact with other hormones—and thus alter various brain processes. We have less or more sensitivity to stimulus, and develop different ways of perceiving that stimulus. The possibilities are endless. It's difficult to say what constitutes "male" or "female" nature, when the neuroplastic brain is constantly responding to external cues and events.

In *Pink Brain Blue Brain*, Lise Eliot takes the reader step-by-step through her journey to evaluate research, most of which attempted to prove that male and female brains contain dissimilar circuitry and even discrete physical structures. The neuroscientist examined hundreds of studies on humans and animals. These included studies that were poorly designed, were not replicable, or clearly showed experimenter bias. Some experimenters looked at prenatal hormones, others looked at postnatal hormones, and still others investigated pubertal hormones. Amniotic fluid was extracted from pregnant mothers and analyzed under a microscope. Readings were taken of pregnant mothers' plasma *in utero*. Blood from pregnant mothers was drawn intravenously and tested for levels of specific hormones. MRIs were used to see which parts of the brains lit up when subjects performed various tasks, and brain functions of males and females were compared. Piles of papers later—much of which yielded contradicting data—Eliot still could not pin down exactly what the differences were between male and female brains. Did the environment make hormone levels rise or fall, or were the hormone levels high or low to begin with? The best we can conclude is that there are *tendencies* toward differences between men's and women's brains, but with a great deal of overlap. Plus, there are always exceptions. As for the differences that are obvious, Eliot remarked, "Who's to say that such differences are caused by nature and not by learning—by the thirty or so years of living as a male or female that any research subject invariably carries into the MRI scanner?"[26]

Knowing that our environment helps shape us—even if we might not be able to identify some of those influences—let's look at several examples of how males and females are thought to differ, even during infancy. While these examples appear to reflect reality, I will be showing how cultural stereotypes can inflate their importance and distort their meaning.

- *Males are much more visually oriented than females, and females are much more auditorily oriented than males.* While this oft-repeated conviction may give men an excuse to ogle women or become addicted to centerfolds ("It's in my nature!"), it's simply not true. In 1974, researchers Eleanor Maccoby and Carol Jacklin conducted an extensive review of nine studies on almost four hundred infants. They found no differences in girls' and boys' attention to a wide variety of colors, shapes, and movements. Another fifty-four experiments, published in thirty-three papers, yielded similar conclusions. As for differences in hearing between the sexes, the difference is not statistically significant—which is why screening for hearing impairment is the same for both sexes (and yields accurate results). Therefore, generalizing that boys learn through seeing and girls learn through hearing is inaccurate. In fact, during early infancy, girls are even more visual than boys, because testosterone may delay the development of 3D vision and the visual cortex in males.[27]

  Leonard Sax, who wrote a book titled *Why Gender Matters*, has often been cited as an authority to support the boys-are-visual-and-girls-are-auditory belief. In fact, he once wrote that "If a male teacher speaks in a tone of voice that seems normal to him, a girl in the front row may feel that he is yelling at her."[28] Although a later edition of Sax's book omitted the passage quoted, that he published it at all reveals the strongly sexist attitudes of some researchers—and illustrates how such beliefs are regarded as "fact" even after the original citation is removed and new information is released. Sax ignored the comprehensive research of Maccoby and Jacklin, which is considered by many authorities to be the "gold standard" of this type of data.

- *Boys are naturally tough because they have a higher pain threshold than girls—and this makes them (desirably) masculine.* A study of two-day-old infants who were pricked in the heel (routinely done on a newborn for blood screening) concluded that the girls experienced more pain than boys because they exhibited more dramatic facial expressions. But there are other indicators of pain that were not measured in the experiment: crying, breathing patterns, neurological arousal, and limb position.[29] Another, later study conducted by Swedish scientists measured pain differently with a noninvasive method that detected cerebral blood flow, an indicator of brain activity. This yielded a very different picture. Boys exhibited greater cortical activation during the heel prick procedure than girls. They weren't more tough. They just didn't register it on their faces as much as girls did.[30] This may have been due to the less developed fine muscle development in infant boys than girls, an already well-known fact.

  It's a fallacy, then, to assume that boys are naturally physically tougher than girls. This study has profound implications for how we treat boys. If we believe that it's natural for boys to be less emotional—and hence more callous—than girls, this may turn into a self-fulfilling prophecy. I will discuss this in depth in the next chapter.

- *Boys are tougher than girls because their brains are wired to enjoy rough play.* Few scientists would dispute that in boys, especially during the first year of life, the senses of smell, hearing and touch mature more slowly than in girls. Also, boys' fine motor and language skills are less developed. However, boys surpass girls in gross motor development: standing, sitting, and walking. A male's higher testosterone level gives him more energy than a female, which is why most boys move more than girls. Therefore, it's no wonder that boys want to chase each other, hit balls, and wrestle. But it's a mistake to use this biological need for higher-energy movement as an excuse to draw conclusions about toughness—and by extension, masculinity. Praising boys for apparent toughness, believing that this makes them desirably masculine, establishes a dangerous precedent. Boys feel pain as much as girls do when they're injured (see prior point); but if they believe that it's unmanly to complain, they will physically and emotionally numb themselves. They'll "grin and bear it," and avoid asking for help when they need it. Letting off steam due to high energy levels is necessary. Learning that it's socially acceptable and more desirable to push beyond their limits to the extent that injuries occur—to themselves and others—is hurtful and counterproductive.

  Although girls don't have as great a need as boys to discharge excess energy, they still require physical outlets in order to grow properly. Unfortunately, the "boys are tougher" mindset has an unwitting counterpart: If boys are tougher, girls are more delicate. As a result, parents tend to be much more protective of girls. "While girls are often easier to care for and more socially aware," writes Eliot, "they do not get as much encouragement as boys for their physical development and emotional independence...Because of baby girls' smaller size, and possibly because of lingering stereotypes, parents tend to be more cautious with infant girls, permitting them less freedom to explore and to push their physical limits. But later on, girls begin falling behind boys in their physicality and spatial skills, and it's clear that girls could benefit from greater physical challenges and earlier opportunities to explore."[31] The physical needs of children leads me to one more, related topic: toys, which almost everywhere are labeled and marketed according to the sex of the child. See below.

- *The toys that are natural for boys are in the "active" category of miniature cars and trucks, balls, and guns; while the toys that are natural for girls are in the "passive" category of dolls, miniature kitchen utensils, and beauty items such as ribbons.* This stereotype is believed by an overwhelming majority. While there's some truth to it, as usual the reality is much more complex.

  Until about age one, boys are attracted to dolls. Then—probably because they are at a higher activity level due to a testosterone surge—they're attracted to balls, trucks, and similar items that they can physically move and manipulate. Nevertheless, environment plays a huge role in children's toy preferences, more than you might think. Let's look at some experiments.

A huge number of studies have been conducted with infants, toddlers, and young children to learn if children's preferences for toys is related to their sex. Some children were shown the toys, others were allowed to play with them, and still others were simply given pictures of the toys. Some of the toys were stereotypically female-oriented, some were stereotypically male-oriented, and still others were considered gender-neutral, such as a stuffed animal or a picture book. The research was conducted all over the world: Sweden, the Netherlands, Canada, and the United States.

The Swedish study was particularly revealing because it followed up on the children when they were one, three, and five years old. This allowed the researchers to chronicle any changes in the children's preferences—which would suggest that input from parents and peers influenced the toys that the children chose. This was indeed the case. The innate preferences of the children were enhanced by social and cultural factors, especially their own growing awareness of whether they were a boy or a girl. According to experts, conscious gender identity emerges between ages two and three, and is cemented in most children by age six or seven. This also happens to be the age at which children form their most heavily stereotyped views of males and females.[32]

One study conducted with 56 children age four to nine years old yielded some alarming results. Toys were presented to the children for their tactile exploration—but with a catch. They were labeled as being for either boys or girls. No matter what the toy was, if the label was for the "wrong" sex, the children explored the toy less and remembered it less than a toy labeled for "their" sex.[33] Another study yielded similar results. Children refrained from exploring the toy, did not ask as many questions about it, and recalled it less, when it was labeled for the opposite sex instead of their own sex or even both sexes.[34] As might be expected, this has huge implications—not just for children but also adults, who are less able to learn if they believe the material is unsuitable for them. This will be explored in depth in the next chapter.

A very revealing and innovative experiment was conducted at a daycare center with children who ranged in age from three to five. Instead of toys, two neutral categories were created. The children were assigned membership in either the "red" or the "blue" social group and were given red or blue T-shirts to wear each day. The control group of children merely wore the colored T-shirts. In the experimental group, teachers used the colors to label the children and organize the classrooms. The children's cubbyholes were decorated with red and blue labels. The teachers would greet the children by their color name and had each color group line up on different sides of the room. Most importantly, they told the red and blue groups which toys were preferred by members of each color. In just three weeks, biases developed. The children wanted to play with the toys corresponding to their own color group.[35]

Once again, we see how strongly our environment influences us. Children's toy choices are based not only on energy level or hard-wired inclination, but also on what they believe they *should* want after being told what their culture, parents and peers deem appropriate. The toys chosen by the children reflect their growing awareness of their sex—and everyone "knows" which toys are for girls and which are for boys! By about age four, this programming becomes cemented and the child is less flexible. Due to intense peer pressure—along with their need for approval—children can be the most severe enforcers of sex role stereotypes. Adherence to the party line continues into adolescence. Only very mature children can see through the biases. For a child, it takes courage and inner strength to play with, or wear, something "belonging" to the other sex.

A story from open-minded psychologist Sandra Bem, who with her husband was very careful to avoid stereotyping of any kind in their household, illustrates the degree to which children can be successfully indoctrinated. Her nursery school-age son Jeremy wanted to wear a barrette to school. She let him, despite her concern that he might be teased. As it turns out, he was. A male classmate called him a girl because, in his mind, only girls wear barrettes. To prove he was a boy and not a girl, Jeremy pulled down his pants. Incredibly, the other boy still insisted that Jeremy was a girl. The classmate thought that everyone had a penis.[36] If this story has a moral, it's this: Children need to understand that differences between males and females do not depend on something external that can change—such as what toys are played with, what fashion is being worn, or what activities are preferred.[37] As I discuss throughout this book, relying on external cues to know who we are gets us in heaps of trouble.

Parents are the most immediately influential purveyors of sex role stereotypes, even if it's unintentional. If their child picks up a toy they consider sex-appropriate (such as a boy with a truck or a girl with a baby doll), they convey approval. But if the child plays with the opposite sex's toy (such as a boy with a baby doll or a girl with a truck), they convey disapproval. Fathers have been observed to be more invested than mothers that their children choose the "correct" sex-linked toys. From dozens of studies that Eliot reviewed, it was clear that young boys were very intimidated by their fathers' disapproval if they selected toys associated with girls. The boys tended to stop playing with the toys, even if they were considered more neutral and the boys were especially fond of them. Interestingly, girls playing with toys associated with boys elicits a less negative response. It's more acceptable for a girl to be a tomboy (have stereotypically masculine traits) than for a boy to be a sissy (have stereotypically feminine traits). Not only are girls' toys—and what they represent—devalued, but many fathers fear that their sons will become homosexual if they gravitate toward interests attributed to girls. Parents can help their children by encouraging their daughters to play ball or build with size-appropriate tools, and by giving their sons dolls or stuffed animals to cuddle—without labeling which sex is supposed to play with which toy. Art supplies, board games, and building blocks tend to lack the stigma of sex-typed labeling. Whatever the toy, though, children will be much less enthusiastic to play with it if it's labeled for the other sex.

In the Swedish study, 97 percent of 3-year-old boys, when given a choice of toys to play with, were more likely to spend time with stereotypical masculine toys than the average girl did. Note, however, that a child's choice of toys does not indicate what interests he or she will develop as an adult. The choice of toy does not—and *cannot*—predict future competency in verbal, mechanical or social skills, or even one's chosen profession.

Not surprisingly, it has been shown that children from homes in which the mothers explicitly sanctioned sex role stereotypes are conscious of their sex several months sooner than those children whose mothers were less traditional and not invested in those stereotypes.[38] But if the parents are enlightened enough to avoid sexism in their own household—let's say a girl is given tools or a boy is given a miniature kitchen set to play with—in most cases it's not enough that the immediate family refrain from stereotyping. Freedom from gender roles needs to be reinforced by the child's school, community, and any media to which the child is exposed. Otherwise, the home might be perceived as an anomaly. This is said not to discourage parents from giving their children the opportunity to explore, but to emphasize the degree of conditioning that everyone deals with every day—even if it's not on a conscious level.

♦ *Males are intrinsically more competitive and risk-taking than females.*[39] The presumably higher rate of competitiveness in males (ascribed to testosterone, naturally) is disproved by many findings. This includes a study showing that one in six elite male athletes has testosterone levels that are actually *below* the range considered normal for non-athlete males—and in some cases, below the average for female elite athletes.[40] Yet no one would think that top male athletes lack a competitive drive. "Contrary to what many might assume," Cordelia Fine writes, "women and men have similar risk attitudes," regardless of age. "For the same subjectively perceived risk and benefit, they are equally likely to tempt fate. When men and women *do* diverge in risk-taking propensity, it is because they perceive the risks and benefits differently." This isn't surprising, because unlike with men, ambition and assertiveness are usually not rewarded in women. A survey of more than 800 managers at a consulting firm found that women were generally less willing to make sacrifices and take risks in their career to be promoted—not because they were less ambitious, but because "they had lower expectations of success, fewer role models, less support, and less confidence" that their company would be fair.[41] Another paper reviewed studies of young Chinese men and women to determine who took risks versus who avoided them. "Imagine you are a woman," the authors wrote, "who lives in a... culture that considers conservativeness and timidity as becoming characteristics of women. Would you demonstrate bravery, adventurousness, and risk taking, or timidity and risk avoiding as mating strategies in front of a desirable potential mate?" In China, the ideal woman is still seen as subordinate, fragile, dutiful, and virginal—hardly the profile of a risk taker! In one study, men who thought they were being observed by an attractive member of the opposite sex increased their risk taking, while women in equivalent circumstances decreased it. But Chinese women equaled their male counterparts in risk taking—defying an antiquated, idealized version of femininity—*when they thought they weren't being observed.*[42] "*Male* risk taking," Fine remarks, "is a norm of masculinity and seen as a more important trait for men than for women."[43]

******

Now that we know more about how our unconscious biases affect babies and young children, what can we do? Based on the different developmental needs of males and females, Dr. Lise Eliot suggests:

> The exact prescription for sensitive, responsive caregiving may differ for girls and boys, or for babies of either sex with different temperaments.
>
> Boys are often more needy as infants than girls are. They are less physically mature and take longer to develop the self-calming skills, such as hand-sucking or pulling into a tightly tucked posture, that help them compensate when overwhelmed. Parents may need to step in sooner with a boy, picking him up, changing his position, or giving him a soothing ring to grasp and suck on. Here is where stereotypes can get in the way. In the general spirit of "toughening them up," parents may let their baby boys fuss and squirm longer, or they may resort to artificial stimuli—videos, electronic swings, and elaborate toy bars—to entertain them without helping them to discover their own self-calming skills.
>
> Girls, on the other hand, can sometimes be too easy. Quiet, complacent babies may not get as much attention as fussier types, and they may actually suffer from a lack of the stimulation and interaction needed to fully develop their motor and cognitive skills. While there are plenty of exceptions, girls fall into this category more often than boys. So...by keeping your baby nearby, you are likelier to interact more—talking to her, pointing out interesting things in the environment, and generally integrating the baby into your daily life, making the most of her waking hours.[44]

The goal is to help each person have the most fulfilling life. "Both sexes have their strengths and vulnerabilities," writes Eliot. "The reason for studying sex differences is not to tally up who's winning or losing but to learn how to compensate for them early on, while children's brains are still at their most malleable....Piecing together the different influences at each state is the only way to truly understand them, equalize opportunity between the sexes, and, ultimately, bring out the best in every child."[45]

One more thing. If you give girls and boys similar activities, their brains will be more similar. Remember neuroplasticity. "Sex isn't a biological dictator that sends gonadal hormones hurtling through the brain, uniformly masculinizing male brains, monotonously feminizing female brains," writes Cordelia Fine. "Sexual differentiation of the brain turns out to be an untidily interactive process, in which multiple factors—genetic, hormonal, environmental, and epigenetic (that is, stable changes in the 'turning on and off' of genes)—all act and interact to affect how sex shapes the entire brain.... A particular environmental factor can have a profound effect on sex differences for one brain characteristic, but the opposite influence, or none, for others."[46] In another book, *Delusions of Gender: How Our Minds, Society, and Neurosexism Create Difference*, Fine cautions us that "when researchers look for sex differences in the brain or the mind, they are hunting a moving target. Both are in continuous interaction with the social context....[N]euroscience is used by some in a way that it has often been used in the past: to reinforce, with all the authority of science, old-fashioned stereotypes and roles."[47] My view is that even *calling* a particular character trait "masculine" or "feminine" is not only biologically inaccurate, but leads us to trouble. This will become especially clear later in the book when I discuss the recruitment tactics of transgender activists.

Some Neurotransmitters and Their Effects

The body produces many other chemicals besides estrogen and testosterone that affect brain organization. In *Why Him? Why Her?*, anthropologist Helen Fisher discusses how four major ones—testosterone, estrogen, dopamine, and what she believes is serotonin[48]—contribute to four distinct personality types in men and women. (Dopamine and serotonin are classified as both neurotransmitters and hormones.) The biochemicals are not based on the person's reproductive organs, but on *biochemical expression in the brain regardless of sex*. According to Fisher, most people's behaviors and attitudes are stimulated by two of the four hormones, one more dominant than the other. Some people express three of the hormones, and a very small number of people are balanced in all four hormones. The activity of these biochemicals depends on many factors, including the number and sensitivity of receptor sites to the hormone, the efficiency of the body's feedback system to the biochemical, and even the availability and potency of the enzymes that help produce the hormone (which determines amounts). Also, the biochemicals don't exist in a vacuum—they work together with other major neurotransmitters and hormones. And, depending on their amounts and even the timing of their secretion, they can produce different effects. Not only that, the variables that help form brain function can change over time. It's very complicated.

"After doing extensive research on the biological underpinnings of personality types," Fisher writes, "I have come to believe that each of us expresses a unique mix of four broad basic personality types."[49] Fisher did not examine how environment and bias influence the expression and amounts of neurotransmitters, but that was not her intended focus. Her research is pertinent here because it not only shows different styles of thinking and behaving, but illustrates how our culture is obsessed with classifying personality traits as masculine or feminine. The following is what Fisher gleaned from the scientific literature. Again, keep in mind that these neurochemicals are dominant in the *brain*, and are independent of the hormones that shape the body and reproductive organs *in utero*.

- *Testosterone tendencies*, what Fisher calls the Director. Many of these traits are the archetype of what Western culture regards as masculinity: focused, energetic, analytical, and emotionally contained (except for the expression of enthusiasm). Such a person would be good in engineering and the sciences, and sports that require brains more than brawn. People with testosterone tendencies are also direct, decisive, logical, tough-minded, exacting, good at strategic thinking, bold, competitive, and excellent at figuring out machines, mathematical formulas, or other rule-based systems.

- *Estrogen tendencies*, what Fisher calls the Negotiator. Many of these traits are the archetype of what Western culture regards as femininity: nurturing, emotionally expressive, intuitive, and sympathetic. Excellent at reading postures, gestures, facial expressions and tones of voice, such a person is able to quickly detect the needs of others and might be drawn to a service profession such as teaching, medicine, psychotherapy, or child care. The individual can also see the big picture and connect disparate facts, which Fisher calls contextual and holistic thinking. Hence, he or she might be drawn to the arts, especially writing. People with estrogen tendencies are also imaginative, verbally skilled, mentally flexible, agreeable, idealistic, and altruistic.

- *Dopamine tendencies*, what Fisher calls the Explorer. Adventurousness, sensation seeking, and a proclivity for the unusual drive these people. They might be passionate about uncommon activities such as skydiving, and engage in the more perilous sports such as football or ice hockey. People with these prominent traits are also drawn to dangerous professions that require risk taking, such as firefighting and police work. Individuals with dopamine tendencies are also high-energy, spontaneous, curious, creative, optimistic, enthusiastic, and mentally flexible.

- *Serotonin tendencies (which may be better ascribed, at least partly, to GABA)*, what Fisher calls the Builder. Such a person is consistent, family-oriented, reliable, responsible, and grounded. People in this category, sometimes called pillars of society, help form the foundation of civilizations. They might not be considered extraordinary or exciting to be around, but they keep everything running. With a strong work ethic, someone in this category will think long and hard before doing something considered unusual. People with serotonin traits are calm, social, cautious but not fearful, persistent, loyal, fond of rules and facts, orderly, guardians of tradition, and skilled at building social networks and managing people in family, business, and social situations.[50]

While Fisher originally conducted this research to determine which combinations of brain chemicals would work best in romantic relationship pairings—there are benefits and pitfalls with each combination—her findings have a much wider application. Clearly, biochemicals other than testosterone and estrogen are involved in brain development. And, because people possess combinations in different amounts at different times in their lives, what you get is a varied, changeable mix of character traits no matter what the body looks like.

Unsurprisingly, in Fisher's paradigm testosterone is dominant in the brains of men who naturally exhibit what's considered stereotypically masculine behavior. A testosteronized body, combined with a brain regarded as testosterone-inclined, produces what our culture considers quintessential, culturally desirable masculinity. It's not the only way to be a man, but when the archetype of "man" is invoked, this is what many people think of. In the sample that Fisher examined, however, most men did not possess this archetypical combination. Of the heterosexual men and women who participated in her study, just 16.3 percent—less than one-fifth of the population—had this brain constellation; and of that percentage, men were two-and-a-half times as likely as women to manifest it. Extrapolated to the general population, we might conclude that males as a group have more "masculine" brains than females as a group. But females can also possess more "masculine" brains, and Fisher emphasized that this is a natural, normal occurrence.

Similarly, it's not difficult to guess that estrogen is regarded as dominant in the brains of women who naturally exhibit what's considered stereotypically feminine behavior. An estrogenized body, combined with a brain regarded as estrogen-inclined, produces what our culture considers quintessential, culturally desirable femininity. It's not the only way to be a woman, but when the archetype of "woman" is invoked, this is what many people think of. According to Fisher, one-quarter of the female population has this brain constellation. The brains of some heterosexual males are also estrogen-dominant. Like their female counterparts, these males tend to be sensitive, empathic, and oriented toward figuring out what others need and then giving it to them. It's perfectly acceptable for males to have more "feminine" brains.

Despite Fisher's apparent concession to sex role stereotypes in some ways, her research does concur with the aforementioned studies showing that human brains contain a "mosaic" of features. There are *degrees* of so-called masculinity and femininity in people's brains, just as in their bodies. One group of biochemicals is no better or worse, or more or less desirable, than another group. But any culture that obsesses over labels of "masculine" or "feminine," applies them to character traits, and imbues those traits with hierarchical meaning, is doing people an enormous disservice. *All* types of brains are needed. Brains don't need to be genderized, and it doesn't matter what bodies those brains are in.

Now let's see what happens when a person's genitals don't correspond to what our culture thinks they're supposed to look like.

Divergences of Sexual Development, Including Intersexuals
Atypical Chromosomes and Hormonal Departures

There's a lot that can happen during the complicated process of growing a baby. The "3G" combination to which some scientists refer—genes, gonads, and genitals—may unexpectedly appear in atypical combinations. If the twenty-third chromosome on either the sperm or egg doesn't fuse the way it normally does, due to biochemical or genetic interruptions, the Y chromosome might be reversed. Or it may move. Under these circumstances, instead of XX (the most common female) or XY (the most common male), there might be the following chromosomal arrangements: X (female, occurring in a few births per thousand), Y (male, occurring in a few births per thousand), XXY (male), XYY (male), and XXXY (male). Evolutionary biologist Colin Wright writes that these unusual combinations "are not new sexes, but rather represent natural variation *within* males and females….The presence of a Y chromosome, or two, or three, etc., *all* result in the development of testes and therefore these individuals are biologically male. Likewise, individuals with additional or fewer X chromosomes, in the absence of a Y, all develop ovaries and are therefore biologically female."[51] In other words, as long as there's a Y chromosome someplace, regardless of how many X chromosomes might also be present, the sex of the person is male. That's because the Y chromosome indicates the existence of testes, testes produce testosterone, and as a result during puberty male secondary sex characteristics develop—except in the extremely rare instances when they don't. Let me explain.

While the "Y equals testosterone" guideline sounds reasonable, and certainly streamlines identification—you can't get any more straightforward than that—there are some exceptions that can occur, for any number of reasons, that cause an ambiguous appearance. The testes might not be producing enough testosterone. Or the receptor sites for testosterone may be too few or unresponsive, and therefore don't sufficiently register the "Make a male!" message that testosterone conveys. Along with scarce or unresponsive testosterone receptors, any estrogen that's present (which is naturally produced by both female and male bodies) may feminize some of the features more than usual. These atypical departures can manifest in different ways. An infant might possess both ovarian and testicular tissue. The child might have external genitalia that appear to be male, while also possessing some internal female structures. Or the child might have external genitalia that appear to be female, while also possessing some internal male structures. Bodies with both male and female gonads (testes and ovaries) may appear not exactly male and not exactly female, may appear to be both male and female, or may appear to be neither. Individuals who have developed in these ways, rather than from the more usual sex differentiation process, are known as *intersex*. The website of the National Library of Medicine gives a clear definition of intersex: "a group of conditions in which there is a discrepancy between the external genitals and the internal genitals (the testes and ovaries)."[52]

Intersexuals aside, sometimes the genitalia are ambiguous even in XX and XY bodies. There might be greater or lesser amounts of certain hormones than are normally present. Or, the receptor sites to those hormones may be partially or completely inactive. These conditions can cause a clitoris to be larger than doctors think it "should" be, or a penis to be smaller than doctors think it "should" be. Sometimes the boy's scrotum is not completely fused, making it reminiscent of the outer labia of a female vagina. Or the girl's labia are fused, visually appearing similar to a male scrotum. Strictly speaking, these variations of genitalia—while potentially hampering the ability to identify a child's sex—do not constitute an intersex person. This is because a person's sex is defined by their reproductive organs and the sperm or egg they are potentially capable of producing.

The existence of both ovarian and testicular tissue is a logical and correct definition for intersexuality. However, this hasn't stopped some people—including misguided academicians and researchers—from expanding the criteria for intersexuality to such a degree that the term is no longer instructive, meaningful, or scientific. One typical definition from Planned Parenthood states that "Intersex is an umbrella term that describes bodies that fall outside the strict male/female binary. There are lots of ways someone can be intersex....a person is born with reproductive or sexual anatomy that doesn't fit the boxes of 'female' or 'male.'"[53] This definition is vague and highly subjective. It indicates that designating someone "intersex" depends on what "female" and "male" look like to the person doing the assessment, rather than on objective scientific criteria.

"Intersex people," states the website of Intersex Human Rights Australia, "share common ground due to the shared experience of stigmatisation of our atypical... physical or anatomical sex characteristics…It is the perceived need for diagnosis and treatment itself that defines the intersex population, and not necessarily a specific and narrow set of causal factors."[54] But defining the intersex population by "a specific and narrow set" of factors (though not necessarily causal) is, in fact, the correct way to determine intersexuality—although I can understand why one might want to broaden the term to include other conditions. People with presumably atypical genitals, or secondary sex characteristics that don't match their perceived sex, suffer ridicule, bullying, shunning, prejudicial psychological labeling, and even medical malpractice. Many are forced to undergo surgery to make their genitals conform to the way doctors think they're supposed to look (discussed shortly). To help bring these cruel and unethical practices to the public's attention, a wide range of people have organized under the intersex umbrella.

True intersexuals—that is, individuals who possess both male and female reproductive organs in whole or part—are quite rare, numbering only about 0.018% of the world's population.[55] But if you accept the definition of intersex to include biological males and biological females with health conditions whose symptoms include atypical genitals, the numbers skyrocket. A popular medical website cites about 1.3 intersex individuals in 1000 babies, which—using the statistic of 7.8 billion people in the world in the year 2020—would make the total intersex population 10,140,000.[56] A similar statistic reports the incidence of intersex births in the United States as almost two for every one hundred, or about 2 percent of the population—about the same odds, we are told, for being born with red hair.[57] Many websites and even some scientists have widely publicized this "red hair" analogy as irrefutable fact.[58]

A website devoted to intersex equality gives an astronomical number of 132,600,000—a little more than 13 times the figure of 1.3 in 1000 infants—based on calculation by Anne Fausto-Sterling.[59] She labels people with various medical conditions as intersex. These include females with Turner Syndrome (they lack a second X chromosome, but are clearly female) and males with Klinefelter Syndrome (possessing XXY chromosomes, but they are clearly male). People with Congenital Adrenal Hyperplasia are also considered intersex, even though it's a well-known medical condition (discussed shortly), and no experienced physician would dream of calling a CAH person "intersex."

In a paper published in 2000, Fausto-Sterling and co-authors expanded the label of intersex to include any person who diverges from the Platonic ideal of physical dimorphism at any level: chromosomal, gonadal, genital, or hormonal. *Physical dimorphism* refers to a markedly different appearance in males and females, which is how you tell them apart. The so-called Platonic ideal (named after teachings of the Greek philosopher Plato) characterizes the features of all things in nature with extremely narrow parameters so that any variations of a basic pattern are seen as different species, not as organic changes or deviations evolving over time. The authors' interpretation of the Platonic ideal for a male consists of XY chromosomes, testes in a scrotal sac that produce functional ejaculate, hormone production ensuring a normal masculinizing puberty, and a penis measuring between 2.5 and 4.5 cm at birth. An ideal female is supposed to have XX chromosomes, functional ovaries that produce eggs and ensure a normal feminizing puberty, oviducts (tubes through which the eggs pass) that connect to a uterus, a vaginal canal connecting the cervix (lower portion of the uterus) to the mouth of the vagina, inner and outer vaginal lips, and a clitoris measuring between 0.20 and 0.85 cm at birth. The authors of the article begin by asking how often male and female development meets these exacting criteria.[60]

How often, indeed? Certainly not as often as one might hope, considering such stringent requirements. Penile and clitoral measurements can vary widely, and a man or woman might possess improperly functioning structures or lack them altogether. Therefore, it's not unreasonable to guess that some people's reproductive apparatus would fall outside this Platonic template. Why, then, were such unreasonably rigid—not to mention unrealistic—criteria used by the authors? Colin Wright offers a levelheaded hypothesis:

> There appear to be two main goals when forwarding this claim—one laudable, the other insidious. The laudable goal is to normalize the existence of intersex people and thereby help facilitate the societal acceptance of a marginalized community who may experience social

ostracism and who have often been victims of medically unnecessary "corrective" cosmetic surgeries as infants. The insidious goal is to plant seeds of doubt in our collective understanding of biological sex and suggest that the categories "male" and "female" may be social constructs or exist on a "spectrum."[61]

Wright takes care to point out that no matter what the percentage of intersexuals is, even if it's "quite low, this by no means justifies any of the mistreatment, whether socially or medically, that many gender activists hope to prevent when they overstate its prevalence. How we treat people, and the rights afforded to them, should not be predicated on their prevalence within a population. And that is the point we should be trying to normalize, rather than false statistics."[62] I agree. The mistreatment that intersexual people endure is inexcusable. But by sacrificing science at the altar of getting people to behave compassionately, the authors of the "Platonic ideal" article end up doing everyone a huge disservice.

Let's take a more detailed look now at the most common variations of sexual development—some of which are genuinely intersex, and some that have been classified under the intersex umbrella. This is not merely an academic exercise. Several of the anatomical variations are the result of serious medical conditions, which if left untreated can be life-threatening.

Some Common Variations

Below are the most common and easily recognized departures from the usual development of males and females. Some of the syndromes overlap, and in many cases the causes are multifaceted.

- *Androgen Insensitivity Syndrome (AIS)*
  This syndrome, occurring in one in 20,000 to one in 64,000 individuals, affects sexual development before birth and during puberty. Children are born with the male XY pattern and testes that make abundant testosterone. However, the body's cells are unable to detect and respond to testosterone (a major androgen hormone), either completely or partially. The testes of all males naturally produce some estrogen during puberty; so if the body's ability to respond to testosterone is exceptionally reduced, feminization will be more pronounced. The individual often develops breasts. The body shape may appear female because the waist narrows and hips widen—so much so, that the person may develop a voluptuous figure. Usually secondary sexual characteristics do not appear, so once puberty starts the child does not develop facial hair. This condition used to be called "testicular feminization syndrome" because often it was not discovered until the adolescents—assumed to be girls due to their appearance—failed to menstruate. Then, after they were examined, it was discovered that some of them had testes instead of ovaries.

  Complete androgen insensitivity causes the person's external genitalia to look like those of a typical female. Milder cases of androgen insensitivity can cause the person's external genital to be more ambiguous in appearance. The organ might only somewhat resemble a typical female's, it can possess both male and female characteristics, or it might even resemble a typical male's.

At this time, conventional medicine has no way of inducing the androgen receptor sites on the cells to start receiving and absorbing testosterone, although some holistic methods might help (see Notes).[63] The medical establishment provides sexual "reassignment" in the form of hormone replacement and genital plastic surgery. Sometimes counseling is offered, but sadly, not often. If the baby's sex is unclear, most doctors immediately advise the parents to "correct" the child's appearance so it is recognizable as either male or female (usually female). Usually, the individual appears female and is raised as a girl.

Some medical authorities consider this an intersex condition while others see it as a medical problem. I agree that this a medical problem because the condition is due to malfunctioning androgen receptors.

♦ *Congenital Adrenal Hyperplasia (Adrenogenital Syndrome)*
Congenital adrenal hyperplasia, or CAH, is not a "one size fits all" disorder. It encompasses a group of disparate medical conditions that are due to a malfunction of the adrenals, the pair of walnut-size glands that sit on top of the kidneys. The adrenals produce cortisol, which regulates the body's response to illness or stress; mineralocorticoids such as aldosterone, which regulate sodium and potassium levels; and testosterone and other androgens, which both males and females produce.[64] How CAH manifests, when it emerges (it can be late-onset), and at what intensity, depends on which gene is expressing and which enzymes or hormones are being produced in insufficient or excessive amounts. Each contributing factor may have more than one name, depending on the source describing it. However, the overall dynamics are widely recognized by medical personnel.

Classic CAH is the most severe and rare form, also known as "salt-wasting." It results from insufficient aldosterone and affects about one in 10,000 to 15,000 people. The body, unable to retain enough sodium, suffers severe, life-threatening problems with the heart, occasionally accompanied by ambiguous changes in the genitals.[65] This clearly medical condition requires treatment for the person's entire lifespan. However, the two manifestations of CAH more relevant to our discussion are considerably less severe, affecting primarily the sexual system: simple virilizing CAH and nonclassic CAH.[66]

Simple virilizing CAH reflects a moderate 21-hydroxylase deficiency and a mild aldosterone deficiency, which in simple language means too little cortisol and too much androgen. Nonclassic CAH is caused by a slight deficiency in 21-hydroxylase (cortisol)—so slight, in fact, that some people with this condition don't know it because the symptoms are so mild.[67] In girls and boys with more challenging issues, there may be a growth spurt at a very early age that culminates in lessened growth as an adult, with occasional infertility.

Otherwise, health is normal. Both CAH types have similarly ambiguous genitalia. Males may display early signs of puberty and an enlarged penis. Females may exhibit an irregular menstrual cycle, facial hair, a deeper voice than usual, and an enlarged clitoris.

Some researchers claim that girls with simple virilizing CAH are less stereotypically feminine and more masculine according to current Western cultural standards. For example, they enjoy playing with trucks and other boy-associated toys instead of dolls, and they're more interested in their careers than in marrying and having children. Other researchers have disputed these findings. None of this matters. The girls will need the love and support of understanding adults if they are to love and accept themselves.

This is not an intersex variation, but a medical condition. Most CAH individuals can live fulfilling lives. They can be treated with feminizing or masculinizing hormones if they are uncomfortable with their appearance.

- *Polycystic Ovary Syndrome (PCOS)*
PCOS is the name for a somewhat complicated condition in women that can have more than one cause. Normally, females produce testosterone and other androgen hormones in small amounts: in the ovaries, adrenal glands, and certain fat cells. (Males produce them in much larger amounts in the testes, and to a much lesser extent in the adrenal glands.) Androgens are responsible for male sexual characteristics and reproductive activity, but in females they also play an important role in more than two hundred bodily functions. This includes the stimulation of hair growth in the pubic and underarm regions, the prevention of bone loss, the regulation of muscles and several organs, and sexual desire and satiety.

In women, the body normally converts the androgens into estrogens. But four to seven percent of women are unable to make the conversion due to a tumor on an ovary or adrenal gland, or a malfunction of the pituitary gland. Possible outcomes include an enlarged clitoris, a decrease in breast size, a more angular figure, an increase of male-pattern body hair (on the face, chin, and/or abdomen), a deepened voice, lack of a menstrual period, and greater muscular strength than the average female. Many women with PCOS are medically treated because this hormonal imbalance can have more severe and harmful effects, including high blood pressure and insulin resistance that leads to diabetes. Sometimes, though, a woman has a much milder case, her more masculine appearance being the chief symptom.

With this condition, there is no question that the individual is female. Hormone imbalances are causing her male secondary sex characteristics, so this is not a true intersex variation. She might be treated with feminizing hormones if she's uncomfortable with her appearance. If there's a tumor on one of her glands, it's probably necessary to surgically remove it.

- *XY with 5-α-Reductase Deficiency*
    The majority of people with an insufficient supply of enzyme 5-α-reductase live in portions of the Dominican Republic and in the Papua, New Guinea highlands, home to the Sambian population. (The geographical specificity suggests a nutrient imbalance in the soil or water, or certain toxins that might interfere with enzymatic reactions in the body.) At birth, XY infants with this enzyme deficiency have ambiguous genitalia: a tiny penis that looks like a clitoris, undescended testes, and a divided scrotum that could easily be mistaken for a vagina. Sometimes the ambiguity of such children is recognized immediately, while other times the children are raised as girls. Most of the time during puberty, when the sex glands—which are functioning normally—produce additional testosterone, the individuals appear more typically male. Testes descend and the divided scrotal lips fuse to form a more typical scrotum. The boys become more muscular and develop hair on the body and face. In the United States, doctors tend to immediately operate on the hapless infant, but in the two areas of the world where this phenomenon is common, the infant is left alone because it's understood that he will change when he hits puberty. Both cultures have a name for such a child. The Dominicans call him *guevedoche*, or "penis at twelve," while the Sambians term the impending transformation *kwolu-aatmwol*, which means "[will transform] into a male thing."[68]

    The outcome is always male. The genitals simply become more developed and recognizable later in life, and the secondary sex characteristics occur later than with typical males. Testes are always present. Therefore, I do not consider this condition intersex. Some medical authorities disagree.

- *De la Chapelle Syndrome (Sex Inversion): Males With XX Chromosomes*
    With this condition, a male possesses XX chromosomes. Known as "sex inversion," 46,XX, or De la Chapelle Syndrome—after the Finnish doctor who first described it—this variation occurs in about one in 20,000 infants. During fertilization, a gene that programs for male development gets moved from where it's normally located. Commonly, a small Y chromosome fragment transposes onto an X chromosome, which produces an XX male.

    Due to the predominance of X traits, the body produces less testosterone than usual. The appearance of XX males can vary. The most common manifestations are small testes, enlarged breast tissue (noncancerous), bone weakness (due to decreases in calcium and phosphate), erectile dysfunction, diminished libido, infertility, and sometimes depression. However, not all XX males manifest all these characteristics. Internal and external genitalia may be ambiguous, unambiguous, or a mixture of the two. Males with De la Chapelle Syndrome have different degrees of masculinization.

    I have not seen recent research on someone with this syndrome who has chosen to live as a woman. British racing driver and World War II fighter pilot Robert Marshall Cowell (1918–2011), who later became Roberta—the first known British subject to undergo sexual "reassignment" surgery—claimed

to have been born with De la Chapelle syndrome. Unlike 80 percent of people with this condition, Cowell was not sterile, having fathered two children with his wife when he lived as Robert.

Hormone and genetic testing can confirm this syndrome. Supplementary testosterone usually corrects the manifestations. Psychosexually, these individuals generally identify as male. If boys are treated with kindness and are given counseling—along with testosterone—early enough to help them cope with their condition, they can live normal and productive lives. Some may choose not to be medically treated.

Medical authorities label De la Chapelle Syndrome an intersex condition.

- *46,XY*

The "46" refers to a chromosome involved in sexual development. There are many possible causes of 46,XY. The person might be unable to completely synthesize testosterone and other androgen hormones. Or the receptor sites to those hormones might be scarce, resistant, or functioning poorly in other ways. Sometimes there's a deficiency of one or more enzymes that are required to produce testosterone—in which case, the amount of testosterone will be scanty, or the hormone won't work as well as it typically does.

The repercussions of this condition are many and varied. The person may appear markedly male, but most often masculinization is weak due to insufficient testosterone. The individual may look male and possess atypical external genitals. The genitals may be ambiguous, incompletely formed as a male micropenis, or even female in appearance. But even if an individual has what appears to be a vagina, there may be an absence of ovaries, Fallopian tubes, and a uterus. Testes might be absent. If they are present, they could be internal—which means they simply haven't descended from the abdominal cavity as they usually do. If the testes are internal and functioning properly, and receptors to the hormone are also working, the person will be masculinized in the usual manner, especially when puberty starts. Alternately, if testes are present they might be abnormally formed. There are as many variations as there are individuals with this syndrome. Olympic track and field runner Caster Semenya has this condition, producing ample testosterone and appearing masculine while living as a woman due to the appearance of an isolated vagina-like structure. The athlete's participation in women's sports is covered in Appendix B.

This condition is rightly considered intersex. Doctors typically "correct" the genitals via surgery when the child is very young. But this is at best a mistake, and at worst unkind. If the individual is surgically manipulated to look like one sex but possesses functioning gonads, ample hormone levels and normal hormonal receptors of the opposite sex, overtly opposite-sex traits will manifest at puberty. Young children, rather than having hormones and surgery forced on them, should be allowed to choose their own path as adults.

- *Simultaneous Male and Female Sex Organs*
  The medical profession used to call this condition "hermaphroditism" or "pseudohermaphroditism" until objections were raised by those who felt stigmatized by the labels. These individuals possess both male and female external genitalia that are visible at the same time. One cause is excessive androgen hormone exposure in female embryos, which results in male-looking genitals. Another cause is delayed testosterone exposure in males, which results in female-looking genitals until puberty.

  Variations of this intersex condition can occur when two fertilized eggs fuse together, giving the fertilized cell or zygote two X chromosomes and one Y chromosome. Some individuals who display such genitalia might have been exposed *in utero* to common agricultural pesticides, which are known to adversely affect hormones (see Chapter 5). Before such pesticides were manufactured, such intersex individuals existed, but they were rare.

Regardless of one's genetic makeup or reproductive organs, everyone deserves to be treated with respect. Unfortunately, not everyone is. See below.

Surgical "Corrections"

What is being done to help children with atypical genitalia? It depends on what kind of help you are talking about, and who is offering. The Western medical establishment, rather than expanding its world view to include variations of human anatomy and respecting an infant's right to bodily autonomy, chooses instead to "fix" the child.

When any child is born, the doctor or midwife checks for general health and examines the genitals to determine the child's sex. If a doctor decides that the genitals don't appear normal—that is, if the testes haven't descended, the vulva doesn't look like other vulvas, the penis is deemed too small or the clitoris is deemed too large—tests are ordered. A genetic evaluation and hormone tests are conducted to ensure that they coincide with each other according to the most usual standards. Then the doctors make sure that their visual inspection of the genitals corresponds to both the chromosomes and the hormones. Based on what the tests reveal, the genitals are surgically altered. Unless the parents intervene, it's usually not a matter of *whether* to perform surgery on the child, it's a question of *which* sex's genitals to use as a template *when* doing the surgery. Surgery is intended to make the child's sex organs match the gold standard for what genitals are supposed to look like, according to the medical profession.

In 2018, Kristina Turner and her 10-year-old intersex child Ori gave a presentation. They showed a chart depicting "optimal" genital sizes, designed to help doctors determine if a newborn's genitals are female or male. If clitoral/penile tissue is under three-eighths of an inch, the child is a girl. If the tissue is above one inch, the child is a boy. The gray area between three-eighths of an inch and one inch is apparently unacceptable and indicates the "need" for surgery.[69]

The problem is, standards for genital size and shape depend on the aesthetic preferences of the doctors, and sometimes the parents too. Surgeons who don't think that the genitals match the child's chromosomal and/or hormonal makeup advise giving the child hormones and surgically reshaping the genitals before the age of two—even though in the vast majority of cases, the infant is perfectly healthy. In the case of intersexual Ori Turner, had mother Kristina succumbed to pressure from the medical establishment and allowed surgery, the doctors would have been faced with quite a dilemma. Ori possesses both XX and XY genetic material. In this case, what is Ori's sex? I have not seen reports of the size and appearance of Ori's genitals—the child has a right to privacy—so it's difficult to say if Ori is fundamentally male or female, neither, or both.

Few infants and children possess Ori's apparent ambiguity. And many CAH girls exhibit only an enlarged clitoris to indicate an internal health issue. Yet doctors tend to push parents to give very young girls "corrective" genital surgery. What, exactly, is being corrected? A perfectly intact clitoris is being mutilated because it doesn't conform to a stereotypical clitoris as envisioned by medical personnel. The surgeon typically cuts off the tip intact, lobs off most of the shaft, and then reattaches the tip to the stump. But when you excise tissue and cut through sensitive nerves, it kills them. This almost guarantees that as an adult, the girl's chance for a healthy and gratifying sex life will be destroyed. She may suffer reduced sensation, or never be able to experience orgasm at all. Then there's the risk of infection from surgery. Any type of alteration to genitals, female or male, that is performed for a reason other than absolute medical neccessity, can and should be regarded as mutilation.[70]

"Some women with CAH," one website advises, "who had surgery as babies wish they had not had it. This risk of surgery needs to be weighed against concerns over parenting a child with unusual genital appearance. Take your time to decide about surgery that is *elective* and not *medically necessary*. There's no reason to rush into elective surgery."[71] Registered nurse Stephani Lohman, whose daughter has a mild (not life-threatening) form of CAH, explains her decision.

> I had noticed right away that my baby's genitals did not look like what any of my other children had. A couple days later, a urologist suggested that we do elective surgery: a clitoroplasty [surgery to reduce the size of a clitoris], and a vaginoplasty [surgery to increase the size of a vagina or create a cavern to imitate a vagina] to make our baby look more "typically female." We argued back, saying that we had done a little research on our own and it didn't seem like this was a good suggestion....They may believe genital differences cause social problems, but that has never been shown, and urologists are not the authority on psychology....[F]or those who do grow up to have a female gender identity, how can we be certain they might not want to grow up with their original bodies, or decide based on how they feel later?...We decided that we would wait and let our child make an informed choice on their own, since it is their body.[72]

Besides destroying sexual pleasure and orgasm, clitoral surgery can cause permanent pain that does not subside, regardless of whether the clitoral tissue is flaccid or erect. Surgery frequently causes necrosis (the death of tissue) because cutting severs the flow of blood to the area. Stenosis—the narrowing or obstruction of a canal, channel or duct—is the most commonly reported complication of surgery for ambiguous genitalia, reports Fausto-Sterling, based on her review of the literature. Scar tissue, often occurring in the vaginal (introital) opening, is a typical cause of this obstruction. The narrowing or outright obstruction causes not only discomfort, but often excruciating pain. Additional surgeries may be required to eliminate the original scar tissue.

Cheryl Chase, Executive Director of the Intersex Society of North America, sent a letter in 1998 to a judge in Columbia, South America about a case involving the unnecessary cutting of girls' genitals. Among her many points, Chase wrote that when a child is older, the genitals are larger and therefore easier for a surgeon to work on without scarring. "One reason for poor surgical outcomes may be that scar tissue is negatively affected by the changes in size and shape that accompany normal growth and pubertal development; surgery performed after puberty would avoid that risk. It is likely that surgical techniques will have improved by the time she has grown; waiting will allow her to benefit from advances in technology....There is good evidence that adults would not choose clitoral surgery for themselves. There are many adult intersex women who express regret and anger that genital surgery was imposed on them."[73]

Morgan Holmes was one unfortunate recipient of such surgery. When Morgan's mother was pregnant with her, to prevent miscarriage doctors prescribed the hormone progestin, which can masculinize the fetus. As a result, Holmes was born with an enlarged clitoris. Doctors "corrected" her genitals with surgery—which she remembers—when she was seven years old. Unfortunately, Morgan Holmes did not have parents like Stephani Lohman to protect her. Although she could still have orgasms, her sexual function was nonetheless severely affected. "If my body had been left intact and my clitoris had grown at the same rate as the rest of my body," she wonders, "what would my lesbian relationships [and]...my current heterosexual relationship be like?...When the doctors initially assured my father that I would grow up to have 'normal sexual function,' they did not mean that they could guarantee that my amputated clitoris would be sensitive or that I would be able to achieve orgasm...What was being guaranteed was that I would not grow up to confuse the issue of who (man) fucks whom (woman)."[74]

Another common surgery for CAH girls involves the urinary tract. Most females have two separate openings at the front of the vagina: the birth canal, and a smaller opening to the urethra which connects to the urinary bladder. CAH females sometimes have a urogenital sinus, which is an area where the urethra and vagina connect inside the body. This means that there's a single opening for fluids to leave the body. "Most children with CAH and genital differences," explains Lohman, "have a urogenital sinus with a low confluence, meaning that the urethra connects with the vagina at a point that is close to the outside of the body instead of higher up toward the bladder." Some doctors claim that failing to perform surgery on a urogenital sinus increases the risk of more urinary tract infections (UTIs). But "this is false and misleading," Lohman writes.

> In fact, children who do not have surgery for a urogenital sinus have no greater risk of UTIs than those who do. It is actually the opposite—it's been shown that surgery itself can increase UTI risk. Surgery can also cause incontinence, or leakage of urine. For most people, urine does not dribble out on its own. The urine stays in your bladder because you have a sphincter: it opens, you urinate, it closes, and you're done. Some people will be incontinent *because of* surgery if the sphincter or the nerves that control it are damaged....Think about it: you opened a sterile region of someone's body, cut tissue, and moved things around. This creates scar tissue that can interfere with urinary function. Afterwards, it makes sense that we'd see UTIs increase.[75]

Boys are not immune, either, from being robbed of their birthright of pleasure. If the child's penis is deemed too small, the doctor will examine the infant rectally to see if the body contains a uterus or prostate gland. If there's no prostate, the decision on how to "correct" this is clear: Create a girl! According to an article on surgery for ambiguous genitalia, fewer than 10 percent of babies born with ambiguous genitals receive surgery to resemble males. This isn't surprising, as it's easier to remove tissue than create and attach a functional appendage. Therefore, with an infant whose penis is considered insufficiently developed—perhaps accompanied by an unfused scrotum, and *especially* if the child also possesses XX genetic material—doctors simply remove the penis, and either form a cavern to resemble a vagina or enlarge an already existing opening. The idea is to raise such boys as girls. But not all boys respond well to such surgery, even if they don't consciously remember it. Later in life they may discover, much to their grief and anger, that they had been violated.[76]

The article "Surgery for intersex," published in 2001 in the *Journal of the Royal Society of Medicine*, discussed the long-term outcome of genitoplasty, a form of plastic surgery to "feminize" the genitals. The author admitted that results from surgery were poor, and often more than one surgery was necessary because sexual intercourse wasn't possible, or was painful. Continued pain or complete lack of sensation, often due to scarring, was common. Also, there were too few long-term follow-up studies because doctors like to perform surgery immediately—which makes it difficult to find a large enough control group of intact females against whom results can be compared.[77] Since the article's publication, the desire has not lessened to "fix" people whose genitals don't look the way doctors or parents think they should. The authors of "Surgical Management of Infants and Children With Ambiguous Genitalia" emphasize how important it will be in the future for their patient to have a "satisfactory appearance when compared with peers....The existence of a normal-sized penis [which of course is their job to surgically correct] in patients assigned a male role is comforting *to the parents*... Conversely, female babies born with an ungainly masculine enlargement of the clitoris evoke grave concern *in their parents.*"[78] [emphasis added][78] Note that the emphasis on having surgery is typically for the comfort of others. The individual's bodily integrity, the right to experience pleasure, and the need to live a life free of pain, are never considered. Few doctors tell parents of the risks of surgery, and the patients are too young to give consent. How many parents would agree to a risky surgical procedure for their child if they knew the dangers—physically, mentally, and emotionally?

People with atypical genitalia who have reached adulthood are now fighting back. They recognize that the mutilation to which they were subjected as infants and children is a human rights violation. In fact, the Nuremberg Code specifically prohibits involuntary surgical procedures designed to alter the genitals for aesthetic rather than medically necessary purposes.

Christiane Völling from Germany is one person who fought back. Born in 1960, she had the medical condition called virilizing adrenal hyperplasia, which gave her ambiguous genitalia. Although she was raised as a boy, Völling had always considered herself female. When she underwent an appendectomy at age 17, her surgeon found that she had a uterus and womb. Although her female reproductive organs were completely intact, he removed them without telling his patient what he had discovered—and without her consent. In 2007, Völling began a two-year lawsuit against the surgeon for damages relating to the nonconsensual surgical intervention. For years, she said, she suffered physical impairments, pain, and psychological problems. She was awarded one hundred thousand pounds by the Regional Court of Cologne, which ruled that the surgeon had acted illegally.[79]

In 2015, Michaela "Micha" Raab sued the Erlangen University Clinic, also in Germany, for a nonconsensual partial clitoris amputation and hormone treatments. The doctor who performed surgery was found not liable—the court said that other doctors were responsible—but the clinic itself was found guilty. That same year, Nils Muižnieks, the Council of Europe Commissioner for Human Rights, published a paper outlining the rights of people with atypical genitals to decide for themselves whether to undergo surgical and hormonal interventions. The document read in part:

> Sex assignment treatment should be available to intersex individuals at an age when they can express their free and fully informed consent. Intersex persons' right not to undergo sex assignment treatment must be respected....National and international medical classifications which pathologise variations in sex characteristics should be reviewed with a view to eliminating obstacles to the effective enjoyment, by intersex persons, of human rights, including the right to the highest attainable standard of health....Intersex persons and their families should be offered interdisciplinary

counselling and support, including peer support. Intersex persons' access to medical records should be ensured.[80]

Malta is the first country to prohibit modifications to sex characteristics without the person's consent. As this issue is given wider publicity, more countries are expected to enact similar laws. As positive as this step is, though, we need to confront the deeper issues that people with atypical genitals elicit.

The underlying concern is that most people are uncomfortable with ambiguous sex organs. At what point do we stop perceiving sexual ambiguities as "variations" and call them statistically unusual "aberrations"? When a woman has a clitoris that's "too long"?[81] When a man has a penis that's "too small"? Or when someone with XY chromosomes has a female-looking body? But why do chromosomes matter now, when they didn't in the past? In real life (except perhaps until recently), before we started dating we didn't ask others about their chromosomal makeup; usually, one look at their appearance sufficed. During a presentation in June 2022, Colin Wright pointed out that throughout human history, we knew what males and females were long before we had microscopes that allowed us to observe the mysterious realm of imperceptible chromosomes. Ironically, there were a lot fewer problems with identifying sex when we didn't have the luxury of delving into microscopic worlds. There's a difference, Wright astutely declared, between "Your sex is *determined* by your chromosomes" and "Your sex is *defined* by your chromosomes."[82]

It's worth noting that before the phrase "Divergences of Sexual Development" was used to describe atypical genitals, the medical term was "*Disorders* of Sexual Development" and sometimes "*Disturbances* of Sexual Development." Some medical professionals still use the old phrases. But even for those who use the politically correct newer terminology, no words can erase how they really feel about genitals that don't conform to their aesthetic criteria. If we believe that such variations are created by genetic *disorders*, it's a small step to then assume that the owners of those genitals are abnormal—and thus need to be fixed. If they require fixing, it's another, small step to seeing them as a bit less than human, because they aren't "real" males or "real" females. Some people equate being "less than human" to being less deserving of compassion, regard, and even basic rights. Compare the condition of non-boilerplate genitals to medical conditions such as arthritis, needing a wheelchair due to amputation of a limb, or having cancer. A compassionate and humane person would never dream of judging someone who's ill as less deserving of respect and care. So why do we do this to those whose genitals fall outside of a certain standard of beauty or so-called normalcy? We would not slash into the genitals of someone who has the flu. So why do we insist on doing it to people whose genitals appear different? Why can't there simply be genital variety? Why not allow individuals to be themselves?[83] As long as they are happy, fulfilled and productive—and their atypical genitals are not presenting medical problems—who cares what their chromosomes are or what their genitals look like?

Unfortunately, some people do care—even though it's none of their business—about whether other people's genitals match their notion of normalcy. If a child presents standard-appearing genitals, then chromosomal and hormonal discrepancies might be overlooked. But the majority of physicians who observe atypical genitals feel compelled to investigate further to ensure that chromosomes, hormones and genitalia are all aligned with the most common template. And most parents of unusual children also seem overly concerned that their child appear "normal." As much as some of us might want to believe that the desire to "normalize" an infant is well-intended and for the child's own good, ultimately that desire is usually for the peace of mind of parents and doctors—not the child. Surgery that alters healthy genitals should be called what it is: mutilation. Let the individual decide as an adult what, if anything, should be done. Damaging a human being so we can make ourselves more comfortable with that person's sex organs is unethical, wrong, and cruel. The only reason to offer medical treatment to an individual with unusual genitals is for potentially life-threatening conditions, such as tumors on the gonads, a hernia, or a salt or other biochemical imbalance due to adrenal malfunction. None of these medical symptoms specifically require interfering with the size or shape of the genitalia.

When a rare albino deer, rhino or buffalo are spotted in nature, we celebrate and marvel at it. We need to apply this appreciation of difference to sexual ambiguity. Rather than changing someone's body, we need to expand our standards of what's acceptable. A provisional identity may be given until the child is old enough to decide what she or he wants to do.

Categorizing Versus Assigning

When a doctor examines a newborn to determine its sex, the medical establishment typically calls this process "*assigning* a sex" to the child. Similarly, when someone undergoes the scalpel to have their genitals repositioned, sculpted and reshaped to approximate the opposite sex's genitalia, modern medicine calls this "sexual *reassignment* surgery." I find both of these phrases very troubling because the sex of a child cannot be "assigned."

The secular, common definition of *assign* is "to appoint to a post or duty," or "to appoint as a duty or task."[84] A reporter at a newspaper is *assigned* to cover an event. A schoolchild is given homework *assignments*. Someone is *assigned* specific duties as part of their job. How is it possible for human beings to "assign" genitals to other humans? Only nature (or God) can "assign" body parts. What we are doing is *observing* the child's sex so we know whether it's male or female. On the other hand, sex *roles*, also known as gender roles, *are* assigned. I'll be discussing sex (gender) role stereotypes in great detail in the next chapter, but right now I will finish my point, which is related to biology and not culture.

Whenever we use the phrase "sexual assignment," this sleight-of-hand with the English language is not only misleading, it's dangerous. It's dangerous because it promotes concepts that are fictitious. If we believe that we can call a child one sex or the other based on our beliefs, then there's no such thing as biology. And without biology, there are no facts; it's all opinion. What we *can* do, though—which *is* consistent with reality—is *categorize* children according to their biological sex. *Categorize* means "to put into a category," and a *category* is "any of several fundamental and distinct classes to which entities or concepts belong."[85] We can reliably place human beings into categories of male or female, based on what type of reproductive cells they produce: eggs (ova) in females, or sperm in males.

Proponents of the "there are more than two sexes" theory like to point out that nature is not as rigid as we might believe. This is true; variety is part of the natural world. Some species of animals share duties. For example, the male seahorse gestates the eggs that the female lays in his pouch. Male penguins stand on the eggs of their offspring, and later, keep the baby birds warm after they've hatched. In a massive transformation, certain species of fish, reptiles and amphibians are able to change their biological sex.[86] But there is never a third sex. Males change into females, and vice-versa. With humans, even when the sex is ambiguous, it's *still* never a third sex. It might be both male *and* female. It could be just slightly reminiscent of one or the other, or of both. Or it could be neither. But even if that ambiguity seems like neither, it still would have differentiated into something resembling male and/or female: It contains the seeds for both. We might possess greater or lesser amounts of "maleness" or greater or lesser amounts of "femaleness," but the reference points are still male and female. We all belong somewhere on the male-female spectrum—there are simply no other choices. Keep in mind that being on the biological spectrum does not mean another species or a different sex. As I mentioned earlier during the discussion of the Platonic ideal, any departures from a basic pattern are variations. The same basic pattern remains and never disappears.

This biological reality notwithstanding, more people than ever—especially those under the 30-year-old age bracket—are claiming that they are "non-binary." They don't want to be categorized as being either male or female, so they are "assigning" themselves a category that they believe somehow neutralizes, negates, or changes their genitals.

Why would some people want to fight so hard against their own biology?

There are many causes. One major reason is the harmful stereotypes that are foisted on people whether they want them or not. You got a small taste of them in this chapter, and the next chapter will be devoted exclusively to all sorts of ways in which we box people in. Our culture promotes the mindset *You're either a man as society defines him, or you're a woman as society defines her. Anything else is unacceptable.* But society's definitions are extremely limiting. Children who don't follow this script—whether physically, behaviorally, mentally, or emotionally—are harshly judged, bullied, and ostracized. Therefore, some people might think that if they renounce their sexual category as a biological male or biological female, they'll be able to fling away the cultural expectations, labels, and pressures that automatically accompany what lies between their legs. But with this magical thinking, these non-binary folks are making a huge error. They're mistaking their biological sex for the *social roles* ascribed to that biology—and because of that, are causing themselves immense and unnecessary heartache.

Sex role stereotypes are so ubiquitous in our culture that they have become invisible. How can we lessen—even if we can't entirely eliminate—some of the pressure people feel to be more stereotypically masculine or more stereotypically feminine? That is what I'll be exploring in the next chapter.

PART II

CULTURE

2

SEX ROLE STEREOTYPES

Clarifying Gender

What is gender? Ever since the word came into existence, its meaning has changed—but only in some circles, and only sometimes. A person might use the word differently on different days. The first thing, then, is to clarify the meaning of the word as I will be using it throughout this book.

Since about the 14th century, *gender* meant "kind, sort, class, a class or kind of persons or things sharing certain traits." An earlier form of the word came from the Old French *gendre* and *genre*, which meant "character" as well as "kind" or "species." All these words are rooted in the much older Latin *genus*, which meant "race, stock, family; kind, rank, order, species," as well as "(male or female) sex." Despite its etymological age, *gender* was rarely uttered. Instead, *sex* was used to describe whether someone was male or female.[1]

The concept of gender *roles* is said to have been introduced in 1955 by a psychologist.[2] But the differences between sex and gender became widely publicized and accepted in 1972 with the publication of *Sex, Gender, and Society* by sociologist Ann Oakley. In her book, Oakley distinguished between *biological sex*, which is determined by one's reproductive organs, and *gender*, based on beliefs about what men and women are capable of and how they ought to behave. Oakley's book was groundbreaking because she explored many cultures. The cross-cultural comparisons of men's and women's roles—which were quite different, depending on the country and even region—demonstrated how characteristics that might have been considered innate were in fact heavily influenced by one's environment. Oakley not only provided clarity about women's issues, she also catalyzed the extensive use of *gender* to mean *sex role stereotypes*.[3] Those phrases, along with *sex roles, gender roles,* and *gender stereotypes* were all used by feminists and some academicians to mean the same thing.

Problems arose when the word "gender" began to be used interchangeably with the word "sex"—and its meaning as *imposed cultural stereotypes* became lost.[4] Today, most people say "gender" when they really mean "sex," thinking that it indicates the biological reality of whether one is male or female.

The fusion of the two words confused more than just the general public. A surprisingly large number of researchers and scientists conflated the terms as well. Editors of a scholarly textbook describe problems they encountered as a result of the shifting terminology.

> One of the first barriers that…[we] faced was the inconsistent and often confusing use of the terms *sex* and *gender* in the scientific literature and the popular press.
>
> Use of *sex* and *gender* varies widely among disciplines and authors. Anthropologists…consider the distinction between *sex* and *gender*…to be very important, as it is possible to determine sex by analyzing skeletal remains and to obtain information on gender roles through the study of artifacts. A 1988 study…demonstrates [that] although the rate of use of the term *sex* in the biomedical literature has not changed significantly since the late 1960s, the rate of use of the term *gender* has increased markedly…[M]ost articles published in the late 1960s and early 1970s made a distinction between *sex* and *gender*. However, among the more recent articles…more than half did not distinguish between the terms….[M]ost published reports are using gender as a synonym for sex…Medical textbooks perpetuate the confusion. *Harrison's Principles of Internal Medicine*, the quintessential internal medicine text, uses sex and gender interchangeably.[5]

Some sources, though, are clear about the distinctions between sex and gender. The differences are so important that the American Psychological Association defines the terms in a pamphlet. "Sex…refers to one's biological status as either male or female, and is associated primarily with physical attributes such as chromosomes, hormone prevalence, and external and internal anatomy. Gender refers to the socially constructed roles, behaviors, activities, and attributes that a given society considers appropriate for boys and men or girls and women. These influence the ways that people act, interact, and feel about themselves."[6]

Even the Office of the High Commissioner of Human Rights (OHCHR) offers a definition: "A gender stereotype is a generalized view or preconception about attributes or characteristics, or the roles that are or ought to be possessed by, or performed by, women and men." The OHCHR also cautions that "A gender stereotype is harmful when it limits women's and men's capacity to develop their personal abilities, pursue their professional careers and/or make choices about their lives."[7] Neuroscientist Lise Eliot warns that stereotypes can induce severe anxiety because they pressure people to conform to society's expectations that might not be compatible with their own desires, needs, and proclivities. Other researchers investigating stereotyping—in this case, of minority racial groups, but it applies to sex-related prejudice as well—write that "Being stereotyped can negatively influence academic performance, memory, leadership aspirations, and self-esteem."[8]

In this book, sex and gender have distinctly separate meanings. *Sex* indicates whether one is male or female, based solely on one's reproductive organs. *Gender* specifies the different cultural expectations imposed on males and females. Except when I quote others, whenever "gender" is used it will always be accompanied by "roles," "stereotypes," or something similar.

How did this one little word come to be so misunderstood? Especially in the scientific arena, where the need for precision is critical, you'd think researchers would get it right. Some believe that by the mid-20th century, the word may have been too closely associated with sexual intercourse and other erotic acts, which is why *gender* became widely used as a substitution for "sex [of a human being]."[9] However, psychiatrist Miriam Grossman believes that the term was deliberately perverted. "The conflation of sex with gender was a critical development, but like so many things it escaped the radar of most. It was a deliberate weaponizing of language, but to what end? Gender, we are told, is subjective, fluid on a spectrum, multidimensional. If sex and gender are interchangeable, then sex is all those things too—subjective, multidimensional, nuanced…In the end, 'male' and 'female' mean nothing. *They [transgender activists] want sex to be synonymous with gender, so they can destroy it.*"[10]

Grossman's assertion is not as far-fetched as it might seem. The very biology of being human *is* in danger, courtesy of sex "reassignment." One of the chief strategies used by trans activists to indoctrinate children is the maintenance, promotion, and exaggeration of sex role stereotypes. This is partly accomplished by language manipulation. Another way is to secure the cooperation of researchers to create and propagate phony science. Let's see how this is done.

Fraudulent Research

When I was growing up, scientists were revered. But today, the image of the earnest, white-coated man or woman who works long hours in a laboratory for the benefit of humankind is obsolete. The truth is, researchers lie. And fabrication is found in all realms of science.

Dr. Marcia Angell is a highly respected medical doctor trained in anatomic pathology and internal medicine. In the past, she has held positions as Senior Lecturer in Social Medicine at Harvard Medical School and Editor-in-Chief of the *New England Journal of Medicine*. One of her most famous publications is her book, *The Truth About the Drug Companies: How They Deceive Us and What to Do About It.* "It is simply no longer possible to believe much of the clinical research that is published, or to rely on the judgment of trusted physicians or authoritative medical guidelines," she wrote in 2009. "I take no pleasure in this conclusion, which I reached slowly and reluctantly over my two decades as an editor of the *New England Journal of Medicine.*"[11]

Angell is not the only physician to conclude this. As far back as 2005, after conducting a review of the literature, the respected Greek epidemiologist and statistician John Ioannidis had written that "for most study designs and settings, it is more likely for a research claim to be false than true."[12] And more recently in April 2015, medical doctor Richard Horton, editor-in-chief of the respected British journal *Lancet*, bluntly stated that "much of the scientific literature, perhaps half, may simply be untrue. Afflicted by studies with small sample sizes, tiny effects, invalid exploratory analyses, and flagrant conflicts of interest...science has taken a turn towards darkness. As one participant put it, 'poor methods get results.'... [S]cientists too often sculpt data to fit their preferred theory of the world. Or they retrofit hypotheses to fit their data. Journal editors deserve their fair share of criticism too. We aid and abet the worst behaviours."[13]

The sad truth is, researchers lie for money, more often than you might think or want to believe. Pharmaceutical companies pay large sums to doctors to claim how effective their drugs are, and the public (and other doctors) falsely assume that these assessments are objective. Some researchers, feeling pressured to publish quickly in order to advance their careers, fail to double-check their findings. Even when authors are discovered to have filled their papers with inaccuracies and shoddy science—let alone outright fibbed—most of them fail to retract due to professional pride. The journals in which they publish usually don't retract inaccuracies, either. Sadly, the bias and outright fabrication from researchers applies to all fields of science. This includes the study of sex differences.

In 2010, Cordelia Fine—then senior research associate at Macquarie University in Australia and Honorary Research Fellow at the University of Melbourne's Department of Psychology—published *Delusions of Gender: How Our Minds, Society, and Neurosexism Create Difference*. Fine was uniquely equipped to sort through the scientific literature, which included hundreds of dry neuroscience journal articles and books. After carefully analyzing the original data, Fine found that a lot of it was alarmingly deceitful. She reported how easy it is for poorly constructed research to become entrenched as irrefutable fact, establishing as "common knowledge" that men, women, boys and girls have certain innate qualities and not others. Just a few of the whimsical titles of her chapters give an idea of what she found: "We Think, Therefore You Are." "The Brain of a Boy in the Body of a Girl...or a Monkey?" "Brain Scams." And don't forget the chapter called "Sex and Premature Speculation."[14]

One example Fine cited was a study by Leonard Sax, who attempted to explain why boys seem ill-equipped to tap into their feelings. According to Sax, older girls, but not boys, process emotion in the brain's cerebral cortex (the outer layer of the cerebrum located at the front of the skull). The cerebral cortex is responsible for many higher brain functions, including voluntary movements, reasoning, and language. Because, Sax theorized, emotion processing and language are located in the same part of the brain *in girls* (but not boys), females can more easily use language to communicate their feelings. This means, he decided, that girls access their emotions more easily than their male counterparts. All of this is nonsense. In reality, it's the brain's *amygdala*—also known as the more primitive reptilian brain—that processes emotions in *both* sexes. As you might imagine, Fine had a few criticisms of Sax's fable.

> The implications for teaching are clear: *girls to the left, phylogenetically primitive ape-brains to the right!* Yet this "fact" about male brains—variants of which I have seen repeated several times in popular media—is based on a small functional neuroimaging study in which children stared passively at fearful faces....The children were not asked to speak or talk about what they were feeling and, critically, brain activity was not even measured in most of the areas of the brain involved in processing emotion and language. As [University of Pennsylvania professor] Mark Liberman has pointed out, "the disproportion between the reported facts and Sax's interpretation is spectacular."...[As for the claim that girls process emotions] "in the cerebral cortex" [it's] a statement so unspecific as to be a bit like saying, "I'll meet you for coffee in the Northern Hemisphere."[15]

Once claims like the above become public, they are eagerly embraced, escalate beyond control, and are then used to justify other untrue notions. The general public is usually ignorant of this because flaws are rarely admitted or publicized by the mainstream press. Fortunately, not all researchers are biased. Some intelligent and objective scholars are finding serious flaws in the experimental designs, data, and conclusions of the initial research. "Arguments from neuroscience are exaggerated, not to say completely bogus," writes Mark Liberman. "I looked into some of the 'science' [from well-known authors]...What I found was shockingly careless, tendentious and even dishonest. Their over-interpretation and mis-interpretation of scientific research is so extreme that it becomes a form of fabrication."[16] Unfortunately, when something is repeated for a long enough period of time, it becomes an unchallenged fact and ultimately common knowledge. The public—the majority of whom do not read journal articles or know how to assess data—must pay the price when lies become time-honored truths.

Any study can be slanted to yield the conclusion that the experimenters want. The best way to maintain objectivity—and obtain factual information—is to learn how the subjects were selected, what was included or omitted in how the study was conducted, and what prejudices the experimenters might have brought to their research. Let's examine some persistent beliefs about gender roles, and see how data can be twisted to correspond to what the experimenters believe.

Masculinity and Femininity

When hearing of a birth or an impending birth, the first thing most people want to know is, "Is it a boy or a girl?" The answer to this question allows us to mentally prepare in advance for the child's expected behaviors, mental capacities, and emotional inclinations. Also, most parents want to paint the nursery the right color, because nowadays pink is for girls and blue is for boys (although this wasn't always the case).[17]

Significantly, categorizing the world according to sex (male or female) is not a worldwide phenomenon. Take the Yoruba people who primarily inhabit Nigeria, Benin, Togo, and part of Ghana in western Africa. These people, who comprise about one-fifth of the population of Nigeria and number about 47 million worldwide, base their social structure around age. Yoruba pronouns don't indicate the sex of the person. They also don't indicate the sex of the word, as is the case with many languages including German, Spanish and French. Rather, Yoruba pronouns specify who is older or younger than the one who is speaking. Contrast this with American culture, where sex/gender is so ingrained into our world view that it's difficult to conceive that other societies could be organized differently.

In the United States and similar cultures based on gender roles, the masculinity of a male and the femininity of a female are very important. These sex-related terms encompass a wide range of traits, both biologically inborn and culturally stereotyped. On the physical side, *masculinity* refers to a male's features that various ratios and levels of hormones have helped to create *in utero*. The most obvious of these are the penis and scrotum of an infant boy. Masculinity also refers to the secondary sex characteristics that males develop during puberty: hair on the body and face, a deep voice, and bigger and stronger muscles than those of a female. However, we also think of a man as masculine when he lifts something heavy, does something heroic (such as rescue trapped orphans from a burning building), or performs at a job that we see as gender-appropriate (such as working at a construction site). *Femininity* refers to a female's features that various ratios and amounts of hormones have helped to create *in utero*. The most obvious of these are the labia of an infant girl, and later enlarged breasts, which develop during puberty along with other secondary sex characteristics such as broader hips and the redistribution of fat that make her body curvy. However, we also think of a woman as feminine when she births a baby, nurses it, or performs at a job that we see as gender-appropriate (such as working in a beauty salon or teaching). Clearly, the adjectives *masculine* and *feminine* designate more than simply biology. They also refer to shared assumptions about reality—the respective sex role stereotypes of behaviors, preferences, skills, and ways of thinking and perceiving that our society has attributed to males as a group and females as a group. In the U.S. and other technologically advanced countries, despite the political and professional advances that women have made in the past several decades, many people still ascribe certain qualities to each sex, even if it's on a subconscious level.

"Gender stereotypes," writes Anne M. Koenig, "have descriptive components, or beliefs about how males and females typically act, as well as prescriptive components, or beliefs about how males and females should act."[18] Surveys listing twenty-one characteristics with a scale from one (very undesirable) to nine (very desirable) have yielded strong sex differences. Women are, and should be, communal and cooperative—that is, warm and sensitive. They should avoid being dominant, aggressive, intimidating, and arrogant. This means refraining from pursuing authoritative roles in business, because they will be disliked. Women are also interested in language, the arts, and helping others. Females are dainty, and wear pink and tight-fitting clothes. Men are, and should be, agentic—that is, self-directed, assertive, competitive, strong, and independent. They should avoid showing insecurity, shyness and emotionality, which are considered weaknesses. Men are also interested in science, technology, and mechanical objects. Males are sturdy in appearance, and wear blue and loose-fitting clothes.

In these surveys, men were judged more harshly for displaying "feminine" behaviors than women were for displaying "masculine" behaviors. The respondents regarded feminine-looking men as homosexual, and homosexuality in men was viewed more negatively than in women. This indicates the premium placed on so-called masculine tendencies. The fear of male homosexuality extended to boys who acted too "girly," while tomboys were viewed more positively. Children were also stereotyped by their choice of toys and appearance. The majority of survey respondents, who were middle-class and white, perceived blacks as a group as more masculine and Asians as more feminine. Elderly people were not expected to rigidly follow gender stereotypes as much as children and younger adults.[19]

Other qualities often ascribed to men include analytical, direct, independent, worldly, self-reliant, invulnerable, self-confident, and demanding. Other qualities often ascribed to women include emotional, indirect, passive, dependent, helpless, vulnerable, and self-sacrificing. When we compare most of the qualities ascribed to each sex, the characteristics of women are similar to those of a child whereas the characteristics of men describe those of an adult. Grownup females are stuck with being viewed as children. Grownup males are viewed as adults.

A recent study, which surveyed 4,344 U.S. Naval Academy students, involved performance evaluations of men and women. Although there were no differences in grades, fitness scores, or class standing in those being evaluated, the subjective biases of the survey participants contradicted the objective findings. In the performance reviews, more positive words were used to describe men and more negative words were used to describe women. Men were judged as analytical, competent, athletic, dependable, confident, versatile, articulate, level-headed, logical, and practical. There were only two negatives: arrogant and irresponsible. In contrast, the women were judged as compassionate, enthusiastic, energetic, and organized. But there were many negatives too: inept, selfish, frivolous, passive, scattered, opportunistic, gossipy, excitable, vain, panicky, indecisive, and temperamental. The adjectives ascribed to men indicated leaders, whereas the adjectives ascribed to women indicated followers.[20]

An analysis of 3.5 million fiction and non-fiction books, conducted by computer scientists in Denmark and the United States, yielded some very interesting statistics about how characters in books are depicted. In general, males are described with words pertaining to behavior and psychosocial qualities while females are described with words associated with physical appearance. Moreover, negative adjectives associated with the body and appearance were used five times more frequently for females than for males. Two adjectives most often used to describe women were "beautiful" and "sexy," whereas commonly used adjectives for men were "rational" and "brave." The lead researcher, Isabelle Augenstein, pointed out that although many of the books were published several decades ago, they are still being read today and influence people's thinking.[21]

"In general," summarize Cecilia Ridgeway and Shelley Correll, "contemporary stereotypes describe women as more communal and men as more agentic [self-directed] and instrumental. In addition…gender beliefs have a hierarchical dimension of status inequality. Men are viewed as more status worthy and competent overall and more competent at the things that 'count most.' Women are seen as less competent in general but 'nicer' and better at communal tasks." However, communal tasks "are less valued."[22] Gender stereotypes represent more than simple differences in attitudes toward males and females. They signify qualities that are deemed more important than others. Notably, each stereotype lacks traits that make up a whole human being, although for the most part the ones attributed to males are for a more desirable, well-rounded, and mature person.

A *myth* is "an unproved or false collective belief that is used to justify a social institution."[23] Some of our often hidden assumptions about gender roles—how women "should" behave and how we believe they think and perform, and how men "should" behave and how we believe *they* think and perform—are myths that become self-fulfilling. As I will discuss throughout this chapter, although studies have shown some innate differences in the attitudes, preferences and behaviors of girls and boys, these differences are often minor. And environment can emphasize or de-emphasize them. There's a huge overlap of traits between the sexes, with even more overlaps than there are extremes. People rarely possess solely "masculine" or "feminine" mental and emotional traits. Moreover, their physical traits might not be solely masculine or feminine. Men whose voices are in a higher register, who are slight of build, aren't super muscular, and don't have much of a beard or body hair, are often denigrated for being too feminine. They might also be assumed to be gay, even if they're not. Likewise, women who are tall, muscular, wear their hair very short, and have deep voices may be denigrated for being too masculine. They might also be assumed to be gay, even if they're not. Not all secondary sex characteristics are at the extreme ends of a continuum. Nevertheless, our culture only values men and women who fall at those very extremes. Anything in the middle is considered less worthy or deficient.

In the U.S., secondary sex characteristics and physical attributes have become merged with mental and emotional traits, aptitudes, behaviors, and other non-physical qualities to form a very rigid ideal of what constitutes acceptable and correct masculinity and femininity. This polarity doesn't leave room for variety or individual uniqueness—which is precisely what the trans agenda is trying to obliterate. The truth is, differences vary more between individuals than along the lines of biological sex. Psychologist Janet Hyde's seminal 2005 study found that over 75 percent of sex-linked "gender differences" between women and men were either incredibly small (0.1 or less) or merely small (0.35 or less). Explained another way by Cordelia Fine, "about 40 percent of the time, *at least*, if you chose a woman and a man at random, the woman's score would be more 'masculine' than the man's or vice versa....These included skills like mathematical problem solving, reading comprehension, and characteristics like negotiator competitiveness and interpersonal leadership style. A recent ten-year follow-up of Hyde's landmark paper...confirmed the gender similarities hypothesis no less emphatically."[24] Hyde's study was a *meta-analysis*, which combines all previous studies about a given topic to obtain an overview. This big picture approach encompasses far more data than what individual studies by themselves can offer. Plus, compiling studies offers far more precision. A piece of data that in a single study might have seemed highly significant can be put into perspective and factored as statistically unimportant when compared and contrasted with data from other studies. Furthermore, Hyde's work synthesized 106 *other* meta-analyses of sex differences—so its accuracy was unimpeachable.

To summarize, males and females share more similarities than differences. And their ways of self-expression are only *possibilities*. The human brain is extraordinarily malleable, especially during infancy and childhood. Let's take a look at how we internalize the beliefs of others, and how those myths can actually change the function and structure of the brain.

Expectations of Stereotyped Gendered Behavior
Epigenetics: Imprinting the Brain

In the last chapter when I discussed the neuroplasticity of the brain, I also mentioned *epigenetics*—the study of how environment influences genetic expression. It has been known for several decades that genes can turn on or off, and even express themselves in distorted ways, depending on what attaches to the receptors on the cell membrane.[25] It's logical that cultural expectations would impact an organism just as a toxic chemical or vitamin would, because all of these factors cause biochemical changes in the body—changes that influence which DNA strand is expressing itself or acts abnormally, which then affects cellular function.

One very interesting experiment, conducted with rats, straightforwardly shows how treatment of male versus female pups causes changes in the brain. Scientists had observed that mother rats lick their newborn male pups more than their female pups. This was not due to a sexist preferences for sons, but because the mother rats are drawn to the higher levels of testosterone that's in the urine of males. Knowing that the amount of maternal care a rat pup receives—including being licked—causes changes in certain receptor sites in the brain, the experimenters replicated maternal licking with a group of newborn female rats by stimulating them regularly with a small paintbrush. This stimulation changed some of the DNA pathways in the female rat brains, resulting in fewer estrogen receptor proteins. Thus the estrogen expression in the female brains matched that of the male rats. This changed their behavior. The researchers reported a decreased ability for social recognition, along with an apparent decrease in anxiety.[26]

That experiment was with rats. What about humans? Love or abuse, attention or neglect, warmth or coldness—all induce changes. These changes might include immune cell number and mobility; types, amounts and ratios of stress and other hormones; and dominance of either the sympathetic (fight-or-flight) or parasympathetic (relaxation) nervous system. In 2019, scientists asked, "Does Gender Leave an Epigenetic Imprint on the Brain?" The authors wanted to find out if—and how much—socially constructed gender identity, as opposed to biological sex, influences the brain's structure and function. "Treating children differently based on their biological sex is an important part of our definition of gender," they wrote. "Thus, exposure to early life stress changes the neural epigenome [the chemical compounds that modify the expression and function of genetic material]....[and] can be a gendered experience."[27] Put another way, the preferences and biases of parents determine how they perceive, value, and behave toward the child. This influences the child's emotional and mental states, which correspond to thousands of biochemical and neurological reactions. "We are just starting to understand and study," remarks professor Nancy Forger, director of the Neuroscience Institute at Georia State University, "the ways in which gender identity, rather than sex, may cause the brain to differ in males and females."[28]

Researchers have long known that parents treat boys and girls differently. It begins in infancy. Boys are most often applauded for what they can do (an active quality), while girls tend to be admired for how they look (a passive quality). Also, because parents are eager to maintain what they consider sex-appropriate behavior—remember, the infant's clothing as well as the nursery walls must be the "right" colors!—boys are discouraged from playing with dolls and girls are discouraged from engaging in activity that the parents fear might incur physical risk.[29] "I've heard enough parents," Fine writes, "openly labeling certain sports, toys, activities, behaviors, and personality traits as being for boys or for girls. In one month alone, I heard people referring to coloring in a dinosaur, playing soccer, being noisy, and wanting to press elevator buttons as boy things."[30]

It can be hard to let go of the idea that girls are dainty dolls. One paper, "Gender Bias in Mothers; Expectations about Infant Crawling," described a study that "examined gender bias in mothers' expectations about their infants' motor development."

Mothers of 11-month-old infants estimated their babies' crawling ability, crawling attempts, and motor decisions in a novel locomotor task-crawling down steep and shallow slopes. Mothers of girls underestimated their performance and mothers of boys overestimated their performance. Mothers' gender bias had no basis in fact. When we tested the infants in the same slope task moments after mothers provided their ratings, girls and boys showed identical levels of motor performance.[31]

Fathers exhibit bias too. In a study of 60 children between ages four and six, researchers observed parents' responses during a game. Fathers paid more attention to their daughters when the girls behaved submissively, but they were more responsive to their sons when the boys were aggressive and had temper tantrums. The children continued to manifest sex-typed behaviors throughout school.[32] What we take in from the environment changes thoughts and beliefs, which affects the structure and function of the brain—which affects our thoughts and beliefs even more, and so on. Another study yielded similar results. Researchers found that fathers sang more to their daughters than their sons. Furthermore, they responded more strongly to their daughters when the girls had happy facial expressions—and responded more strongly to their sons when the boys registered neutral facial expressions. Physical contact was sex-typed too. Fathers engaged in rougher play with their sons than their daughters. (So do mothers.) Moreover, the orientation of language was heavily linked to concepts of masculinity and femininity. Fathers used more achievement-oriented language ("win" and "proud") with their sons, and language related to emotion ("sad" and "happy"), as well as words relating to the body, with their daughters. Boys were encouraged to be more competitive while girls were encouraged to be more empathic. The men's behavior and even brain function changed according to the sex of the child. Conversely, children's behavior and brain function was based on how they were treated by their fathers.[33]

One interesting experiment involved the kinds of praise that boys and girls receive. Boys are usually praised for their efforts, hard work, and ingenuity at solving a problem or creating something (acts, or *effort attributions*). Girls are usually praised for their assumed inherent qualities, such as "niceness," or an aspect of their appearance (traits, or *ability attributions*). Acknowledging someone's resourcefulness and initiative (effort attributions) is known as *process praise*. Acknowledging someone's looks or natural aptitudes (ability attributions) is known as *person praise*. Even if boys and girls are praised for equal amounts of time, they are given different types of praise. Boys typically receive process praise for *what they accomplish*, while girls receive person praise for *how they look and what they are*—or how they are perceived to be.

The differences between the two types of praise are significant, and their end results are profound. The process praise that boys receive encourages them to believe in themselves and, most importantly, pursue their interests. The person praise that girls receive discourages them from believing in themselves. You'd think that if a girl was told how smart she is, that would be a positive thing—but there's a hitch. Her intelligence, it's implied, is a fixed trait. Therefore, no matter how much effort she exerts she'll always remain the same level of smart, and nothing she does can affect her ability to improve. So if a girl who's praised for her intelligence fails at a task, she'll attribute those mistakes to her inferior innate ability. Moreover, she won't bother to try to make things better because predetermined ability means that the outcome will always be the same. On the other hand, if a girl is told that *she's doing a good job* (process praise), this is an act over which she has control—because if she applies herself, she can do better.

"We asked," wrote the authors of the study, "whether the types of praise that parents give their young children at home play a role in the development of children's beliefs about the malleability of traits, [their] motivation to pursue challenging tasks...[predictions] for success and failure, and [the children's] ability to generate strategies for improvement." It's not difficult to guess that boys got the better deal. Process praise comprised 24.4 percent of the praise boys received, whereas for girls it comprised only 10 percent. The researchers measured the process praise given to children up to 38 months of age, because children are likely to be praised in the home environment before they receive formal schooling. By age seven or eight, boys were significantly more likely than girls to be confident that they could improve their abilities and performance.[34] It's easy to see why. Effort attributions indicate the capacity to influence the environment and oneself, while ability attributions indicate the *in*capacity to influence the environment and oneself. The former helps with self-mastery and authority. The latter suggests defeat and a lack of empowerment (because remember, the person is dealing with predetermined characteristics that cannot be changed). These two attitudes and ways of treating children lead them to manifest stereotyped masculine and feminine traits that remain with them far into adulthood. Boys, who develop confidence that they'll be able to master their environment, learn to be assertive. Girls, who lack confidence that they'll be able to master their environment, learn to be passive. Once a woman's persistence and motivation are reduced, her ability to perform in stereotypically male domains such as mathematics and science are markedly lower. We will see examples of this shortly.

As adults, both males and females—even if they grew up with process praise—can be highly susceptible to other people's negative opinions of their abilities. In a highly revealing account, Jan Morris, a male-to-female transgender, wrote, "The more I was treated as a [stereotyped] woman, the more woman I became.... If I was assumed to be incompetent at reversing cars, or opening bottles, oddly incompetent I found myself becoming. If a case was thought too heavy for me, inexplicably I found it so myself."[35] It's human to respond negatively to being stereotyped. Most of the time, the neuroplastic brain will oblige and go along with what's expected of us.

There's a lot we can do to help children grow up to become confident, competent adults. An equality survey, conducted by the children's newspaper *First News*, interviewed 1,000 children age nine through fourteen. Children know when they're being treated unfairly, and understandably they don't like it. The young people who were interviewed were quite vocal about their likes and dislikes. Half of the children said that girls were more likely to be judged for their looks than boys, 70 percent of the girls and 60 percent of the boys reported overhearing sexist remarks made about their friends, and many of the children said that both sexes suffered from gender stereotyping. A 10-year-old boy told researchers, "Once I heard a boy say to another boy, 'don't be such a wimp, you are more like a girl!' when they backed out of a task." A 10-year-old girl recounted, "There are set things that girls are expected to do and it isn't fair. I love football but our school is a girls' school so apparently we can't play football. I've been told to act more ladylike, and often questioned it. Why do girls have to be like this?" One girl (age unknown), when asked to respond to the use of the phrase "ladies first," responded, "You could just say 'you first' or something, but 'ladies first' makes people think that you always need to be more polite around women when really, you should be polite around everyone."[36] Children can demonstrate a great deal of common sense. We need to listen to them.

Girls and Boys in School

From the beginning of life, we group children according to their sex. This tendency to categorize continues when the child starts school: *Girls line up on the left, boys on the right. In this spelling bee, girls against the boys.* Clothing and accessories further exacerbate this division based on sex. Lise Eliot points out that very young children tend to categorize themselves by sex (or, as it's erroneously called, gender) because unlike adults, children are not defined by common social categories such as a club membership or particular profession. Lacking other labels that help them identify themselves and give them the feeling of group support, children's only sense of belonging is knowing whether they are a boy or a girl. Thus, a boy or girl will emphatically adhere to culturally boyish or girlish clothing and behavior, even if parents try to discourage it.

Teacher bias is powerful and commonplace. Hundreds of studies show how large number of teachers are guilty of expecting different aptitudes and behavior from their students based on sex. Media critic Soraya Chemaly writes:

> The impact of unconscious teacher bias is long understood and well-documented...[N]ew research confirms decades of work done by Myra and David Sadker and Karen Zittleman....They, as others have, found that teachers spend up to two thirds of their time talking to male students; they also are more likely to interrupt girls but allow boys to talk over them. Teachers also tend to acknowledge girls but praise and encourage boys. They spend more time prompting boys to seek deeper answers while rewarding girls for being quiet. Boys are also more frequently called to the front of the class for demonstrations. When teachers ask questions, they direct their gaze

towards boys more often, especially when the questions are open-ended. Biases such as these are at the root of why the United States has one of the world's largest gender gaps in math and science performance. Until they view their videotaped interactions, teachers believe they are being balanced in their exchanges.[37]

As already mentioned, far too often girls hear comments about their appearance instead of their scholarly aptitude. This unconscious bias is the reason that some parents send their daughters to a girls-only school. Free from being rudely interrupted or distracted, and without being made to feel self-conscious or intimidated, many girls blossom to become outstanding students.

In the 2006 essay "Does Gender Matter?" neuroscientist Ben Barres cited an abundance of scientific evidence showing "no compelling evidence for *relevant* innate gender [sex] differences in cognition. There is [however] overwhelming evidence for severe gender prejudice. Both men and women often deny gender-based bias; we all have a strong desire to believe that the world is fair. When faculty tell their students that they are innately inferior based on race or gender [sex] they are crossing a line that should not be crossed—the line that divides responsible free speech from verbal violence. In a culture where women's abilities are not respected, women cannot effectively learn, advance, lead, or participate in society in a fulfilling way."[38] Barr was in a unique position to discuss bias against females. In Chapter 5, I will explain why.

Boys also suffer from negative expectations in the schoolroom, although their experiences are very different from those of girls. College teacher Matt Pinkett—who, with assistant principal and college teacher Mark Roberts, wrote *Boys Don't Try*—said to an interviewer, "There's a 'boys will be boys' attitude . . . boys produce more testosterone, and that's why they fight and punch, that's why they don't sit quietly in lessons, that's why they're harder to control, that's why we have different expectations about what they can do." This "anti-school mindset [is] fuelled by stereotypical masculinity" Roberts added, which includes "the stereotype that schoolwork is something girls 'naturally' do best."[39] (This pertains to girls' greater ability to sit quietly and do schoolwork, separate from their reticence later to go into the math and science professions.) Boys generally do have a greater need than girls to be in motion. But they should be given appropriate outlets for their energy, rather than being forced to endure negative attitudes about whether or not they can learn.

Another problem is that boys and girls are set up to see each other not only as strangers, but as adversaries. To illustrate this point, Pinkett told of an encounter he once had with a female colleague. They were discussing a poem and what it meant to them. She commented that his interpretation was based on the fact that, as a man, he thought about sex all the time. The colleague had made an assumption about him based on the stereotype of men as sex-crazed animals! "It was acceptable sexism, because it was directed at a man [and] not a woman," Pinkett remarked. "And it made me realize that, though girls and women undoubtedly come off worse as a result of sexist assumptions, boys and men are damaged by them, too."[40] In this case, a woman was expressing her bias about males to a mature, adult man who was psychologically secure enough to correct her assumptions. But had this exchange taken place with a young, impressionable male student, she would have been guilty of actively encouraging a male to be sexist—while unintentionally contributing to her own subjugation.

If boys and girls are ever going to relate to each other as real human beings, what's taught in schools—in addition to how it's taught—needs to change. As Pinkett has pointed out, the "English curriculum is unfairly and disproportionately dominated by men, and many of them are deplorable men like Macbeth and Dr. Jekyll. And Dickens: a lot of his writing is unsavoury. So we need to challenge that in school, and we need to think about...sexist male behaviour and violence in the texts they're reading."[41] Significantly, the stories to which Pinkett refers are called "classics." An interesting sidebar to all this is Chemaly's report that teachers subtly undermine boys' interest in the arts and language, assuming that those fields are "feminine."

Reading materials play an important role in either reinforcing stereotypes or opening students to more expansive possibilities. Books for younger children contain a hugely disproportionate number of male compared to female characters, regardless of whether the main characters are humans or animals. Several researchers have not only counted the number of characters, but also reviewed the book titles and examined the pictures in the books to see the male-to-female ratio of representation. Sociologist Janet McCabe reviewed almost 6,000 books published from 1900 to 2000 and found that main characters were male in 57 percent of books published in a given year, while female characters were in only 31 percent. Male animals were central characters in 23 percent of books in any year, while female animals comprised 7.5 percent. Only 33 percent of children's books contained central characters that were adult women or female animals, while adult men and male animals as central characters appeared in 100 percent of the books. Also, there were twice as many males as females in the titles.[42] A researcher who had conducted a study of older books—which found that almost one-third contained no female characters at all—summed up the attitude of authors: "Children scanning the list of titles of what have been designated as the very best children's books are bound to receive the impression that girls are not very important because no one has bothered to write books about them."[43]

A more recent study of 3,280 books for children up to 16 years of age, published between 1960 and 2020, found that "although the proportion of female protagonists has increased over this 60-year period, male protagonists remain overrepresented even in recent years."[44] Books that featured non-human characters were even more biased toward male characters than books featuring humans.[45] Children's book characters that have been beloved by generations—such as Cat in the Hat and other personalities from Dr. Seuss, Babar the Elephant, and Peter Rabbit—although heartwarming, have also helped convince little girls that females are incidental, supplementary or an afterthought, because all those wonderful animal characters are male. Non-fiction books are also problematic, as they're far more likely to be about men than women. The worse offender may be Golden Books, which publishes large picture books for very young children. The animals tend to be male unless a situation specific to females is portrayed, such as a mother duck searching for her lost babies. Parents who read to their young children compound the problem. "Mothers almost always label gender-neutral characters in picture books as male," remarks Cordelia Fine. "If it doesn't look like a female, it's male....[W]e have a tendency to think of people or creatures as male unless otherwise indicated. In other words, as has been long observed, men are people, but women are women."[46] Simply put, male is the default sex.[47]

In 2022, a different type of study was conducted—this time, at the University of Southern California's Viterbi School of Engineering. Three thousand books from the Gutenberg Project were analyzed. Genres included adventure, science fiction, romance, and mystery. The study used software to perform three main functions: to identify male and female pronouns, to determine how many females were main characters, and to examine the descriptions used for the characters. There were four times as many male as female characters. Akarsh Nagaraj, one of the researchers, stated that adjectives associated with women included "weak," "pretty," "amiable," and sometimes even "stupid." Words associated with male characters included "power," "strength," "leadership," and "politics." Mayank Kejriwal, the co-researcher, remarked that "Gender bias is very real, and when we see females four times less in literature, it has a subliminal impact on people consuming the culture. We quantitatively revealed an indirect way in which bias persists in culture."[48]

Unwanted sexual attention is also a serious problem in school. Matt Pinkett estimated that one-third of girls experience this. That's a huge number. "It breaks my heart that's how boys prove their masculinity—by using sexual language and bravado in which girls, and female teachers, become the victims."[49] We can help remedy this problem by teaching girls to be more assertive and not please others at their own expense. Girls also need support to accept their bodies. This includes eliminating shame about having sexual desire, while at the same time maintaining strong emotional and physical boundaries.

Schools are not the only sphere needing change. But they're a good place to start because children spend so much time there. It's easier to teach young children to be kind and aware than to try instilling major attitudinal changes once those children reach adulthood, and are less mentally and emotionally flexible.

The Math Myth

It's popularly "known" that girls aren't as good in math as their male counterparts. The title of this journal article says it all: "'How good are you in math?' The effect of gender stereotypes on students' recollection of their school marks." The authors reviewed two studies that examined how well French students recalled their grades in the stereotypically masculine domain of mathematics and the stereotypically feminine domain of the arts. As it turned out, gender stereotypes influenced the students' recollections of how well they performed. In the first study, the more that students embraced sex role stereotypes, the more biased their recall was when they reported their grades (compared to what their actual grades were). As might be expected, what they recalled was consistent with sexual stereotypes. Female students underestimated how well they performed in math, while male students underestimated how well they performed in the arts. The second study produced similar results.[50] The female students falsely recalled doing better in the arts than they actually had, while the male students falsely recalled doing better in mathematics than they actually had. The difference was three percent. "This might not seem like a large effect," comments Cordelia Fine, "but it's not impossible to imagine two young people considering different occupational paths when, with gender in mind, a boy sees himself as an A student while an equally successful girl thinks she's only a B [student]."[51] As sociologist Shelley Correll put it, "boys do not pursue mathematical activities at a higher rate than girls do because they are better at mathematics. They do so, at least partially, because they *think* they are better.... Cultural beliefs about gender...contain specific expectations for competence"[52]—or lack of it. Although the study was conducted in France, it could easily apply to the U.S. and many other countries. The mind can be manipulated into a false belief even when that belief is directly contradicted by a person's actual experience.

The powerful effect of cultural beliefs and expectations was shown in another study with over 100 students at the City University of New York who were given a math test. The researchers had assessed the students as excellent mathematicians who would succeed in either the math or science professions. The young men and women were divided into two groups, each given an identical test accompanied by different information. One group, known to experimenters as the "stereotype threat" group, was told that the test was designed to measure their math ability so researchers could understand why some people were better at math than others. As might be expected, the female students—whose upbringing had very likely made them self-conscious about being successful in math and the sciences—became even more self-conscious when it was publicly implied that they might not do as well as the male students. Their scores reflected their fear—they scored way below their male peers. A very different story emerged with the other students, known to experimenters as the "nonthreat" group. They were told that thousands of students had been tested, and no differences in ability between males and females had been found. The researchers (and you and I) might have guessed that this encouragement—subtly conveyed under the guise of "information"—would cause the women to perform as well as the men. But surprisingly, the women performed even *better* than their male counterparts! When stereotyped expectations are explicitly removed, people's ability to reach their potential can be even greater than we might have imagined.[53]

Women's fear of math can be catalyzed by the most unexpected sources. In 1992, Barbie was implanted with an electronic chip that allowed her to talk. The Mattel toy company, which makes the doll, came under fire for such sexist (and consumerist) declarations as "Let's go shopping" and "Will we ever have enough clothes?" But the one that aroused the most ire from parents and teachers was "Math class is tough." As if girls didn't have enough problems fighting a stereotype, here they actually paid good money to be given negative reinforcement. Mattel eventually removed the math remark but kept the consumerist comments, which undoubtedly were great for business.

Like Barbie, commercials can also exert a huge influence, often without one's knowledge. After being shown television commercials, two groups of college students answered questionnaires about their professional aspirations. The control group saw ads for insurance, a cell phone, and a pharmacy. The targeted group saw commercials in which women were stereotypically portrayed. They gushed over a skin care product and expressed eagerness to try a new recipe. Viewing just *three minutes* of the stereotyped TV commercials was enough to discourage the female students from stating an interest in engineering and computer science careers. Instead, they opted for jobs in the communications industry. Women who viewed the gender-neutral ads expressed a stronger interest in those professions that required mathematics ability. The commercials didn't even refer to math—so imagine what the students' professional choices might have been if mathematics *had* been mentioned.[54]

Earlier I discussed how process praise instills confidence and encourages effort, while person praise introduces doubt and discourages effort. Person praise has been found to be directly responsible for women's underperformance in mathematics. In another study of 66 female undergraduates who were given a math exam, the young women who were encouraged to do a good job by applying themselves (process praise) tried harder and performed better than their counterparts, whose static ability was implied (they received person praise).[55]

One research paper showed that positive role modeling, even if it's indirect, can give women more confidence and improve their math scores. The experimenters wondered if either direct or indirect role modeling from a woman in math-related domains would affect female students' standardized math test scores. This role modeling was offered in three ways. In the first study, a woman rather than a man gave the test. The female students performed better. In the second study, simply the *perception* that a female experimenter was competent helped motivate the female students to do better. It wasn't even necessary that the experimenter be in the room. In the third study, although the female subjects negatively assessed their mathematics abilities, the perceived competence of a female experimenter helped bolster their confidence so much that their performance on a difficult math test was enhanced.[56]

What all of the above experiments have in common is the power of familiarity. The more that competent women are visible in a discipline that's typically ascribed to men, the more natural it seems. This encourages women to feel more relaxed and self-confident, and thus perform better. The more visible that women are in a given field, the greater the chances are that women will choose that field in the future. The researchers were optimistic that "increasing the number of female role models in math and engineering classes may allow female students to view the negative gender stereotypes that confront them as surmountable barriers rather than ones that are insurmountable and therefore potentially inspire more women, who may not be initially identified with math, to pursue careers in these academic areas."[57]

Schools are directly responsible for reinforcing the fable that females aren't as good as boys at math. Teachers routinely give girls lower grades on math tests than they give boys. We know about this bias because when those same tests are graded by outside teachers who don't know the sex of the student, the grades of the girls always increase. A *Time* magazine article, "All Teachers Should Be Trained To Overcome Their Hidden Biases," stated, "Researchers found that girls often score higher than boys on name-blind math tests, but once presented with recognizable boy and girl names on the same tests, teachers award higher scores to boys."[58]

If the girl isn't white, and she's poor, the odds are stacked even more against her. Boys of color, and those born into poverty, don't do well either. Consider a 2019 research study, "Teachers' Bias Against the Mathematical Ability of Female, Black, and Hispanic Students." The findings were more complex because the authors dealt with multiple combinations of girls of color, boys of color, white girls, and white boys. When assessing correct answers without knowing who had taken the test, teachers did not display any bias. However, once the race and sex of the students were known, the teachers' estimation of the students' abilities revealed huge bias. Hispanic and black female students were judged more harshly than white girls, although all girls were assumed to have poorer math skills than boys. The white teachers in the study (who happened to be primarily female) believed that boys were better at math than girls. Interestingly, non-white teachers believed that white boys and girls were better at math than students of color.[59] Note that Asian girls—who are not subjected to the same negative expectations that they cannot do well in the sciences—are noted for their success in various scientific fields, sometimes when they are still teenagers.

Verbal Virtuosity and Spatial Skill

A 2017 article summarizes a common assumption that females have superior verbal proficiency while males are better at spatial perception.

> Women excel in several measures of verbal ability—pretty much all of them, except for verbal analogies. Women's reading comprehension and writing ability consistently exceed that of men, on average. They out-perform men in tests of fine-motor coordination…Men, on average, can more easily juggle items in working memory. They have superior visuospatial skills: They're

better at visualizing what happens when a complicated two- or three-dimensional shape is rotated in space, at correctly determining angles from the horizontal, at tracking moving objects and at aiming projectiles.[60]

Women may have better fine motor control than men do, but that's women as a group. Many men have excellent fine motor control. If they didn't, they couldn't do watch and jewelry repair. Now let's look at language skills.

To determine verbal fluency, scientists have conducted all kinds of experiments. They've measured the effects of six hormones in women at various times of the month, charting menstrual estrogen fluctuations. They've hypothesized the amount of tissue in the planum temporale—the brain area devoted to understanding language—of both sexes. They have measured which sides of the cerebral cortex are used for a given function in their search for sex differences in brain lateralization. Some researchers found that women's brains have slightly longer dendrites (the "legs" of the nerve cells). But because education is also associated with longer dendrite length, this could be a case of epigenetics: A learning environment has already caused nerve cells and other brain structures to change by the time scientists get a chance to examine them. Some scientists have measured the skull. Others have tried to find answers by dissecting brain tissue—as if looking at inert tissue outside a living body can yield usable information! So far, such experiments have proven unreliable due to inconsistent results.

To make a very long and meandering story short, we really don't know how, or to what extent, hormones contribute to verbal virtuosity, or if the contribution is statistically significant. One study that initially showed promise—women's brains have 11 percent greater density of neurons in the language processing center—cannot be considered valid because only nine subjects were studied. This happens a lot. Fewer than a dozen people are examined and the results are extrapolated to include the entire population of the planet. Lise Eliot theorizes that if women as a group do possess greater neuron density, this may have evolved to make up for their slightly smaller brain size (which *has* been verified, even after taking into account body size).[61] This is a good example of what I discussed in the first chapter—that different neural components of males and females, rather than creating differences, help them reach the same goal in very different bodies.

Many legitimate researchers contest the claim that there's any significant neurological basis for the ways in which the sexes use language. Linguist Mark Liberman has extensively criticized the sloppy work of numerous authors—including Leonard Sax, whose data was riddled with major errors. Liberman not only discussed Sax's use of improper terminology, but he also criticized Sax for reporting test results that were actually the opposite of what the original material had concluded. "We move from carelessness to misrepresentation," he posted on his University of Pennsylvania website. "He [Sax] should stop pretending that he's got science on his side, or else he should start paying some minimal attention to what the science actually says."[62] This advice should be heeded by all researchers.

Do girls talk more than boys? A common gender stereotype is that females are chatterboxes, while males emit a few grunts now and then, unable to get a word in edgewise. Girls do speak more words in a given period than boys, but the difference is slight. Because girls speak faster than boys—they are better at hearing nuances in phonation and pronouncing syllables—it gives the impression of a lot more words than there actually are. However, the circumstances of the conversation can change all this. In mixed company, men tend to dominate conversations, due to their status.[63] Also, men tend to speak to impart information or exert dominance (assertive speech), while women tend to speak to develop relationships, and accommodate and support others (affiliative speech). Women also use more qualifiers, prefacing a remark with "I'm not sure," "I might be wrong," "This is only my opinion," or "I may not be the best judge of this, but." Men are far less tentative, and instead speak with directness and authority. [64, 65]

A 6-year-old girl is generally a few months ahead of the average 6-year-old boy in verbal fluency, , but this isn't statistically significant and boys can catch up. Nevertheless, this doesn't stop sexist researchers from offering opinions based on fiction. "When [researcher] Michael Gurian warns parents," remarks Eliot, "that because of their 'biological tendencies,' boys are as much as a year and a half behind girls in reading and writing, not only is he focusing on the most extreme measures, he's also setting up enormously different expectations for their [boys'] performance."[66]

The foundation of literacy is verbal communication. Girls do have a slightly better vocabulary than boys, but the difference is not considered statistically significant. And while girls are a bit more proficient than boys in reading and spelling, and are somewhat better writers—probably because they read more than their male classmates—this doesn't mean that boys cannot be accomplished in those areas. Most gaps in verbal skills and literacy can be eliminated if boys are helped early enough at home and in school. Reading scores are impacted by many factors, including whether the parents read to their children, the socioeconomic status of the family, and whether the children read for pleasure (those who do, score higher on literacy tests). Girls, who are less active than boys, tend to read more. Research shows that cross-culturally, parents expect more reading fluency with their daughters than their sons, which widens the gap further. If consistent attention is paid to boys at a young age to get them to express themselves and read more often—and if they are talked to more as infants and as children—their chances for excellent verbal and literary fluency improve.

Let's look now at spatiality. The belief that males have superior spatial abilities and females have superior social cognition skills has been repeated so often, it feels like common knowledge. One often-cited 2014 study is "Sex differences in the structural connectome of the human brain." *Connectome* is a comprehensive map of the brain's neural connections. The authors concluded that male brains are designed to "facilitate connectivity between perception and coordinated action, whereas female brains are designed to facilitate communication between analytical and intuitive processing modes." Males were presumed to have greater connectivity *within* a single hemisphere of the brain, while females were believed to have greater connectivity *between* the two hemispheres.[67] (See Chapter 1; these are the same conclusions that scientists had after studying the corpus callosum.) If there's any truth to these findings, remember that the 949 people who were studied were 8- to 22-year-olds. This allows plenty of time for stereotyped beliefs and expectations about sex-based capabilities to amplify and solidify already existing tendencies—thus causing permanent structural changes in the brain that would support the researchers' conclusions. Human beings, with their neuroplastic brains, are incredibly complex. Most studies fail to take this into account.

The most common test of spatial skills uses silhouetted shapes on a sheet of paper. The subject is shown an unfamiliar three-dimensional shape comprised of small cubes, and four other similar shapes. Two of those are the same as the original but have been rotated in three-dimensional space, and the other two are mirror images. The subject must decide which two are the same as the original. "Mental rotation performance is the largest and most reliable gender difference in cognition," Cordelia Fine explains. "In a typical sample, about 75 percent of people who score above average are male....[Some people claim] that male superiority in this domain plays a significant role in explaining males' better representation in science, engineering, and math."[68] However, in one experiment something very interesting happened when psychology was used. Men who were told that excellent performance in mental rotation tasks were linked with success in aviation or nuclear propulsion engineering, navigation, and undersea approach and evasion, performed well. But when the men were told that excellent performance was linked to talent in interior design and decoration, clothing design, decorative needlepoint, crocheting, sewing, knitting, and flower arrangement, "this emasculating list of activities had a draining effect on male performance."[69]

As for testosterone, by now it should be evident that the hormone doesn't offer the guarantee that might have been assumed (or hoped). Some researchers found that higher testosterone levels are associated with better mental rotation performance, but others found no difference. As it turns out, though, *practice* has the biggest impact for developing spatial skill. Playing computer games can improve mental rotation scores for everyone, but the improvement in scores for women is greater than for men.[70] People can, and do, learn—if they have a supportive environment. But as long as boys are expected to be more inherently capable at spatially related tasks than girls, girls won't be given a chance to practice so they can get better at it. It would also help girls greatly if they received process praise for learning better rotational skills.

Human beings are resilient, but in some ways we are very fragile too. Belief systems can make or break us when we're trying to learn. One experimenter showed the power of belief in a unique study of mental rotation skills. Male and female students were told to complete ten items from the Purdue Visualization of Rotations Test. Those who read that other students had previously completed the tasks satisfactorily proved not only more self-confident, but they actually performed better on the ten rotations than students who had merely read about the tasks without learning that others could also do them well. Interestingly, there were no differences in performance between males and females. The moral is, role models—even if they are one's peers—can help boost confidence.[71] (I cannot rule out the possible impetus of competition as well.) Another interesting finding is that whereas boys from economically privileged backgrounds outperformed their female counterparts in spatial skills, boys who were economically disadvantaged performed the same as economically disadvantaged girls.[72] If abilities we're born with are not encouraged, they remain undeveloped—and soon they're not only unremarkable, they can even atrophy and eventually disappear.

By the way, the United States military disagrees that boys have better spatial perception—a critical skill for soldiers. In fact, women are known to be excellent sharpshooters. Although one might argue that women with superior visuospatial abilities would be attracted and accepted to serve, this is still worth noting. For a more cross-cultural comparison, decades ago anthropologists studied Eskimo people living on the Baffin Islands of eastern Canada. They found no sex-based difference in spatial skills. The women and men, who shared the hunting, had to plot their course over sea and barren terrain that lacked easily recognizable landmarks. The women and men excelled equally at this task.[73]

Just as boys face prejudice when dealing with myths about their verbal skills, girls are at a disadvantage when advised that they are deficient in spatial skills. And just as it's vital to encourage boys to read more and develop their verbal acumen, we need to give girls better opportunities to develop spatial proficiency. Both sexes can augment their skills as long as they receive positive input from their environment. So far, all that scientists have managed to prove is that there may be *tendencies* for some differences between the sexes in these departments. While we still don't know the causes, we *do* know that skills cannot be so glibly ascribed to the presence or absence of a given hormone. Social conditioning plays a huge role—more than we might think, because so much of that conditioning is unconscious. Ultimately, we need to focus on how we can best help each individual in areas where he or she requires the most support.

Most of all, we need to stop calling these "masculine" or "feminine" attributes. Everyone will achieve more if we stop gendering talents and skills.

Boys Aren't Good at Feelings

One of the most troubling stereotypes is the belief that males are not as emotional as females. In fact, in our culture it's considered desirable for males *not* to feel, and *not* to express their emotions. Intense emotions can make us vulnerable. We don't like vulnerability in males because being vulnerable is equated with weakness—and men shouldn't be weak. It's downright unmanly.

Modern Western civilizations denigrate men for crying, among other emotional displays. But according to research by Sandra Newman, "the gender gap in crying seems to be a recent development. Historical and literary evidence suggests that in the past not only did men cry in public, but no one saw it as feminine or shameful. In fact, male weeping was regarded as normal in almost every part of the world for most of recorded history." Accounts from the Middle Ages indicate that men cried in public. "In chronicles of the period, we find one ambassador repeatedly bursting into tears when addressing Philip the Good, and the entire audience at a peace congress throwing themselves on the ground, sobbing and groaning as they listen to the speeches."[74] Fiction mirrored real life. In Homer's *Iliad*, the ancient Greek army cried profusely. And in an 11th century French epic, a poet described how noble it was for twenty thousand knights to swoon from grief. "Remarkably, there's no mention of the men in these stories trying to restrain or hide their tears," Newman remarks. "No one pretends to have something in his eye. No one makes an excuse to leave the room. They cry in a crowded hall with their heads held high. Nor do their companions make fun of this public blubbing; it's universally regarded as an admirable expression of feeling."[75] With the exception of Scandinavia, the world found no shame in men's crying in public until the 18th century at the earliest. Newman hypothesizes that this shift occurred when societies converted from agrarian to industrial. Whereas Medieval kings "routinely conducted business from their beds, at the foot of which their favourite servants slept at night,"[76] the factories that eventually arrived—which required efficient, orderly, fast production—could not afford to permit public displays of intrusive emotions.

The mechanistic mentality that allowed factories to exist has suffused modern science. Today, researchers want to put everyone and everything under a microscope, and emotions are no different. Some studies have used MRIs to map which parts of the brain appear active in men and women according to the emotions they experience. The results have shown that there are some differences. But you cannot research someone in a vacuum. Researchers are mapping not only biology, but also a lifetime of beliefs, experiences, and habits based on stereotyping—which affects hormones, the brain's circuitry, and even physical structures. Still, scientists insist on putting the entire body, not to mention pieces of it—including portions of the brain they think are involved in emotions—under a microscope. If they took the trouble to look up once in a while, away from the eyepiece, they might achieve a broader and more accurate overview.

A broader overview is what Lise Eliot and some of her colleagues were seeking when they conducted a meta-analysis involving the amygdala, the part of the brain that deals with emotions. You may recall that a meta-analysis is a big picture review of all previous research that eliminates what's not significant and ties together the data that's important. Their findings were quite revealing. A lot of the data from individual studies conflicted. But when the differences were more thoroughly analyzed, they were found to be insignificant. Despite oft-repeated claims that males as a group have larger amygdalas than females as a group, the meta-analysis authors discovered this to be untrue. While freely conceding that there might be subtle differences in the amygdalas of males and females, the authors could in no way accurately call the human amygdala sexually dimorphic.[77] *Sexual dimorphism*, which technically means "two different forms," indicates fundamental differences between males and females unrelated to their reproductive organs. In this case, an amygdala belonging to one sex was indistinguishable from that of the other. "There is no categorically 'male brain' or 'female brain,'" declares a press release from a medical university. In fact, there's "much more overlap than difference between genders...Despite the common impression that men and women are profoundly different, large analyses of brain measures are finding far more similarity than difference."[78]

There are, however, differences in the emotions that males and females tend to articulate. With girls and women it's sadness, while with boys and men it's anger. Men's naturally higher levels of testosterone is usually given as the reason for their heightened expression of aggression and anger.[79] But in truth, gender stereotyping better explains why men gravitate to anger more often than other emotions such as sadness or embarrassment. Psychologist Sean Haldane writes:

> More men than women have difficulty in crying. And more women than men have difficulty in expressing anger. The causes are not hard to find. Most small boys are told it is not manly to cry; whereas most small girls are expected to cry easily. Most small boys can get away with angry behavior, even to the point of nastiness—"boys will be boys"; whereas most small girls when angry are seen as exhibiting unladylike and ill-mannered behavior. These attitudes survive into adulthood. Many men feel it would be soft to cry; so, of course, they cannot allow themselves to be soft in any circumstances—not in playing with children, making love, or responding to affection. But women are expected to cry frequently, even to "sob hysterically." Many men take out their tension in anger at those around them, and are forgiven as being "under stress." A woman doing the same thing will probably be labeled "bitchy."[80]

Studies have shown that the more men fear tender emotions and expressions of vulnerability, the greater their chances are of articulating anger—their default emotion.[81] One very revealing slur aimed at boys who cry or get upset is, "Don't be such a girl!" This is typically articulated by peers, but male adults use that admonishment too. In a sex-stereotyped society, a large part of what makes a boy a boy (or a man a man) is precisely what he *isn't*: a girl (or woman). Maleness is the very absence of femaleness. So if girls are perceived as being emotionally expressive, it's vitally important that boys *not* be. Another common remark is the contemptuous "You're throwing like a girl," even though girls and women can be quite capable athletes. Again, our culture makes it very clear to boys that being a girl, or exhibiting a trait perceived as girlish, is an affliction—and a threat to their very masculinity (read: personhood). If a boy is sensitive and quiet, enjoys playing with dolls, or engages in other pursuits commonly regarded as feminine, he receives even worse treatment: He's sneeringly referred to as a sissy, and perhaps a homosexual, which in this paradigm is the worst insult imaginable. In contrast, when a girl acts like a boy, engaging in rough-and-tumble games or playing with toys categorized as masculine, she may be accepted or even admired as a tomboy—though not always. It can be dangerous to break the rules and push beyond the limits of one's prescribed role.

Regardless of what behavior is exhibited, and by whom, every day girls are given the message that who they are is undesirable and inferior—and therefore, they deserve to be ridiculed. As damaging as this mindset is to girls, it also hurts boys. How can males be expected to develop healthy, cordial and intimate relationships with females if they're constantly being told, overtly or covertly, that girls are inferior to boys? Equally important, the stereotype of hyper-masculinity blunts boys' ability to express most emotions. Without free expression, after a while emotions become less accessible, and then boys become incapable of knowing what they're feeling. Without ready access to what they are feeling, boys' capacity for empathy—and ultimately, their humanity—is reduced. Instead of talking about what's really going on internally, they cope by making snide remarks, teasing, and physically roughhousing with other boys.

"Imagine being a young boy," writes counselor Henry A. Montero, "crying over a painful injury or an emotional heartbreak that feels like the end of the world, and then being told to 'man up,' instead of being gently asked what's making you cry, how you feel about it, and what you think you can do about it" (good advice!).[82] Boys may be taught to hide their emotional responses, but it doesn't mean they don't feel them. Lise Eliot cites a comprehensive laboratory study in which men responded even more strongly than women to intense emotional and physical stimuli, such as a violent movie or an anticipated electric shock. The men's reactions—considerably more severe than women's—included rapid heartbeat, increased sweating, and elevated blood pressure. It's possible that men exhibit these elevated physiological responses *because* they have not mastered the ability to recognize, acknowledge, and release emotions. By age 16, boys are 40 percent less likely to cry than girls. This difference cannot be explained solely by pubertal hormones, because the frequency and intensity of boys' crying continues to decline after puberty has completed.[83] Socialization, along with role modeling by fathers, teachers and other authority figures, plays a significant role. One study of adolescent boys reports that they equate appearing stoic and tough with manliness, and thus avoid expressing physical or emotional pain. Plus, they believe that exhibiting worry, hurt, and concern for others is not only "girly," but means that they might be homosexual. Taunting, mocking and rough jostling, even if hurtful, are considered acceptable because these behaviors are regarded as reinforcing masculinity.[84]

Haldane writes that in his experience, "emotional differences between men and women are largely socially conditioned, not innate....Men and women are physically similar in those parts of the body which most participate in emotion: the face which expresses it, and the throat and lungs and trunk from which breathing fuels and drives it....I have seen hundreds of men and women in [psycho]therapy. Their rage, fear, joy and crying are in no way different."[85]

As we have seen, autonomy and self-sufficiency are very much attributed to being male. But although these traits are desirable in any adult, when you add stoicism and an attempt at invulnerability to the mix, the combination becomes a damaging masculine stereotype. How to cultivate meaningful relationships can be taught—but in order to have them, boys as well as girls must allow themselves to be honest about their feelings. This requires letting go of the notion that being vulnerable is the equivalent of weakness. "We can no longer afford to support the false idea that boys are less emotional than girls," writes the stay-at-home father of a 4-year-old boy who freely expressed his joy at seeing a friend by tightly embracing him and pressing their cheeks together. "This wrongheaded belief… creates a culture in which girls are encouraged to express emotion, while boys are left behind with no access to the resources and relationships they need to grow." The title of the article says it all: "The key to letting boys actually be boys? See them as the emotional beings they are."[86]

The message that males must not be weak at any cost, even if it kills them, has proven prophetic. Ignoring emotions means risking an earlier death from a variety of causes, including cancer.[87] The authors of "Consequences of Repression of Emotion: Physical Health, Mental Health and General Well Being" advise that even a healthful diet and suitable activity levels are not as important as good mental health for ensuring wellness and longevity.[88] (Men's suicide rate used to be much higher than women's, but women are quickly catching up.) Chapter 9 discusses in detail the harmful physiological, biochemical, and psychological effects of suppressing emotions.

Despite the damage caused by numbing our emotions, this culture still insists on training boys to hold back their feelings. Many fathers are still uncomfortable when their young sons cry; they urge them to "act like a man." But mothers also contribute to boys' lack of emotionality. "While differences between the sexes in sociability and emotional expression are not obvious at birth," writes Eliot, "they grow significantly during early infancy. The differences probably originate in boys' greater fussiness and [developmental] immaturity, but they are amplified by the way that parents respond to these differences, as well as our preconceived notions of what boys and girls are like. By ignoring boys' expressions of pain, mothers may be trying to 'toughen up' their sons, while by ignoring girls' expressions of anger, mothers may be attempting to dampen their assertiveness."[89]

A review of a psychological test on emotional expressiveness administered to Gen Z young people age 22 years and younger—2,089 boys and 3,307 girls—showed a statistically significant difference in most areas. Girls were better at identifying emotions in themselves, and were more willing to be flexible and compromise. Not surprisingly, then, they proved more adept at conflict resolution. In addition, they exhibited better social skills, empathy, insight, and the ability to read body language. But there were two areas in which boys excelled over the girls: the ability to let go of minor issues, and to pick their battles wisely.[90] Girls have been so heavily socialized to *be* emotional—sometimes to the point of irrationality—that they are frequently seen as unable to be objective. They are also perceived as becoming embroiled too often in relatively unimportant issues. There is such a thing as being a slave to one's emotions, and here girls could learn a great deal about beneficial self-control from their male peers.

In general, boys have been severely shortchanged in the name of masculinity. Boys, and the men they grow into, are being taught, encouraged, and even rewarded for being emotional cripples. Boys will feel much safer to deeply connect to others if we eliminate the demand that in order to be acceptable, they must cut themselves off from some of the best qualities that make us human. This means discarding outdated stereotypes of what it means to be masculine and male, and what it means to be feminine and female.

Girls Aren't Good at Science

In comparison to half a century ago, there are more women in male-dominated professions today. It's becoming much more common to see female doctors and even male nurses. However, the belief that men and women are inherently suited to different jobs still persists. What seem to be genuine choices may actually be default decisions made even before students graduate from school.

The title of a 2017 article, "Gender stereotypes about intellectual ability emerge early and influence children's interests," concisely summarizes the problem. The authors reviewed many studies of children's attitudes toward themselves and their peers regarding intelligence and ability. Seventy-five percent of the children were white and mostly from middle-class backgrounds. Until age five, the children made no distinction between the sexes as intelligent. But by age six, girls avoided games they perceived were only for those who were "really, really smart." Sadly, the children characterized females as "really, really nice," compared to males who were "really, really smart." The girls believed that boys were more intelligent, despite the fact that girls generally receive higher grades in school. The perception of intelligence heavily influenced the children's choice of activities. Girls were less interested than boys in games they believed were meant for smart kids. The authors concluded that many young children believe that being intelligent is a quality reserved exclusively for males—and furthermore, this stereotyped belief markedly restricts children's interests and greatly impedes the career choices they will make later in life.[91]

Even if a girl manages to enter high school intact, all it takes is one biased teacher to wreck her career plans. A teacher's bias, albeit unconscious, is the main reason that relatively few girls have careers in engineering and the sciences. Studies conducted with girls and the sciences, similar to those with girls and math, have yielded similar results. Because girls are discouraged from even considering those careers—and this occurs even in all-girl classrooms—their lower participation in male-dominated professions is not a true choice based on preference, but a concession based on avoidance. "Any factor that causes a teacher to have higher expectations for some of their students and lower expectations for others," states a website devoted to learning, "is bound to create results to match....Teachers' belief in their students' academic skills and potential is a vital ingredient for student success because it is linked to students' beliefs about how far they will progress in school, their attitudes toward school, and their academic achievement." But more than academic success is at stake. "When teachers underestimate their students, it affects not just that one student-teacher relationship [and their grade point average] but the student's entire self-concept."[92]

In 2006, forty-three global companies in the private sector conducted a research project on women with degrees in SET (an acronym for *science, engineering and technology*) to see if the women had reached, or were reaching, their career goals—and if not, what was preventing them from doing so. Over the period of a year and a half, four extensive surveys were sent to men and women in major cities all over the world, including in the United States, Hong Kong, England, Russia, Switzerland, and China. The findings were very revealing. The dropout rate for women was huge, at 25 percent, due to hostile work environments and excessive job pressures. What constituted "hostile"? Sixty-three percent of the SET women experienced sexual harassment. Many found themselves to be the only woman on a team or at a site, which made it difficult for 45 percent to find mentors and 83 percent to find sponsors. Overall, the women felt isolated, bombarded by "macho" attitudes and behaviors of their male colleagues.[93]

The late neuroscientist Ben Barres wrote an excellent description of what it was like:

> What all of these folks [male scientists and deans of colleges]...as well as many of the other highly successful white men who have made the same arguments throughout history—strongly believe is that, although more men may be innately better suited for science and engineering than women, there of course should be an individual meritocracy for those women who are as good as or better than men. But what they also entirely fail to see is that individual merit cannot and will not be recognized in the face of pervasive negative stereotyping....At present, the evidence that gender-based stereotyping is holding back women's careers is overwhelming, and I am quite tired of hearing unscientifically supported claims from successful white men (unaware of their benefits from their privileged status that continuously fuels their success) that women are innately less able. Given this pervasive negative stereotyping, all of us (male and female) need to be constantly working hard to make the environment more diverse and supportive.[94]

In the past decade, feature films, articles and books have been released about women, largely unknown to the general public, who made major contributions in science and mathematics. I will mention just a few here.

In the 1800s, mathematician, astronomer and inventor Janet Taylor ran a manufacturing business for nautical instruments, many of which she designed herself. Eventually she won a patent for her Mariner's Calculator as well as three gold medals and grants from different countries. In the 1900s, Cecilia Payne-Gaposchkin was the first woman to receive a Ph.D. from Radcliffe College, become a professor at Harvard, and discover the composition of stars. In the early 1900s, chemist Alice Augusta Ball developed a cure for leprosy. Between 1929 and 1939, Inge Lehmann discovered the composition of Earth's core. Lise Meitner—to whom Albert Einstein once referred as Germany's own Marie Curie—was regarded as the foremost nuclear scientist in Germany, contributing to the discovery of nuclear fission. Chemist Dorothy Hodgkin (born in 1910) won a Nobel Prize for Chemistry in 1964 for "her determinations by X-ray techniques of the structures of important biochemical substances," which included cholesterol, insulin, and penicillin.[95]

Another scientist was Rosalind Franklin. In the 1950s, her X-ray data confirmed the 3D and helical structure of DNA, as well as its structural changes when exposed to high levels of moisture. Franklin's research helped three other scientists (all men) win the Nobel Prize. Franklin neither received credit nor was included as a Nobel Prize recipient. After her death, James Watson, one of the well-known prizewinners, remarked that he never would have published a famous paper or won the Nobel Prize if he hadn't had access to Franklin's research.[96]

Mathematician and aeronautical engineer Mary Jackson was one of many women who starting working as human computers for the space program in the 1950s. She was not well known at the time. Her shoddy treatment is even more poignant because she and other computing women—many of whom were black—were working in the segregated southern United States, where they had to walk a great distance to use the only segregated bathroom available to them. Al Harrison, director of the Space Task Group, eventually removed the "Colored Ladies Bathroom" sign to end bathroom segregation at NASA.[97] Katherine Johnson, another black woman who worked with NASA, calculated the trajectories for astronaut John Glenn's historic Friendship 7 mission.

Despite the recent publicity about these and other remarkable women, we still have a long way to go. Anne Fausto-Sterling shares a personal experience of bias:

> In grade school, a teacher told me that women could be nurses but not doctors after I had announced my intention to become the latter. When, as a young Assistant Professor, I joined the faculty at Brown, a Full Professor in the History Department told me kindly, but with great authority, that history showed that there had never been any women geniuses in either the sciences or the field of letters. We were, it seemed, born to be mediocre. [W]hen I returned from scientific meetings, emotionally shaken by my inability to break into the all-male conclaves, where the true scientific exchanges occurred (chatting at the socials and at meals), I read that "men in

groups" was a natural outcome of male bonding that had evolved from prehistoric hunting behaviors. Nothing, really, was to be done about it. I now understand that I experienced the political power of science.[98]

Not all female professionals in the math and science fields are treated like outsiders. In Armenia, about half of the employees who work in computer science are women. Hasmik Gharibyan, Full Professor in the Computer Science department at California Polytechnic State University, explained to attendees at a conference that in Armenia, the "society, culture, and education system in many ways are quite different from the USA's and therefore may contain factors that positively affect women and attract them to CS [computer science]." The only Armenian university computer science department in the country in the 1980s and 1990s, she reported, contained at least 75 percent women. Now the percentage is between 45 and 60 percent—not because women are less interested, but "due to the growing popularity of CS among men....Interestingly, the decrease of the female population in CS programs gave a boost to the number of women entering the Math programs....apparently, women who can't get into CS programs pick the closest related field, which in Armenia is considered to be Math, with the intention to take additional Computer Science courses and join the CS workforce after graduation."[99]

Ironically, women were among the first computer programmers in the U.S. Yet when modern historian and computer programmer Kathy Kleiman found photos from the 1940s of women configuring wires on the first general-purpose electronic wall-size computer, she said, "I had been told they were models. And of course, they're not." They were the first U.S. computer coders, who received public recognition only after most of them were in their 70s.[100] Similarly, it has become public knowledge just within the past decade that during World War II at Bletchley Park in Great Britain, women played a major role in operating some of the first computational machines used for code-breaking Nazi battle plans. It's also not well known, as Brynn Holland reports, that in the 1950s, "NASA was starting to work with what we now know as computers—but most male engineers and scientists did not trust these machines, believing them to be unreliable in comparison to human calculations. Dismissing computer programming as 'women's work,' the men gave the new IBMs to the women of JPL [Jet Propulsion Laboratory in California], providing them with a unique opportunity to work with and learn to code computers. It comes as no surprise then that the first computer programmers in the JPL lab were women."[101] But later, it was the men working alongside them who received recognition in the form of print and photo credits.

Perhaps not surprisingly, once programming began to be equated with low-level clerical work like typing or filing, it was regarded as women's work even if men did it. Programmer Grace Hopper, who invented the first computer language compiler (which converted mathematical code into a system readable by a computer), stated, "Programming requires patience and the ability to handle detail.

Women are 'naturals' at computer programming." But now that computing jobs pay more, and geeky men are seen as "naturals" for this field, women are hesitant to apply for work they fear they are too incompetent or stupid to perform.[102] In contrast to the self-confident Armenian girls, almost 91 percent of American girls—when asked if they would consider themselves good candidates for a job in computer science—all had similar negative responses. "It's too hard." "It's geeky." "I don't belong." "I feel judged." "No one ever encouraged me." "I'm the only girl in the class." "I don't know any female engineers." And inevitably, "It's a boy's career."[103] If something seems too difficult or impossible, it can help to look beyond our immediate environment to other possibilities—whether they're back in time, or halfway across the globe.

The "Niceness" Syndrome

Despite more recent generous attitudes about raising girls, there is still a bias that females must be "nice." The mandate to be nice, to the exclusion of ambition and drive, unfortunately follows girls into adulthood and also into the professions they choose. It's true that there's an increase of women in professions that used to be perceived as the sole domain of men—which is why many people choose to ignore, or disbelieve entirely, the fact that women can still experience extreme prejudice in the workplace. But insisting that sexism on the job is a thing of the past doesn't make it so. Ambitious women who want to succeed in certain careers, including those in the business world, must battle other people's biases about who they are and how they're supposed to act. The refusal of their peers to evaluate them fairly and objectively for what they can do is still a major problem.

A psychology journal article cites studies that illustrate this dilemma clearly. If a woman is in a high-stress managerial position and exhibits the requisite qualities of discipline, competence, self-confidence and leadership, evaluators consider her domineering, manipulative, autocratic, intimidating, ruthless, and unsympathetic. She is also criticized for lacking interpersonal skills, and is thus judged undesirable as an employee. On the other hand, when a man in that same managerial position exhibits identical qualities, evaluators believe that he's simply doing his job. The fact that he might be lacking in interpersonal skills is either seen as an aberration or is not perceived as a problem. Now let's take another woman in that same managerial position who chooses a different approach. If she attempts to foster an inclusive, participatory, more "gentle" atmosphere, she's generally perceived as having a more pleasant personality but is also considered unqualified for the job. The authors use the word *agentic*, which indicates the ability to be self-organizing, proactive, and leadership-oriented. These are desirable qualities for executives—as long as they are men. But businesswomen are criticized harshly for having these qualities because it means they aren't being "nice." There's such a strong cultural expectation for women to be "nice"—certainly "nicer" than men—that they are more likely to be judged harshly, and even punished, if they fail to meet this standard. In fact, if a woman appears to lack social skills, it's perceived as more of a breach than if she were incompetent at her job.[104]

In one of the above studies, a fictitious male employee—with the same character traits and behaviors as a fictitious female employee—was presented to the same group of evaluators. The evaluators recommended not firing him from his position because they could find nothing wrong with either his performance or attitudes. His counterpart met a worse fate: She was not "nice." The article authors comment that high-status individuals (who tend to be men) are given much more latitude than lower-status individuals (who tend to be women), even if they break the law or violate cultural rules. Not surprisingly, the mandate that women be "nice" means that they're constantly obliged to reinforce their own subordination.[105] But wait—that study was published in 1999. Surely things have gotten better? A 2015 *Forbes* article indicates that not much has changed: "Gender Bias Is Real: Women's Perceived Competency Drops Significantly When Judged As Being Forceful."[106] And a 2021 journal article states bluntly, "Gender stereotyping is considered to be a significant issue obstructing the career progressions of women in management."[107]

In business, forcing a woman to choose between being either a polite pushover or a bitchy boss is clearly not a fair option. Although females are now represented more in business than they were several decades ago, hidden prejudice still pervades the marketplace. Cordelia Fine remarks:

> Unlike men in the same position, women leaders have to continue to walk the fine line between appearing incompetent and nice and competent but cold. Experimental studies find that, unlike men, when they try to negotiate greater compensation they are disliked. When they try out intimidation tactics they are disliked. When they succeed in a male occupation they are disliked. When they fail to perform the altruistic acts that are optional for men, they are disliked. When they *do* go beyond the call of duty they are not, as men are, liked more for it. When they criticize, they are disparaged. Even when they merely offer an opinion, people look displeased. The perceptive reader will notice a certain pattern emerging. The same behavior that enhances *his* status simply makes *her* less popular. It's not hard to see that this makes the goal of getting ahead in the workplace distinctly more challenging for a woman. This perceived dislikability often drives economic and promotional penalties.[108]

"Niceness" in women is linked to being a caregiver, and both directly impact salary. To say that so-called feminine tasks are undervalued—or not valued at all—is an understatement. "Breadwinner Bonus and Caregiver Penalty in Workplace Rewards for Men and Women" cites two studies that examine people's perceptions of economic worth. The first looks at male and female parents in the workforce. Mothers are considered caregivers while fathers are considered breadwinners, even though both work outside the home. Fathers are offered much higher salaries while mothers are offered more flexible schedules, but lower salaries. The second study examines various combinations: men and women who aren't parents, men and women who are parents but whose roles are unspecified, parents who are caregivers, and parents who are breadwinners. The outcome of the study favors the male sex role stereotype. Of all the women, those seen as breadwinners receive the highest salaries (equal to the men's) and leadership training offers. But women who are labeled caregivers or have unspecified roles are financially at risk. Caregivers of both sexes are penalized with decreased salaries, although caregiver males (but not caregiver females) are given leadership training. Mothers are awarded a greater salary only if they are perceived as the family breadwinners.[109] We still have a long way to go. Women as breadwinners is a difficult role for some people to accept. And sadly, both sexes suffer financial losses for being parents.

The corporate double standard points to a larger issue. The model of most businesses in the larger world is still based on values that a gender-based society considers masculine: competitiveness, making the most money, and extracting the most labor possible from underpaid employees. Cooperation, consensus and compassion—values that a gender-based society considers feminine—are not often extolled or encouraged as an ideal business model, even though more fair and humane standards usually provide an incentive to work harder. It's time to stop ascribing traits to one sex or the other, and begin promoting qualities that benefit individuals *and* the larger society. We can take the best from so-called masculine and so-called feminine traits, and call them desirably human.

Empathy Quotient, Motherhood, and Fatherhood

Empathy is the ability to understand or identify with someone else's feelings, internal states, thoughts, or situation. Different types of studies, some dating to over half a century ago, have been conducted to assess empathy by itself, and to compare empathy levels in men and women. There is a widespread assumption that females are more empathetic than males. This belief is used to justify relegating women to service-oriented and caregiving professions such as nursing, childcare, and office assistant—all of which require overt nurturing—and barring them from leadership and managerial positions. This assumption of women's superior ability to empathize is also used to excuse men from the need to be sensitive to the feelings and wishes of others. In fact, some people still regard a man's display of empathy and sensitivity as weak.

As you might guess, the majority of studies have attempted to prove that woman are natural nurturers—and the only sex capable of truly nurturing. One article, "Empathy: Gender effects in brain and behavior," hypothesizes that women's sensitivity to others is hardwired because they give birth to, breastfeed, and care for vulnerable infants whose very survival depends on the ability of others to respond to their signals and needs. The basis for this hardwiring of mothers, the authors believe, lies in evolutionary biology.[110] At face value, this conclusion makes sense. After a mother has given birth, the hypothalamus in her brain produces the hormone oxytocin, which is then released into the bloodstream. *Oxytocin* is often regarded as the "maternal" or "feminine" hormone because it's created during labor contractions, and again when breast milk is produced. It's well known that nursing an infant helps a mother bond with the baby due to augmented oxytocin levels. But oxytocin is also produced by both sexes when they feel empathy, are involved in cooperative social ventures, experience romantic love, and engage in sexual activity—particularly when that activity leads to orgasm. Feelings of closeness that oxytocin induces have led people to label it the "bonding hormone," "love hormone," and "cuddle chemical."

Most importantly, oxytocin is also produced by men who are attached to their babies. Fathers' baseline oxytocin levels are similar to that of mothers. When parents care for their infants, their estrogen levels rise (estrogen is naturally produced in small amounts by the testes), which triggers the production and storage of oxytocin. While this occurs, testosterone and stress-related cortisol levels drop. As with mothers, when fathers bond with their infants they produce oxytocin, which creates a stronger ability to bond, which in turn produces even more oxytocin, and so on. Magnetic resonance imaging shows changes linked to oxytocin in the brains of both parents. MRIs have also verified that certain portions of a man's brain are more active when he hears his child cry, and that a father is as accurate as a mother in identifying the unique sound of his baby crying.[111]

Fathers who share equally in raising their children bond closely with infants in ways that our society normally associates with motherhood. The importance of a man's influence cannot be underestimated, as it strongly affects the baby. When a father's (or mother's) system is flooded with oxytocin, the infant's oxytocin levels also rise—significantly, as compared to a placebo. The higher levels help improve the infant's social behavior.[112] As parents and infants influence each other, the infant's very DNA is changed—a perfect example of epigenetics. Unfortunately, our cultural conditioning still causes us to equate oxytocin with femininity. Cordelia Fine discusses the power of oxytocin in an experiment with rats.

> Male rats don't experience the hormonal changes that trigger maternal behavior in female rats. They *never* normally participate in infant care. Yet put a baby rat in a cage with a male adult and after a few days he will be caring for the baby almost as if he were its mother. He'll pick it up, nestle it close to him as a nursing female would, keep the baby rat clean and comforted, and even build a comfy nest for it. The parenting circuits are there in the male brain, even in a species in which paternal care doesn't normally exist. If a male *rat*...can be inspired to parent then I would suggest that the prospects for human fathers are pretty good.[113]

Another hormone typically labeled as maternal is *prolactin*. Made by the pituitary gland in the brain, prolactin causes a woman's breasts to grow and produce milk. The more frequently and intensely an infant suckles at the breast, the more milk is available. Prolactin helps mother and infant bond. However, what many people don't know is that the hormone also helps fathers bond with the baby—because in new fathers, prolactin levels also rise even though the man isn't nursing. Prolactin should be considered the hormone of parenthood, not just motherhood. (Elevated prolactin levels in both parents also decrease libido, ensuring that both mother and father invest more energy in caring for the infant than in having sex with each other.)[114]

Some researchers believe that oxytocin induces a "different set of parenting behaviors" in fathers than in mothers. According to one paper, mothers exhibit "maternal affectionate touch, talking in 'motherese' and mutual gazing," while fathers display "a 'paternal' way of interaction—highly arousing play, focus on joint exploration, and stimulatory touch."[115] But we have already seen that sex role conditioning heavily influences the different ways in which fathers and mothers interact with their children. Also, conclusions such as the above are drawn from observing fathers in the U.S., Europe, and some countries in Asia. In other parts of the world, a father's role and behaviors in family life are quite different.

Knowing that cultural conditioning and hormones interact with each other, anthropologist Lee Gettler decided to find out how this might relate to fatherhood. He reasoned that because the *roles* of fathers vary across cultures, so might the *biology* of fatherhood. During a trip to the BaYaka society in the Republic of the Congo, he and his colleagues found that this was indeed the case. "BaYaka fathers are not playmates with their children like men are in the U.S. and other large-scale, industrialized societies," reported a team member. "They spend more time in hands-on care, holding their babies, taking their older children with them to work in the forest, co-sleeping all together as a family at night. But fathers are also part of [a] larger, cooperative community."[116] Gettler also visited the Bondongo people in the Republic of the Congo. Whereas BaYaka fathers are valued for their cooperative values, the Bondongo culture values males for their ability to provide for their families. The men hunt, fish, and clear land for farming. But they don't directly participate in the nurturing of their children. When the anthropology team compared the men's testosterone levels in both groups, the Bondongo males were found to have much higher levels. "The data in the BaYaka/Bondongo study are correlational," writes the reporter who covered the story, "meaning the researchers do not know if good sharers' generous behavior leads to low levels of testosterone, or if low levels of testosterone lead to increased sharing."[117] With these populations, there would not have been any "before" or "after" testosterone levels to obtain, because their behaviors were already established. However, we have already seen from other studies that tender caregiving causes testosterone levels in men to decrease, which further augments the ability to be empathic.

What about empathy unrelated to parenting? Studies on empathy have varied widely due to a number of factors: who was being studied (sometimes it was animals), the ways in which the data was collected or interpreted (hidden biases can be built in to both the methodology and the analysis), and unexpected variables (such as whether the same amount of empathy was exhibited toward strangers as with people whom the subjects knew). Because some researchers divide empathy into two categories—the promotion of cooperative social behavior versus the ability to understand or predict the behavior of others—even the very definitions and assumed purposes of empathy can yield different results between studies.[118] In a final, reductionist attempt to scrutinize what would be better left alone, scientists have tried to map which portions of the brain are involved with empathic responses. The problem with this approach is that there is no "one place," or even a few places, where empathy "resides." The neuroplastic brain has plenty of time to make structural and neurochemical adjustments based on what it learns about people's needs and their environment.

All of the above variables, which yielded many flaws in empathy studies, were well known to Nancy Eisenberg and Randy Lennon of Arizona State University when they wrote "Sex Differences in Empathy and Related Capacities." They knew, for instance, that when women were described as having more empathy, it was because of what *they themselves* reported, rather than what researchers could objectively observe. When, on the other hand, empathy was measured by the experimenters—either as quantifiable physiological responses or from direct observations of the subjects' responses to the emotions of others—no differences between the sexes were found. Interestingly, few sex differences for empathy were found in children.[119] So after reviewing all the data on empathy thus far, and examining flaws in data collection and analysis, Eisenberg and Lennon approached the subject in a unique, two-part manner. Rather than measuring hormone levels, they had subjects answer questionnaires about their own empathy levels. Then Eisenberg and Lennon viewed the subjects under a variety of conditions to see if the self-reported levels matched what they observed.

You'd be correct if you guessed that the answers to the questionnaires didn't reflect reality. Women—who *know* that they are expected to be more empathic—reported having high levels of empathy even if they were later observed by researchers in a controlled setting to exhibit less empathy in their interactions with others than they had reported. Men—who aren't burdened with the requirements that they be nice, sensitive or understanding—tended to self-report more accurately. Females had much lower empathy scores when it wasn't apparent from the questions that empathy was being assessed.[120] Results from other studies, along with meta-analyses, have either contradicted each other, or been inconclusive as to which sex feels or displays empathy more strongly.

Some very interesting data from William Ickes showed that when women are reminded that they *should* be empathic—no doubt due to their reputation—their motivation to *be* empathic increases. Apparently, motivation is everything. Ickes found that when men were motivated, they performed as well as women did.[121] Significantly, what motivated men wasn't to please others—which is a typical gender role script for women—but money. Cordelia Fine discusses a study in which the subjects were given two dollars for every correct answer that accurately reflected their empathy levels. "This financial incentive," she remarks drily, "leveled the performance of women and men, showing that when it literally 'pays to understand,' male insensitivity is curiously easily overcome."[122]

Despite the research proving that women can be just as callous as men—or that men can be just as receptive and sensitive as women—the myth of women's superior empathy continues to exist. Why? Children do almost anything to gain love and approval from their parents. From infancy, women are socialized to be other-directed to receive that love and approval, so a female child will hone and emphasize her empathy antennae. This pattern follows her into adulthood. Women tend to be habitual caregivers of others, even to their own detriment. The many books on the market advising women to put their own needs first, or risk suffering burnout, indicates the degree to which females have been heavily socialized to help everyone else except themselves.

Clothes Make the Man—and Woman

Clothing is a major vehicle that defines gender. Men are expected to wear pants, while until recently women were expected to wear dresses or skirts. Although styles of women's clothing have greatly relaxed during the past century so that women are now free to wear pants, men have not been accorded the same right. In fact, in most circles men would be ridiculed if they wore dresses (or obvious amounts of makeup). A man in so-called women's clothing is perceived at best as strange, and at worst as a deviant or pervert. "As is the case with toys," Lise Eliot comments, "boys more fervently reject girl-like clothes than girls reject boy-like clothes, both because girls see a wider spectrum of dress in adult women and because the status difference between men and women makes boys realize quite early that they have much to lose by being mistaken for females."[123] A girl who wears clothing allocated for boys is far more tolerated than a boy who wears clothing allocated for girls.

In the United States, a man is denigrated as "feminine" if he wears what is thought of as women's garb; but other regions have different dress codes. Robust men in the Scottish Highlands still don traditional skirt-like kilts. And monks, Catholic priests during ceremonies, yogis, and desert dwellers wear long, flowing, dress-like robes. Much of what we regard as fixed and innate, according to one's sex, is actually a cultural construct.

Women's clothing is typically more colorful, and has more patterns, than men's clothing. But it's also less utilitarian, as it's often made from cheaper fabric and usually has fewer and shallower pockets—if any. This is a holdover of women being perceived as adornment, while not too long ago men were recognized for their worldly skills and required tools at their fingertips if necessary. What women wear for formal attire, and what they are admired for, is impractical on yet another level: The fancy (often low-cut, and sometimes backless) dresses do not warm the lower legs or upper body in cold weather. Fancier dresses, specifically designed to reveal and accentuate cleavage and curves, are frequently made with many layers of flimsy delicate material that offers little protection and instead must itself be protected. In order to safeguard their clothing, women are obliged to restrict their movements.

High heels heavily confine women's mobility and may be viewed as the less extreme, Western equivalent of the ancient Chinese custom of foot binding. Heels that are especially long, thin and spiky offer little support. Women must practice walking in them to avoid wobbling or falling. All high heels distort the natural curvature of the spine, thus altering the normal gait. For this reason, many women find high heels uncomfortable. Yet men—and even quite a number of women—have been conditioned to view the restructured pelvic tilt of a body on high heels as sexy.

Makeup is another component of "beauty" that almost half the female population uses—and which all women in acting, modeling, and other high-profile professions are seen wearing.[124] Color on the face and eyes highlights features that females want to emphasize, and draws attention away from features they consider undesirable. From an early age, girls are taught to believe that their own natural features are not adequate or beautiful enough, so they spend extra time "putting on their face" or "fixing their face"—was it broken to begin with?—before showing those faces to the world. Most makeup contains toxic chemicals that seep through the pores of the skin and lodge in the body's tissues. A surprisingly high number of these chemicals are verified carcinogens.

When women wear makeup and impractical clothes, they are exhibiting acceptable and even expected behavior. They are admired, not only for how they look but also for following their assigned script. Yet if men wear makeup and fancy sequined dresses, they are ridiculed. They are likely assumed to be homosexual. If they wear such clothing in public, they might be referred to as "being in drag." In fact, men who do this for a living are called *female impersonators* or *drag queens.*

There is one possible aesthetic reason why women and not men should be the sex that wears dresses: The flowing lines of a dress reinforce and complement the curves of a typical female body. Similarly, the straight lines of pants and jackets work well on the straighter, more angular male body. However, dresses might look okay on a less muscled male body, just as a pants suit might look better than a dress on a woman with a more boyish figure. Thus one might inherently look better in gender-defined clothing because of how the fabric drapes. However, an aesthetic preference is not the same as labeling clothing according to who we think should wear it. Note that I'm not referring to similar styles of pants or shirts made specifically for men or for women. Such garments are rightly designated for the respective sex not because of the fabric, style, colors or patterns, but because the natural lines and curves of each sex's body are different, and the garments are appropriately fitted to follow each sex's distinct bodily contours.

Hairstyles are also associated with a given sex. Historically, though, fashion has varied widely. In Egypt 4000–3000 BC, both men and women of noble birth shaved their heads and bodies and wore wigs. In Athens 150 BC, some hairdressing salons catered to only men and curled their hair. In Europe from 900–1250 AD, lower-class women wore short hair. In Europe from 1250–1500 AD, women wore hats and kept their hair hidden. In the Baroque period (17th and early 18th centuries), many women wore their hair piled on the head while men wore wigs of long, wavy hair. In the 1970s, both men and women had long or short hair. Today, either men or women can sport long or short hair, and men with long hair and beards is again in style. Hair length and fashion do not seem to be consistent factors in even a gendered society—especially if criteria for other stereotypes are met. If a traveler took a time machine back to the days of George Washington, the curly-haired wigs worn by 18th century men might be regarded as feminine. Context changes everything.

Sex Role Nonconformity: Homosexuals, Lesbians and Bisexuals

The terms *gay, homosexual, lesbian* and *bisexual* are common today. But historically, those terms did not always exist because the concepts didn't exist. Opposite-sex attraction was so strongly regarded as the natural order of things that it wasn't even seen as a preference. There was no other option, so anything other than heterosexuality was invisible. And because the only sexual orientation was heterosexuality, even the idea of heterosexuals didn't exist.

In 1871, the terms *homosexual* and *heterosexual* appeared in two nonfiction works by the Hungarian writer Daniel von Kászony, who is thought to have borrowed the concepts from Austrian writer Károly Mária Kertbeny after Kertbeny used the terms in a private letter dated 1868.[125] Around that time, the control of sexual matters was shifting from the clergy to medical professionals, who regarded all sexual behaviors other than married heterosexual intercourse as illnesses. In 1886, psychologist Richard von Krafft-Ebing discussed homosexuality—which he categorized as abnormal—in his book *Psychopathia Sexualis*.[126] After that, the idea spread that it was possible for there to be a sexual orientation other than heterosexuality. Between 1898 and 1908 alone, over one thousand publications on homosexuality were written by physicians.[127]

"The emerging definitions of homo- and heterosexuality," explains Anne Fausto-Sterling, "were built on a two-sex model of masculinity and femininity. The Victorians...contrasted the sexually aggressive male with the sexually indifferent female. But this created a mystery. If only men felt active desire, how could two women develop a mutual sexual interest? The answer: one of the women had to be an *invert*, someone with markedly masculine attributes. This same logic applied to male homosexuals, who were seen as more effeminate than heterosexual men."[128]

When the idea of same-sex attraction first reached the public's awareness, few questioned that male homosexuals were men and female homosexuals were women. They might have been different types of men or different types of woman, but they were still perceived as their natal sex. I believe that a change in attitude corresponded to advancements in the field of surgery, when doctors started experimenting to radically alter the human body.

The first recorded sex "change" operation (as it used to be called) was performed at German sexologist Magnus Hirschfeld's clinic in 1926 and 1930.[129] But it was George William Jorgensen Jr. who brought transgenderism to the general public's awareness in the United States. In 1952, Jorgensen underwent a series of major medical procedures—first in Denmark, where he had been stationed while in the military and learned about the procedure, and later in U.S. hospitals. By age 26, he was famous as the first American to "become" the opposite sex. The surgically altered Christine Jorgensen emerged as an advocate and spokesperson for transgenders, bolstered by careers as an actor, writer, and nightclub entertainer. In *Christine Jorgensen: A Personal Autobiography*, the author wrote, "As you can see by the enclosed photos, taken just before the operation, I have changed a great deal. But it is the other changes that are so much more important. Remember the shy, miserable person who left America? Well, that person is no more and, as you can see, I'm in marvelous spirits."[130]

The truth, though, was that Jorgensen was miserably unhappy. Sheila Jeffreys points out that "in a letter to a psychiatrist in 1950/1951 [before his surgery], Jorgensen had described himself as a 'homosexual' with a 'large amount of femininity.'...His preference was to consider himself a woman, perhaps because he considered homosexuality immoral: 'it was a thing deeply alien to my religious attitudes.'"[131] What the public saw, and for the most part celebrated, was a man who "became" a woman. An individual unable to perform according to his culturally assigned masculine role was transformed into an entertaining, somewhat flamboyant, happy curiosity thanks to the miracle of modern medicine. Notably absent was any in-depth analysis or effort to question what would make a homosexual unable to accept himself as he was—and why undergoing such a radical transformation was not only acceptable, but necessary. The message could not have been any clearer: Homosexuality was not okay, but surgery to eliminate the *appearance* of homosexuality, *was*.

Today, homosexuality is becoming more accepted, at least in industrialized Western countries. Statistics from 2020 show that in North America, Western Europe, Scandinavia and Australia, the percentage of the population that believes homosexuality should be accepted by society is a minimum of 72 percent (the United States) to 94 percent (Sweden). In Italy it's 75 percent, in Australia it's 81 percent, and in Canada it's 85 percent. The UK, Germany, and France all score at 86 percent, while in Spain it's 89 percent and in the Netherlands it's 92 percent.[132] Nevertheless, in many places gay men and women are still stigmatized, ostracized and threatened because their very existence challenges the idea that heterosexuality is the normal (or only) way to be in a pair bond. Additionally, some people believe that same-sex attraction is a crime against nature. So although public homophobia may not be as prevalent or overt, it nonetheless exists.

Sadly, many gay men and lesbians suffer from internalized homophobia. They see themselves as deficient, as not masculine or feminine enough—and therefore as not-quite-men or not-quite-women. This makes them especially susceptible to the trans agenda, whose subtext is: *If a man is attracted to other men, he must really be a woman. And if a woman is attracted to other women, she must really be a man.* From there, it's a short step to believing *I must have been born into the wrong body.* Of course this isn't logical, because by definition gay relationships require two members of the same sex—so how can one member of the couple still be their natal sex while the other one isn't? But being shamed and intimidated doesn't foster logic.

Compared to the general population, a disproportionate number of gays and lesbians believe they are transgender. As I mention throughout this book, even though trans activists associate themselves with the letters LGB, they are definitely not aligned with, or even remotely sympathetic to, gay people. In fact, trans activists are intensifying their message to gays and lesbians that if you love the same sex, you need to radically alter your body. Homosexual men and women are still receiving the message (albeit in another way) that there is something wrong with same-sex attraction. But I must ask: Is it preferable that two people be in a fulfilling gay relationship, or for one member of the couple to radically alter their body with drugs and perhaps surgery so that the couple might appear more superficially "normal"? Relaxing sex role stereotypes would eliminate the "need" for hormones and surgery.

As I have shown, the potential mental and emotional differences between men and women have become so exaggerated in our culture that by now they are firmly entrenched caricatures. These caricatures are viewed as genuine. But stereotypes are not real people. By expecting others to adhere to rigid stereotypes, we are asking them to be inauthentic. And by trying to adhere to such rigid stereotypes ourselves, we are not allowing ourselves to be authentic, either.

In the next chapter, I describe in detail the harm inflicted when, in order to conform to sex role stereotypes, people change their bodies instead of changing their minds.

PART III

THE TRANS AGENDA

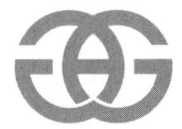

3

BECOMING TRANSGENDER

Gender "Reassignment" Basics

Overview

People who consider themselves transgender typically report feeling as though they are the wrong "gender," or have a different "gender identity" than what they think belongs with their body. "I feel like a girl/woman, but I'm in a boy's/man's body" or "I feel like a boy/man, but I'm in a girl's/woman's body." Statements like these have been made by children as young as two years old and by adults in their 50s, securing them the medical diagnosis of *gender dysphoria*. Based solely on these subjective feelings, the individuals take steps to *transition*, or change their appearance to resemble the opposite sex. Transitioning can never actually *transform* someone into the opposite sex, of course, because that state of being is fixed. But many people believe that switching sexes is possible.

Transitioning involves a number of steps. The person first obtains a prescription for cross-sex hormones. *Cross-sex* refers to hormones that the opposite sex naturally produces in much higher amounts than the person who wants to transition. Then there's alteration of the body. Women who want to be men often have their breasts removed, and men who want to be women receive breast implants. Some people also opt for surgery to their genitals and other areas of the body so they can resemble the opposite sex as much as possible. A male who changes his appearance to approximate a female is known as male-to-female (MtF), while a female who changes her appearance to approximate a male is known as female-to-male (FtM).

The transition process is performed in clinics and hospitals dedicated to *gender reassignment*. The phrase is deliberately deceptive. It suggests that changing one's sex is as simple as checking a box marked "M" or "F," or standing in line under a pink or blue flag. As I discussed in Chapter 1, one's sex cannot be "assigned"; it simply *is*. Recently, the phrase *gender-affirming care* has arisen to replace "gender reassignment" when describing treatments for transgenders. But there's nothing "affirming" about it. If people were truly being "affirmed," they would be encouraged to be who they are without the need to radically alter their physical bodies.

In some circles the word "transgender" is used as a verb—as in "to transgender," or the person "was transgendered" or "is transgendering." This suggests that being transgender is not fixed, but involves a conscious choice to become something other than what one actually is. Trans activists object to this language because in their eyes, being transgender is an immutable state. But while innately being transgender may be true for the tiniest minority (usually very young boys, discussed shortly), for most people it is not. Transgenders are not born, they are created. As I will show throughout this book, many cultural and psychological factors play a role in convincing someone to transition.

What Should Happen

"For mild or intermittent gender dysphoria," says psychiatrist Ray Blanchard, "counseling or cognitive behavior therapy may be sufficient to help the patient through 'flare-ups' of dysphoric feelings. This would be a logical choice of treatment if the [male] patient has a marriage that he wants to maintain or a valued career that would inevitably suffer if he attempted to transition to the female role." However, Blanchard concedes that "For sustained and severe gender dysphoria, hormonal treatment and sex reassignment surgery may offer the best chance of bringing the patient peace of mind and an improved quality of life."[1]

Sexual "reassignment" for people who wish to transgender is a complex process. It should be implemented in carefully structured, multiple-phase steps that take place over the course of several years. The minimal basic stages for a complete transformation are:

- Psychotherapy (to make sure the person is a suitable candidate for the change)
- Complete medical workup (to ensure there are no underlying medical conditions that would make it dangerous to take high-dose hormones or receive surgery)
- Living as the opposite sex (including wearing opposite-sex clothing)
- Cross-sex hormones (which the person must take for life)
- Surgery (or surgeries) on face, breasts, body, and genitals
- More psychotherapy (for help the person adjust to their new life)

The psychotherapy that the transition candidate is supposed to receive first consists of a psychological evaluation, after which regular therapy sessions are conducted over a period of one to two years. This is for the U.S. Some countries require only two to three months of mental health treatment. The lengthy schedule is meant for the individual's benefit, so he or she understands that any deep-seated mental or emotional issues will not magically improve or disappear just because a different appearance is constructed. It's tempting to want to escape problems by becoming someone else, but underneath a surgically altered body is the same person with the same issues that will ultimately resurface. In Blanchard's protocol, a responsible clinician requires the patient to live for a "significant period of time in the cross-gender role before approving them for surgery. One year is a bare minimum, but I think that two years is preferable."[2] Blanchard's slow, cautious approach is wise. He wants to do everything possible first to avoid radical alteration of the body—but if this cannot be avoided, the person's emotional well-being and ability to adjust to these new conditions are supported.

The medical examination of the client is critical because cross-sex hormones can trigger many dangerous and even life-threatening conditions such as heart attacks and cancer. Those transgenders who choose to undergo surgery (not all of them do) hope that the removal and reshaping of various body parts will make their body more closely approximate the physique of the opposite sex. Any surgery involves a certain amount of risk, however. Genital surgery is particularly traumatic and intensely painful. The person must be able to tolerate any painkilling medications that will be needed and withstand whatever pain the drugs won't be able to mask. For such individuals, post-operative psychotherapy is always a good idea to help with any issues that may arise—whether they stem from the individual's psyche or relate to problems with family, friends, or employers who have difficulty with the transformation.

What Really Happens

I have just described the optimal scenario. In reality, the protocol for helping people transition is far different. Those who are eager to transition can receive plenty of advice on how to do it without ever leaving their homes, as long as they own a computer or smart phone. Online support groups, chat rooms, and videos promote escape from discomfort and pain if one is only willing to admit being born into the wrong body. Vulnerable people are routinely counseled to tell gender "reassignment" clinic personnel that they have felt gender dysphoric all their lives—even if this is a lie—so they can immediately be given cross-sex hormones. In the United States, it takes just an hour or less for a client to be given a prescription for powerful drugs whose effects cannot be reversed if those drugs are taken for a long enough period. When discussing testosterone administered to healthy young teenage girls, *Irreversible Damage* author Abigail Shrier points out that the endocrinologists or nurse practitioners who prescribe it are "in the position of hair stylists, who aim to satisfy...[the client's] desired physical appearance... rather than [being] medical professionals who seek to cure....Although alleviation of gender dysphoria was supposed to be its justification, doctors administering T [testosterone] very often seem less interested in treating 'gender dysphoria' than in giving trans-identified patients the look they want."[3]

How young people characterize their treatment by the medical community is much different from the spin offered by trans activists. Responding to a survey, German men and women age 17 to 24 shared their experience of being denied support when they needed it the most. Many were unable to find a psychotherapist who supported their quest to find alternatives to transitioning. The therapists were solely invested in helping them transition, even if the clients themselves questioned whether transitioning would solve their gender dysphoria (or what they thought might be gender dysphoria). Moreover, some therapists did not distinguish between gender dysphoria and self-hatred due to internalized homophobia or misogyny.[4]

Physician-scientist Dr. Lisa Littman focuses on people who aren't sure if they are "truly transgender," and on those who, after transitioning, decide to return to appearing as their natal sex—if they can. She pointed out the abysmal care that children received, based on 256 parent surveys.

> [Over 70 percent] reported the clinician did not explore issues of mental health, previous trauma, or any alternative causes of gender dysphoria before proceeding and 70.0% report that the clinician did not request any medical records before proceeding....And two participants described how the clinician treating their child's gender dysphoria refused to speak with the patients' primary care physicians....[O]f those who knew the content of their child's visit, 84.3% of the parent respondents were reasonably sure or positive that their child had misrepresented or omitted parts of their history.[5]

Most people have a hard time facing painful issues and selectively filter what they remember or disclose. Therefore it's the psychotherapist's job to not automatically accept what the client says, but uncover past and present problems by asking questions. A good therapist probes so the client can make connections between their experiences and traumas and subsequent reactions and choices. However, these "gender-affirming" clinicians in Littman's survey did not take the time to properly evaluate the children psychologically *or* medically. They accepted what their young charges told them without question—apparently eager to promote their plan to start the children on cross-sex hormones right away.

Littman coined the phrase *rapid-onset gender dysphoria (ROGD)*[6] to describe a phenomenon chiefly seen in adolescent girls, who elect to be trans because they don't want the heartache that puberty can bring. Their desire is encouraged and amplified by peer pressure—in person, and from social media—and the seduction of belonging to an exclusive club. "As a therapist," writes Jungian analyst Lisa Marchiano,

> I have spoken with hundreds of parents of teens who have announced a trans identity "out of the blue," and I can corroborate Littman's initial findings. The majority of these parents have a daughter aged

14 or 15—an age at which teens are particularly susceptible to peer influence. These teens often have one or more of the following factors that contribute to their social struggles: they are academically gifted; they are on the autism spectrum; they are same-sex attracted; they have experienced trauma or major disruption; they have other mental health diagnoses such as anxiety or depression; they have a learning disability. Parents often report that their child made a sudden announcement about being transgender after spending increased time on social media sites focused on trans issues, and/or having one or more peers come out as trans. Some teens have even admitted to their parents that they have come out as trans "to fit in."

Since the majority of teens presenting at gender clinics are natal females, we might also consider that many girls feel uncomfortable with gender roles, and that discomfort with one's body is an experience shared by 90% of adolescent females. Teen girls are often very preoccupied with fitting in socially, and are generally more likely than teen boys to manifest emotional problems. Could teen girls be latching on to the narrative supplied online and in the media to construct a story about themselves that serves to explain their feelings of difference while offering a path to transformation?[7]

The influx of preteen and teenage girls into the trans community is so high that some regard it as an epidemic of sorts—which is why the phenomenon is also known as *social contagion*. Children are being fast-tracked to treat their presumed gender dysphoria. On their very first visit they're asked if they want to transition. If the answer is yes, usually after only 45 minutes or one hour they are prescribed cross-sex hormones. Stephanie Winn, a licensed marriage and family therapist in Oregon, used to work with trans-identifying children. "We're just told that if someone tells you they identify in this way, that's the end of the story," she said to a reporter. "Don't ask any questions, just affirm, just agree, and then usher them along this path of medicalization....Many of my colleagues have abandoned our duty of care, either due to ignorance or cowardice....We're expected to tell parents that they must let their children lead, even though children need structure, rules, discipline and boundaries." If the parents don't do what the children say they want, Winn continued, they're accused of being "bigots."[8]

Sometimes the client is evaluated solely on the basis of whether the counselor believes she or he can *pass*—the term used for being able to convince others that one was born a member of the opposite sex. Then the person lives as the opposite sex while taking cross-sex hormones.

Hormones can be injected, taken transdermally (rubbed onto the skin as a cream or lotion, or worn as patches), or swallowed in pill or tablet form. Even minuscule amounts of these chemicals are incredibly powerful, and their effects on the body and brain should not be underestimated. Normally, in both males and females, hormones produced by the reproductive glands are organically involved in a complex feedback loop with different portions of the brain. But when exogenous (outside the body) hormones are taken, the functions of the brain's hypothalamus and pituitary gland are drastically altered. That is why there are substantial "side" effects[9] from such drugs (details of which will follow shortly).

Hormone treatment for transgenders is called *hormone replacement therapy* or *HRT* for short. But HRT is not therapy; there's nothing therapeutic about it. Transitioners are not being given substances to replace what their presumably defective bodies are failing to produce—they are taking unnaturally high doses of substances that their bodies normally produce at much lower levels. The excessively high amounts of hormones exert such radical changes that the hormones are rightly regarded as drugs—which is why one cannot legally obtain them without a doctor's prescription. Therefore, HRT should more accurately be called "HF" for "hormone *forcing*" or "hormone *flooding*." Because HRT is the common nomenclature I will use it for ease of reading, but make no mistake about it: The word "replacement" is a lie. In a healthy biological male body, there is no excess estrogen to "replace." And in a healthy biological female body, there is no excess testosterone to "replace." To maintain focus, I will not be discussing the slightly different effects of various hormone delivery systems, or hormones that might be administered other than estrogen and testosterone.

The final stage of transition, which inexplicably is considered optional for a transgendered person, is to have the genitalia altered to more closely approximate the appearance of the opposite sex's genitals. This is called *bottom surgery*. Bottom surgery is considered corrective, but use of this term is also a lie. For comparison, sewing up tears in a woman's vagina after a difficult childbirth with a large baby is corrective. But the surgery performed on transgenders is mutilation—a creative and imaginative feat of anatomical engineering, but mutilation nonetheless. The fabricated genitalia are imprecise, clumsy, superficial copies of the real ones. Because their structure is not rooted in biology, they can never function like the genitals they were designed to emulate.

Standard of care in medicine refers to diagnoses and treatments that a physician is expected to follow for patients or illnesses, based on what other reasonable and competent medical professionals do when dealing with similar issues. But transgendering is not "reasonable." In no other area of medicine do doctors so easily prescribe drugs or perform surgery, based simply on a patient's declaration that he or she wants them. If a 14-year-old went to a physician and said, "Doc, I have diagnosed myself for cancer, so please operate on my lung to remove the tumor—and by the way, give me such-and-such drugs too," would the doctor automatically comply? Of course not! Tests would be run and options would be discussed. Yet when the medical treatment is related to something we call "gender," many medical professionals eagerly dispense drugs and perform life-altering surgeries. In fact, an opinion piece in *Newsweek* is titled, "There's No Standard for Care When it Comes to Trans Medicine." "I had the most supportive possible environment for transitioning: easy access to hormones, an affirming community and insurance coverage," the author wrote. "What I didn't have was a therapist who could help me scrutinize the underlying issues I had before I undertook serious medical decisions [while in my early 20s]. Instead, I was diagnosed with gender dysphoria and given the green light to start transition by my doctor on the first visit....One year later, I would be curled in my bed, clutching my double-mastectomy scars and sobbing with regret."[10]

Parents As Enemies

In order to fast-track a dependent child or teen into transitioning, it's necessary to eliminate parents from the decision-making process. This means convincing the child to mistrust the parents. The trans community and most mainstream media vilify parents as unsupportive and hostile to the child's goals. If parents question the wisdom of taking cross-sex hormones or slicing off healthy parts of the body—or even if they just ask questions about the procedures—this means, according to trans activists, that the parents do not have the child's best interests at heart and/or are transphobic. A *phobia* is an exaggerated and illogical fear or dislike of something. *Transphobic* means afraid of, prejudiced toward, or unfriendly to trans people. With increasing frequency, parents are being portrayed as being hostile to the LGBTQ+ community—even though being gay or bisexual is not at all the same as being transgender.

Psychotherapist Lisa Marchiano says there's no evidence to support claims by trans activists—who expect the public to simply accept their declarations—that "parents are rejecting their gender nonconforming children in heretofore unseen numbers against the promptings of parental instincts evolved over the eons." She points to how the media "continues to cultivate a narrative of widespread parental rejection and abuse," despite a 2015 study by the Pew Research Center which reported that a "majority" of American parents stated that they would not be upset if their child was gay. Moreover, most gay and lesbian children who disclosed their sexual orientation to their parents felt that their relationship with their parents was either unaffected or grew even stronger. Only a minority said that their relationships with their parents became worse. "Parental acceptance rates have been steadily rising since the 1980s and continue to inch up year by year."[11]

"The literature laments that some families reject their children," Marchiano adds, "but it does not mention the patients' rejection of their families." She also relates what happened when a girl had been "gender affirmed" at school with a boy's name without the mother's knowledge. "The mother received a phone call from the school one day stating that there had been an accident, and her son 'X' (boy name) had been injured. The mother replied that the school was mistaken, as she did not have a son, nor a child named 'X.' Of course, the medical emergency had in fact involved her child, but she only found out later."[12] In a separate incident, another girl who had been similarly "affirmed" took her college entrance exams under her male name, but later resumed her own name. She had problems when applying to colleges, as her test scores had been sent under her false name.

The assumption that all parents are biased and incompetent is part of the radical trans strategy to force dependent, impressionable children to rely on the trans community for support rather than confide in their parents. More than one girl has stated, "I thought I couldn't trust my own mother" because she was led "to believe that parental alienation was inevitable." Marchiano reports that in her experience, in almost every instance it's the child who rejects the parents, not vice-versa. "I have known multiple families in which trans identified young people cut off all contact with their families simply because the parents suggested to their child that a cautious approach to medical transition might be best or shared some academic journal articles about the side effects of treatment."[13]

To parents who still have some emotional connection with their children, child psychiatrist Miriam Grossman advises, "Teach them that like the Earth, their bodies are delicate ecologic systems to be honored and preserved. High-dose estrogen in a boy and [high-dose] testosterone in a girl clash with the instructions in each cell. It's a war against themselves, and they'll pay a price....Yes, hormones will masculinize a girl and feminize a boy but the result is a synthetic persona, not the real thing, and maintaining it will require a lifetime of drugs."[14]

The human brain doesn't mature until age 25 (which parents of adolescents bemoan). A child whose brain is still developing is not in a position to make decisions that can permanently impact him or her in such a profound way. With so much childhood angst and rebellion to work through, it's understandable that a son or daughter might view a parent's disagreements with their choices—or just the act of simply asking questions—as wrong and unreasonable. Marchiano points out that many parents define "support" differently from their children.

> The parents I speak with overwhelmingly love their children. They are interested in supporting their children in growing to adulthood with healthy bodies. They want to support their child's emerging identity by allowing wide-ranging exploration of different orientations and interests. And they want to guide their child in weighing long-term consequences so that he or she can make wise decisions. Many parents who support their child in this way find that their child moves through her period of gender exploration without feeling the need to make permanent changes to her body. Young people with parents who supported their gender nonconformity while encouraging them to accept their bodies often express gratitude for this kind of parental support.[15]

Of course not all children have loving parents with an open line of communication. Some parents are outright abusive. Children with troubled family relationships are especially in danger of being seduced. Once their family connections are severed, it's easier to convince them to keep their transitioning a secret. Dr. Grossman, who has treated countless children, describes how she deals with issues that underlie presumed gender dysphoria. In her book *Lost in Trans Nation: A Child Psychiatrist's Guide Out of the Madness*, Grossman helps parents navigate the psychological and legal difficulties of gently separating a child from the trans agenda. This requires a lot of awareness and effort, because trans activism is relentless and insidious. She writes:

> After practicing psychiatry for forty years, and making it into my seventh decade of life, I have more knowledge and wisdom than my young patients....I'm curious about everything: their family, school, and friends, as well as their worries and dreams. Everything is connected to everything, and nothing is unimportant. Their new [trans] identity serves a purpose, and together we unravel what it is. We slowly explore the source of their distress, and I guide them toward self-acceptance. That's what therapists were once trained to do before gender ideology laid siege to the mental health profession.[16]

Now let's explore what's actually involved in HRT along with many types of surgeries.

Hormones that Give Males Some Features of Females

The hormones given to transitioning males is based on the same HRT (hormone replacement therapy) that was originally developed by pharmaceutical companies for women who have gone through menopause. In women, the loss of natural estrogen—whose production markedly declines after they pass childbearing age—can cause night sweats, low sex drive, fatigue, bloating, weight gain, mood swings, thinning hair, and bone loss or brittleness. A particularly bothersome symptom is pain and other discomfort during sexual intercourse due to vaginal dryness and burning (for which progesterone is often a better choice than estrogen).

HRT for natal women is not without risk. Whether a woman takes synthetic estrogen or bio-identical estradiol (which has the same molecular structure as the hormone naturally produced by the female body), she may suffer digestive issues including nausea, stomach cramps and bloating; breast tenderness; leg cramps; gallstones (for which gallbladder removal is suggested); at least a 30 percent increased risk of heart attacks, stroke and blood clots; and an increased risk of both endometrial and breast cancers.[17] It should not be surprising, then, that health risks are similar for males who take estrogen. But doctors who prescribe feminizing drugs for men rarely disclose the so-called side effects. Compared to biological males not on cross-sex hormones, MtFs have a 200 to 400 percent increase of risk for myocardial infarction.[18] In order for MtFs to obtain feminizing effects from estrogen, they have to take it in doses *two to three times higher than what postmenopausal women receive.*[19] Plus, their testosterone levels need to be lowered. However, according to the Endocrine Society, only one-quarter of MtF individuals reach the goal of reducing testosterone so that it falls within the range of what would be normal for a biological woman.[20]

One of the most obvious and important changes for a MtF on estrogen is body fat, which is redistributed to the hips, buttocks and thighs. But this more hourglass figure is only an approximation of a female body because the skeletal structure remains fixed. The waist is still that of a male—below the navel, rather than above it. Also, the gait will be that of a male, due to the angle of the leg bones to the hip.

The high levels of estrogen in MtFs produce softer and smoother skin. Muscle mass decreases, although not substantially. The breasts grow, although most men find that the increase in size is not enough for their aspirations and they may choose to augment their chests with surgical implants. Balding on the scalp may be slowed or halted. Hair on the arms, legs and trunk will decrease, although the face still retains its beard and many sessions of electrolysis are needed to achieve a smooth face. The size of the penis often decreases. Erections are less frequent, and in some cases they stop entirely. The ejaculate fluid lessens or disappears, due to the shrinkage and poor function of the prostate gland. Sterility always results.

Males who take estrogen will probably gain weight and undergo bloating. Their libido often decreases. Older MtFs especially are more at risk for breast cancer, deep vein thrombosis (blood clots), and osteoporosis.[21] They're also at risk for impaired liver function. The liver's job is to convert toxic chemicals into benign substances. If it cannot perform this vital function, the person has lower immunity than usual and is susceptible to more diseases.

Estrogen affects males psychologically and emotionally as well as physically, although there's not as much data about the emotional states of MtFs as there is for FtMs. Some men report feeling calmer and less obsessive. Many state that their emotions are more accessible, and they cry much more easily than before their treatment. (Does the need to be emotionally vulnerable and feel more deeply influence some men's desire to start taking high doses of estrogen?) However, MtFs on estrogen also experience much more irritability and depression compared to the general population. A 1989 Dutch study of 425 transsexual patients (as transgenders were then called) showed that the number of deaths in men who transitioned was five times the number expected when compared to a control group of non-trans men. Some of the deaths were due to suicide.[22] That is why researchers later wrote, in *The Journal of Clinical Endocrinology & Metabolism*, that "gender reassignment, although effective in relieving the gender dysporia, should not be considered a cure" for depression.[23]

Contributing to a MtF transitioner's success is the ability to pass. Not every MtF can do this. If he transitions after puberty, when secondary sex characteristics have become entrenched, it's much more difficult to "de-masculinize" a man. Even if the individual has had extensive plastic surgery on the face and elsewhere, others might still notice that something's not quite right—and guess that attempts at "reassignment" surgery have been made.

Psychiatrist Paul McHugh (born in 1931)—who published many books about sexual pathologies and stopped the transgender surgery program at Johns Hopkins University forty years ago (although the practice was recently resumed)—has decades of experiences with people who want to be the opposite sex. Based on his many sessions with MtFs, McHugh is not convinced that feminizing hormones and surgical treatments truly bring happiness. "They wore high heels, copious makeup, and flamboyant clothing," he said of his patients. "The post-surgical subjects struck me as caricatures of women."[24]

Hormones that Give Females Some Features of Males

Normal biological men produce 15 times the amount of circulating testosterone than women of any age.[25] In order for females to obtain masculinizing effects from testosterone, they must take it in a dosage *at least ten to forty times greater* than what their bodies normally produce. The testosterone levels for FtMs are even higher than what a woman with polycystic ovary syndrome would produce.

One of the most obvious and important changes for a FtM on testosterone is body fat distribution. Instead of lodging under the arms, and on the thighs and hips, the fat moves to the abdomen and surrounds the internal organs. This straighter figure, though, is only an approximation of a male body because the skeletal structure remains fixed. The waist is still that of a female—above the navel, rather than below it—and the gait will be that of a female, due to the non-parallel angle of the leg bones to the hip.

FtM transitioners on testosterone see an increase in muscle mass. Existing hair becomes coarser, and hair now grows where previously there had been none: on the face, chest, stomach, neck, arms, legs, and even the ears and nose. The skin becomes thicker and often turns more oily, causing acne. Menstruation gradually stops. There may be an increase in appetite as well as libido. Hair loss and baldness are common. The vaginal opening and passage become drier and more fragile. And the clitoris usually becomes larger. A two-inch gain in length is not uncommon, and is referred to as a micropenis.

Females who take testosterone to have more male-looking bodies are at greater risk for high blood pressure, insulin resistance (which leads to carbohydrate intolerance and diabetes), weight gain, and abnormalities in body fat that play a role in the development of heart disease.[26] In fact, biological women on FtM doses of testosterone are almost five times more likely to suffer a heart attack than non-trans women, and almost two-and-one-half times more likely to have a heart attack than men.[27] One follow-up study of short-term consequences showed an abnormal increase in red blood cells. This increase unnaturally thickens the blood. Combined with other factors, it increases the risk of phlebitis (inflammation of the veins), blood clots in a vein, and again, heart attacks[28]—all known in medical circles as cardiac "events." During a thromboembolytic "event," a clot in a blood vessel breaks loose and is carried by the bloodstream to other areas of the body where it can block a vessel in a lung or kidney, the brain, a leg, or the gastrointestinal tract. Liver enzyme abnormalities might also develop, increasing the risk of cancer.[29]

High-dose testosterone also causes psychological and emotional changes. It suppresses anxiety, elevates courage, and lifts depression—all of which can cause or contribute to more reckless behavior. But it also reduces short-term memory, and increases irritability and moodiness. Some FtMs report feeling clearer-headed and hyper-focused, while others report suffering from brain fog. Many FtMs who report a sharper mental focus from testosterone also experience a blunting of emotions. A good example is the actor Chaz Bono (born Chastity). Bono, who began transitioning at age 40, reported being hyper-focused but also less emotionally warm after starting testosterone. Chaz's then-girlfriend—saddened that "there is a softness that is gone" as she watched "the female essence leave his body"—had a difficult time adjusting to this change and ended the relationship as a result.[30] Endocrinologist Walter Futterweit, a specialist in transgenderism, finds that FtMs experience more psychiatric problems including fluctuating moods, hypersexuality, psychotic symptoms, and depression.[31] Lisa Marchiano writes that in her therapy practice—where she frequently treats girls in their teens and early twenties who have started to transition or have already transitioned—she has seen a huge increase in aggression, volatility, and hospitalization for mood disorders.[32] Could these sudden outbursts of irrational anger and rage be caused by unnaturally high levels of testosterone flooding their bodies? More mass shootings of innocent bystanders in public spaces are being committed by FtM trans persons. Yet mainstream media has been reluctant to disclose that the person was taking high-dose testosterone. Why?

Puberty Blockers for Children

Puberty is a complex process to "block." In almost all children, at the start of puberty the hypothalamus in the brain produces gonadotropin-releasing hormone (GnRH). This causes the anterior pituitary gland to release larger than usual quantities of follicle-stimulating hormone (FSH) and luteinizing hormone (LH). The end result of this cascade of hormones (whose biochemistry is slightly different for each sex) is the eventual stimulation of the reproductive glands, which produce effects all too familiar to many a horrified adolescent.

Males experience the first stage of puberty roughly between age 9 and 12. There's an increase in height, and the scrotum and testicles grow a bit more. At the second stage of puberty—usually around age 12 or 13—the testicles continue to grow, which means that more testosterone is being produced in the body, which will then lead to further changes. The boy continues to grow in height and the body shape becomes more defined as masculine. The third stage of puberty, generally at age 13 or 14, produces darker and denser pubic hair, as well as an enlargement of both the testicles and penis (which causes more erections). During the final, fourth stage, which takes place at about age 14 or 15, the boy begins to sprout facial hair and more body hair, including in the armpits. (The hair follicles in the armpits contain glands that produce pheromones, biochemicals that are sexually enticing usually to the opposite sex.) The voice deepens, due to the lengthening and thickening of the vocal cords in a larger larynx. The boy will continue to grow even more in height. His muscles will become larger and their fibers, thicker.

The shoulders will also broaden. Most important, the face will change shape. The chin will become longer and the nose, thicker. A boy with an androgynous appearance—that is, who could be perceived as either male or female—starts to appear unmistakably male. Many boys continue to grow well into their 20s.

Females experience the first stage of puberty roughly around age 10 or 11, although it can come later. Before menstruation begins, wisps of pubic hair appear. The second stage of puberty takes place at age 11 or 12. Breasts start to bud with additional tissue, and the areola (the ring around the nipples) darkens. The breasts may feel tender or uncomfortable due to an intense influx of hormones, which leads to another growth spurt. The third stage of puberty, generally occurring at age 12 or 13, continues the growth of breast tissue and hair in the armpits and pubic area. (As with boys, the hair follicles in a girl's armpits contain glands that produce pheromones, biochemicals that are sexually enticing usually to the opposite sex.) The first menstrual period often follows within six months of the first major growth cycle, when a girl's height may increase as much as three-and-a-half inches. The average age of the first period is 12 years, but usually girls are incapable of conceiving babies until two years after the onset of menstruation. Typically, if menstruation starts after age 13, the ovulation cycles will tend to be more irregular until the age of 18 or 19. The beginning of the menstrual cycle corresponds to the development of milk glands, ducts, and fat tissue inside the breast. The first menstrual period also corresponds to weight gain and major bone growth. The bones have widened and lengthened, but because they aren't yet fully mineralized, they're more vulnerable to fractures. During the fourth stage of puberty, at around age 13 or 14, the girl's accelerated height will slow. She will accumulate more body fat around her hips and thighs. Hair in the genital and underarm regions will continue to grow and become coarser. Unlike boys, girls have five stages of puberty. The fifth stage usually occurs between age 14 and 17, although it could happen later. The breasts achieve their final size. Pubic hair is fully developed, as are the cardiovascular, skeletal, and muscular systems. With a more curvy figure and obvious breasts, any girl who may have had an androgynous appearance now appears unmistakably female.

It's important to remember that for each sex, pubertal changes occur in the brain as well as in the body. The prefrontal cortex, located just behind the forehead, is the rational, self-regulatory part of the brain responsible for cognitive analysis, abstract thought, and impulse control. As many parents of impulsive teenagers already know, the prefrontal cortex is the last region to reach maturation. Typically, the brain doesn't stop growing until the person reaches about age 25.

What if the child is not permitted to experience this natural maturation process? Increasing numbers of young children are being diagnosed with gender dysphoria, after which they are given puberty blocking pharmaceuticals to stop secondary sex characteristics from appearing.

Puberty blockers are synthetic hormone analogues that prevent the pituitary gland from doing its job. Because the ultimate effect on males is the reduction of androgen hormones—which leads to diminished masculinization, including the ability to have erections—puberty blockers were initially created for violent sex offenders. The rationale was that these criminals wouldn't be able to harm children if they were unable to have erections. The drugs also cause the penis and testicles to shrink, along with reduced or absent sexual desire. Breast tissue growth in males (a condition known as *gynecomastia*) is another result, which may be desirable for MtFs but not any other male. Still more effects, which no one wants, will be discussed shortly. In view of their original intended use, these drugs used to be called *chemical castrators*.

One drug that's frequently used to halt normal puberty is Lupron (generic name, leuprolide acetate). It was originally developed for grown women to treat uterine fibroids as well as endometriosis (when the uterine lining spreads to the outside of the uterus). This class of drugs is also used for prostate cancer in men, although its effectiveness has never been proven. Lupron has not been approved by the FDA for use in children. As with all chemical castration pharmaceuticals, Lupron is used to prevent the onset of puberty because it reduces what should be normal levels of testosterone and estrogen in both men and women. Although many complete studies on the drug have been conducted, most of them remain unpublished, although one study did manage to make its way into a 2019 issue of the *British Medical Journal*. The authors criticized the Gender Identity Development Service (GIDS)—England's sole provider of treatment for young people with gender dysphoria—for using Lupron.[33] Other acknowledged "side" effects—found on numerous websites devoted to Lupron—include bone brittleness and breakage, convulsions, hypertension (high blood pressure, including in the brain), blurred vision, loss of vision, eye pain (behind the eye, or pain with eye movement), tinnitus (ringing in the ears), dizziness, injection site swelling and abscesses, headache and migraines, diarrhea, abdominal pain, hot flashes, night sweats, hemorrhage, vaginal discharge and infections, nausea and vomiting, anal itching, pain in extremities, rash, back pain, ligament sprain, increased weight, bone fractures, breast tenderness, insomnia, chest pain, fever, and weight gain. Some of these symptoms appear after only one month of being on the drug.[34] Consumers are told that there may be even more effects, and to contact their doctor to learn about the ones that aren't listed on the websites. Even the FDA warned, in 2022, that puberty blocking drugs could cause the brain to swell, resulting in nausea, severe headaches, double vision, and even permanent loss of vision.[35]

All chemical castration/puberty-blocking drugs have similar effects. And all cause infertility. There are psychological consequences as well: decreased libido; unstable, wild fluctuations in emotions, including crying, irritability, impatience and anger; and augmented aggression. Depression is common, which can lead not only to suicidal ideation, but also actual suicide. I'll discuss suicidal ideation and actual drug-induced suicides in detail in the next chapter.

Children—who are given these drugs simply because they say they need them—are in no position to comprehend the drugs' permanent negative effects, assuming they're even told about them. Parents are hardly ever informed. If they were, they might fight harder to prevent their children from taking those drugs. The number and type of "side" effects from puberty blockers is not surprising, considering the number of processes that are being interfered with. As you can see, much more is involved than merely causing or stopping facial hair to grow.

Depending on when they're administered, these drugs either suppress the body's release of sex hormones altogether, or obstruct the receptor sites for sex hormones—which prevents the hormones from reaching the tissues and catalyzing changes. Although puberty blockers are meant to be taken before puberty starts (so that the development of secondary sex characteristics is halted), the drugs can also be dispensed later to stop the secondary sex characteristics from continuing, including menstrual periods in females.

The rationale for giving puberty blockers to very young children who claim (or are assumed) to be gender dysphoric is simple: Why go to all the trouble to reverse secondary sexual characteristics that the children insist they don't want, if you can prevent those traits from manifesting in the first place? Preventing puberty not only makes it easier for the individual to pass, but it also lessens the possibility of violence, because transgenders who don't appear natural have a greater chance of being physically assaulted. After the puberty blockers have done their job, the children can immediately be put on cross-sex hormones, which will help produce an even more convincing opposite-sex appearance.

Early intervention to help with the ability to pass may seem like a logical and positive step, but it's not. As you have seen, puberty is a complex process that involves more than the reproductive organs. Virtually every system in the body, including the brain, undergoes preparation for optimal functioning as an adult. These drugs don't simply prevent facial hair from appearing in a boy, or breasts from budding in a girl. Puberty blockers slow down—and in some instances completely stop—overall growth. They negatively impact height, strength, and bone density, to name just a few basic elements. Considering that these drugs alter the body so radically, it would be naïve to deny their mental and emotional effects. It has already been observed that children on puberty blockers can experience mood fluctuations. Studies of brain function show that among children whose puberty is halted, cognition and operational memory may be impaired, resulting in a lower IQ.[36] The drugs also appear to interfere with the structure and function of the brain's neural circuits, preventing them from completely developing. Neuroplasticity is impeded as well.[37] Dr. Hilary Cass, former President of the Royal College of Paediatrics and Child Health, addressed these impairments in her July 2022 letter to England's National Health Service:

> [Naturally occurring] adolescent sex hormone surges may trigger the opening of a critical period for experience-dependent rewiring of neural circuits underlying executive function (i.e. maturation of the part of the brain concerned with planning, decision making

and judgement). If this is the case, brain maturation may be temporarily or permanently disrupted by puberty blockers, which could have significant impact on the ability to make complex risk-laden decisions, as well as possible longer-term neuropsychological consequences. To date, there has been very limited research on the short-, medium- or longer-term impact of puberty-blockers on neurocognitive development.[38]

Cass used many qualifiers, such as "*may* trigger," "*may* be...disrupted," and "*could* have significant impact." Did she think the NHS would listen more if she understated her case? Not only are trans-agenda doctors unlikely to admit or disclose the physical and psychological dangers of these drugs; they also don't tell parents that after puberty blockers do their work, *nothing*—not even the administration of natal hormones—can re-establish growth and height, strengthen bones, improve cardiovascular health, support optimal immune response, repair impeded brain function, or restore fertility. That is why no *responsible* endocrinologist advocates putting children on puberty blockers. Yet children are routinely being given these dangerous drugs in the name of treating "gender dysphoria"—which almost all will overcome, if they're allowed to grow up normally.

"The use of puberty suppression and cross-sex hormones for minors," wrote three researchers in 2017—including psychiatrist Paul McHugh, who has a great deal of experience treating transgenders and people diagnosed as dysphoric—"is a radical step that presumes a great deal of knowledge and competence on the part of the children assenting to these procedures, on the part of the parents or guardians being asked to give legal consent to them, and on the part of the scientists and physicians who are developing and administering them."

> We frequently hear from neuroscientists that the adolescent brain is too immature to make reliably rational decisions, but we are supposed to expect emotionally troubled adolescents to make decisions about their gender identities and about serious medical treatments at the age of 12 or younger....The claim that puberty-blocking treatments are fully reversible makes them appear less drastic, but *this claim is not supported by scientific evidence*.... Furthermore, we do not fully understand the psychological consequences of using puberty suppression to treat young people with gender dysphoria. [emphasis added][39]

In 2019, five academics and physicians—some specializing in endocrinology—emphasized the negative long-term effects of puberty blockers in *The Journal of Clinical Endocrinology & Metabolism*. The authors pointed out that no laboratory, imaging, or other objective tests exist that can diagnose a verifiably transgender child—and furthermore, there's no way to predict who will grow out of the condition (desist) and who will remain dysphoric. There's no justification whatsoever, they insisted, to administer any drug whose effects include sexual dysfunction, cardiovascular disease, blood clots, and sterility—and whose long-term effects have never been studied. Furthermore, the authors pointed out, studies have shown that so far, gender transition fails to lower the risk of suicide. Bottom line, if the child is not ill, why would a physician be willing to cause illness with such a drastic medical intervention? To give some perspective, the authors compared FtM testosterone levels due to high-dose hormones—amounts recommended by the Endocrine Society—with known medical conditions. FtM testosterone levels are even higher than what is normally produced by women who have androgen-secreting tumors. And testosterone levels in the ovaries of FtMs who haven't had their ovaries removed correspond to those found in polycystic ovary syndrome (PCOS)—a high-risk situation associated with increases in ovarian cancer and metabolic aberrations. As for MtFs on high-dose estrogen, the risk of venous thromboembolism is 500 percent greater than normal.

In their brief letter, the authors scolded their fellow doctors.

> How can a child, adolescent, or even parent provide genuine consent to such a treatment? How can the physician ethically administer GAT [gender-affirming treatment] knowing that a significant number of patients will be irreversibly harmed?... Existing care models based on psychological therapy have been shown to alleviate GD [gender dysphoria] in children, thus avoiding the radical changes and health risks of GAT. This is an obvious and preferred therapy, as it does the least harm with the most benefit.[40]

At least two of the doctors who signed their name to the article are on the transgender movement's radar as being transphobic. Their concern about the unwanted consequences of powerful drugs is obviously unwelcome.

When doing research for this book, I asked a psychiatrist friend, who also specializes in neurology, if he would ever approve puberty blockers or cross-sex hormones for a teenager. "Absolutely not!" he exclaimed. "That's child abuse. The outpouring of sexual hormones during puberty cause huge changes in both the body and mind. Children undergo a massive growth spurt but they also have thousands of chemical reactions in their brains that impact their behavior as adults. This is a natural process that I would never deny someone. If he or she decides to change after they're fully developed, that's another issue—but to do that to a child is criminal." When asked if I could credit him with the quote he declined, fearing that he'd lose his job if his medical opinion were known.

I already mentioned that the FDA never approved of Lupron for its off-label use as a puberty blocker. Is this because thousands of deaths have been linked to those chemical castrators? Between 2013 and June 2019, 41,213 adverse events were reported, including 25,645 "serious" reactions and 6,379 deaths.[41] How ironic, then, that the use of chemical castration to shut off the normal function of the pituitary gland and cause a cascade of abnormal reactions is called "affirming." In the future, should doctors be legally prevented from using Lupron to stop puberty—or if it's removed from the market entirely—other drugs will most certainly be manufactured to take its place. In the UK, some endocrinologists prescribe the GnRH analog Triptorelin. Although slightly different from Lupron,

Triptorelin has similar effects on the body and thus causes equivalent damage—as any chemical castration drug would. No matter what drug is taken, as long as such a significant natural biological process is being tampered with, an unlimited number of systems will be involved.[42]

There's one more devastating effect of puberty blockers that's hardly ever mentioned by medical personnel. Children who are prevented from going through their normal pubertal maturation process are incapable of having orgasms. Dr. Marci Bowers, a MtF surgeon who transitioned at age 38, bluntly stated at a virtual conference hosted by Duke University, "Every single child or adolescent who was truly blocked at Tanner stage two has never experienced orgasm. I mean, it's really about zero."[43] The Tanner stages are sexual maturity ratings named after the child development expert who first identified the visible stages of sexual maturation as children grow into adolescence and adulthood. Stage two designates preparatory hormones but no discernable physical changes, while stage five designates the beginning of full-blown maturation. At Tanner stage two, the reproductive organs of both sexes are still immature—frozen in a childlike state. The child's secondary sex characteristics are becoming visible, but just barely. In females, the breasts are beginning to bud but the ovaries are pre-fertile. And in males, although the testicles and scrotum are starting to grow, they are still very small and obviously belong to a young child. If these secondary sex characteristics are prevented from occurring at stage two, the person will be unable to climax sexually. "Why," asked a reporter who covered the Duke University conference, "are medical experts encouraging young children to embark on massively disruptive procedures that could prevent them from enjoying some of the greatest pleasures of living?"[44]

An orgasm is more than a good feeling. A full release helps discharge pent-up energy and involves all bodily systems. Blood flow increases and pain-relieving endorphins are produced. Oxytocin levels rise, which not only helps us feel connected to our partner and friends, but imparts pleasure. The amygdala or reptilian brain—which is the locus of fear and anxiety—shows little or no activity. This further promotes relaxation and the dissipation of stress. Having regular orgasms even helps relieve insomnia. The immune system also works better when people sexually climax with a full, pleasurable release. Those who cannot experience this type of discharge are more prone to melancholy and depression.

Human beings were made to have orgasms; the body's neurological pathways are designed for it. Sexual fulfillment is a vitally important part of a rewarding life—so much so, that adults who are unable to sexually climax seek psychotherapeutic or medical treatment. Children robbed of this intense pleasure are being denied their humanity. Moreover, blockages in the body's energy cause, as well as reflect, blocked emotions. I will be discussing this in greater depth in Chapter 9.

As the five aforementioned physicians wrote in *The Journal of Clinical Endocrinology & Metabolism*, "In our opinion, physicians need to start examining GAT [gender-"affirming" therapy] through the objective eye of the scientist-clinician rather than the ideological lens of the social activist."[45]

Surgeries for Males Who Want to Resemble Females (MtF)

Surgery is a major procedure that in theory is supposed to occur at least two years after the individual has received the first psychological evaluation, and has been on cross-sex hormones for at least one year. All operations involve lots of cutting, the removal and assembling of tissue—and then months of recovery.

Men who want the approximation of female bodies are given breast implants. Sometimes they receive plastic surgery on the face so their features might be construed as more feminine. Any part of the face can be involved: nose, jaw, chin, cheeks, lips, eyebrows, and more. In many cases, their prominent Adam's apple is reduced in size through surgical shaving. They also undergo laser or electrolysis removal of hair from the body, while the hairline on the head might be augmented with hair from other areas.

Those who elect to receive bottom surgery have the scrotum and testicles removed. The penis is sliced in half, turned inside out, cut some more, and remodeled into a cavity. During MtF surgery, the urethra in the urinary tract must be moved and integrated with the design of the new cavern. The body perceives the cavity as a wound, and naturally tries to close it. Therefore, to maintain this passageway, the person must mechanically keep it open—either with cylinders called stents, or regular sexual activity, during which a penis or similarly-shaped object is inserted into the cavern. If the male who transitions is a young boy who was not allowed to naturally go through puberty, there are additional problems with trying to create a cavity. The child's penis, not having been exposed to a huge pubertal surge of testosterone, is inconveniently small. Therefore, points out Miriam Grossman, "There will be insufficient tissue to create a faux vagina, and the surgeons will have to harvest it from elsewhere" such as the arm, leg, abdomen, or even colon. She mentions MtF Jazz Jennings, who transitioned before puberty and therefore "needed to go under the knife three additional times following the original surgery."[46]

One MtF reported problems with the new genitals. "One day I was making love and something didn't feel right. There was this little ball of hair like a Brillo pad in my vagina [sic]." The surgeon pulled the hair out, but warned that it would grow back. "He said it would always be there because I hadn't had electrolysis on my scrotum before the sex change made it part of my vagina. When I heard that, I just sat and cried."[47]

"The new orifice is not a vagina in the biological sense," Sheila Jeffreys explains.

> Vaginas are connected into the reproductive system of the female body rather than being simply an external cavity, and they are self-cleansing mechanisms. The newly carved out orifices of male-bodied transgenders do not resemble vaginas; rather they create new microbial habitats in which infections develop and cause serious smell issues for their owners. The problem of bad smell is a commonly occurring discussion thread on transgender advice websites. The medical evidence is that a bad smell exists and is

associated with faecal bacteria common to those male-bodied transgenders who engaged in "heterosexual" coitus...The neovaginas lack the lactobacilli connected with vaginal health in females.[48]

"Frequent episodes of malodorous discharge," corroborate other medical researchers, "were reported by one in four [transgender] women and malodour was even more frequently observed upon gynaecological examination, which in turn might relate to the presence of faecal bacterial vaginosis-like microflora"[49]— in other words, pathogens similar to those present in actual women who suffer from vaginal infections. It's not surprising that a fetid odor is such a problem. If the cavern is constructed from colon tissue, an unpleasant odor seems guaranteed.

After this surgical manipulation, some MtF individuals sense a "phantom" penis—similar to how someone with an amputated limb might feel—as though the original tissue were still present. They feel for the organ, but it's not there. They also suffer emotionally. Grief and loss are common.

What is the health of MtF individuals after surgery? In a French journal article, plastic surgeons followed up 189 patients for a minimum of one year and a maximum of five. The authors reported "a 2.6% of rectovaginal wall perforations. In 37% of patients we had repeated compressive dressings and 15% of them required blood transfusions. Eighteen percent of patients presented with hematoma [severe bruising due to injury, where blood collects under the skin] and 27% with early infectious complications. Delayed short-depth neovagina occurred in 21% of patients [meaning the cavern was not deep enough], requiring additional hard dilatation [expansion], with a 95.5% success rate. Total secondary vaginoplasty rate was 6.3% (4.7% skin graft and 3.7% bowel plasty). Secondary functional meatoplasty [enlargement of an opening to allow urine to pass though] occurred in 1% of cases. Other secondary cosmetic surgery rates ranged between 3 to 20%."[50]

Most MtF transgenders never have their genitals remodeled. According to the 2015 *U.S. Transgender Survey*, only 10 percent reported having any type of genital surgery.[51] However, incongruously they still regard themselves as women, and live according to how they think a woman would live.

Despite all these efforts—and even if the person has been operated on by the best of surgeons—some adult MtFs fail to easily pass as women. The effects of testosterone, to which they were exposed earlier in life, overwhelm any attempts to eliminate their inherently masculine physique. Because of this inability to pass, these masculine-appearing MtF transgenders suffer more discrimination and violence than those who have a more conventionally feminine appearance. The perpetrators who commit violent and discriminatory acts are upset because non-passing trans individuals fail to meet their requirements of what a woman is supposed to look like. They, too, have fallen prey to sex role stereotyping—and they unfairly and cruelly unleash their aggression on MtF transgenders.

Surgeries for Females Who Want to Resemble Males (FtM)

As with MtFs, surgery for FtMs is a major procedure that in theory is supposed to occur at least two years after the individual has received the first psychological evaluation, and has been on cross-sex hormones for a minimum of one year. Bottom surgery for women who want to resemble men is even more complicated than surgery for MtFs. I'll get to that in a moment.

In the transitional phase when living as men, women bind their breasts with a tight compression fabric that squashes the blood and lymph vessels, connective tissue, and breast ligaments. Besides deforming the breast tissue, this compression usually causes severe back pain, bruised or even fractured ribs, and sometimes collapsed or punctured lungs. It should go without saying that women who wear binders also have great difficulty breathing.[52]

Women who want male bodies sometimes have their breasts removed, though not always. The 2015 *U.S. Transgender Survey* states that 21 percent of FtMs receive chest reduction or reconstruction.[53] Most who forego surgery keep binding their breasts. Removal of the female breast consists of eliminating breast tissue and skin, and repositioning the nipples—which usually reduces nipple sensation. Sometimes the person receives plastic surgery on the face so the features appear more masculine. Any part of the face can be involved: nose, jaw, chin, cheeks, lips, eyebrows, and more. After they take testosterone, the voices of FtMs sound more like men than the voices of MtFs sound like women. Once that hormone has coursed through the body of either sex for a long enough period of time, the voice is permanently lowered. A "long enough" time depends on the individual. Even just six months can cause permanent changes.[54]

There are two kinds of bottom surgery for FtMs: phalloplasty and metoidioplasty. Phalloplasty is a more complex and engineered procedure, which involves the complete construction of a penis-like appendage. It's much more difficult to create a penis-like extension from a woman's genitals than it is to carve a cavity using a man's genitals. MtF surgery requires "only" the removal and rearrangement of tissue, but for a FtM, additional tissue is required. Therefore, a FtM who wants a more complex phalloplasty must undergo the simultaneous surgical removal of tissue elsewhere on the body to provide material for the penis-like appendage. To create a penile shaft and urethra, the surgeon removes skin tissue, usually from the forearm, and then connects nerves to the graft site to impart sensation. This requires considerable skill that many surgeons lack—which accounts for many reports of bungled phalloplasties that cause numerous unforeseen medical complications. Because this organ is artificial, it cannot achieve a natural erection. A future surgery might be scheduled so the surgeon can implant a prosthesis into the appendage to more closely approximate an erection during sexual intercourse. One prosthesis consists of a pump inserted into the shaft. Saline water, held in a bag in the stomach, is propelled into the penis-like appendage through a prosthetic testicle.

By comparison, metoidioplasty bottom surgery is simple. The ligaments around the erectile tissue of the clitoris are cut to give the shaft greater length so it hangs down, resembling a tiny penis. But it will never become erect the way the penis of a biological male does. And with cutting, there's always the risk of nerve damage and loss of sensation. With both types of bottom surgery, the urethra in the urinary tract must be moved and integrated with the design of the new genitalia. Sometimes FtMs have the uterus, ovaries, and fallopian tubes removed.

A 2022 article in *Sexual Medical Reviews* analyzed all data thus far on phalloplasty patients. The conclusion of the authors was that in spite of the most modern advances in surgical techniques, the results were inconsistent, much to the disappointment of the patients who expected infinitely better outcomes. Medical problems that directly resulted from the surgery were an astonishingly high 76.5 percent. In every group, complications involving the urethra (urinary tube) were likewise high. The occurrence of urethral fistula—an abnormal connection between the urethra and rectum—was 34.1 percent, which led to a leakage of urine into the rectum and the migration of feces into the bladder. (Fistulas account for a high risk of infection in bottom surgeries for both sexes.) Urethral stricture rate for FtMs was 25.4 percent. This means that during bottom surgery, the urethra can become injured and its delicate mucosa may become overgrown with scar tissue—which then requires at least one more surgery to repair.[55]

With all the potential risk involved in the attempt to create a facsimile of male genitalia, it's easy to understand why most FtM individuals choose not to have their genitals remodeled. In the 2015 *U.S. Transgender Survey*, only 2 percent reported having any type of genital surgery.[56] Nevertheless, they still consider themselves men, and live according to how they think a man would live.

Despite having had the best of surgeons, some FtM individuals may keep enough of their inborn cosmetic characteristics that they fail to easily pass as men. This inability to pass invites more discrimination and violence than those who have a more conventionally masculine appearance. However, due to the intense and permanent masculinizing power of testosterone, in general FtM individuals have an easier time passing than MtF individuals, and are less likely to encounter violence than their MtF counterparts.

I began this chapter with the sentence, "People who consider themselves transgender typically report feeling as though they are the wrong 'gender,' or have a different 'gender identity' than what they think belongs with their body." Let us reframe the problem. *People who consider themselves transgender typically report feeling as though the wrong gender, or sex role, is being imposed on their particular body.* Fair enough. But to remedy this dilemma, do we change the body via hormones and surgeries? Or do we relax our rigid requirements, and expand our definitions of what it means to be male and female?

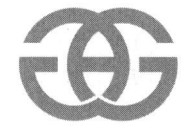

4

GENDER DYSPHORIA AND MENTAL ILLNESS

Fallout of the "Wrong Body" Myth

"Gender dysphoria...belongs in the family of similarly disordered assumptions about the body, such as anorexia nervosa and body dysmorphic disorder," psychiatrist Paul McHugh once remarked.[1] *Body dysmorphic disorder* is the preoccupation with an imagined physical defect or minor flaw that is not obvious to others. But the radical trans mantra, that people are "born into the wrong body," is stated as though such a phenomenon is real. Mental health organizations legitimize this feeling by providing a diagnosis: *gender dysphoria*. The American Psychiatric Association's description of this state of mind is typical.

> Gender dysphoria involves a conflict between a person's physical or assigned gender and the gender with which he/she/they identify. People with gender dysphoria may be very uncomfortable with the gender they were assigned, sometimes described as being uncomfortable with their body (particularly developments during puberty) or being uncomfortable with the expected roles of their assigned gender.
>
> People with gender dysphoria may often experience significant distress and/or problems functioning associated with this conflict between the way they feel and think of themselves (referred to as experienced or expressed gender) and their physical or assigned gender.
>
> The gender conflict affects people in different ways. It can change the way a person wants to express their gender and can influence

behavior, dress and self-image. Some people may cross-dress, some may want to socially transition, others may want to medically transition with sex-change surgery and/or hormone treatment. Socially transitioning primarily involves transitioning into the affirmed gender's pronouns and bathrooms.[2]

A very troubling aspect of this definition is the APA's acceptance of gender as an immutable, biological fact rather than a socially reinforced ideal. If we call gender what it truly is—*sex role stereotyping*—and substitute that phrase everywhere the word "gender" appears, a very different picture emerges. The APA correctly observes that some people (I would say *many* people) have difficulty embracing their assigned gender role. Yet the APA supports the position that gender stereotypes are natural, normal and reasonable, rather than being two-dimensional, limiting, and often demeaning. As discussed in Chapter 2, both females and males are often made to feel inadequate or wrong if they want to break free from their social roles and have more choice in their lives. Instead of recognizing that these stressful stereotypes can easily contribute to mental illness, and calling for the elimination of such roles, the APA recommends that the body be pumped full of cross-sex hormones, that the person take hormones *and* submit to mutilating surgery, or that the person simply declare membership in the opposite-sex camp while wearing its clothing—as evidenced by the suggestion to "cross-dress" or "socially transition." Then, of course, there are the outright dangers to the general public of allowing transgenders to visit the bathrooms of natal men and especially women. I'll discuss this in detail shortly.

What I find almost unbelievable about the above guidelines is the assertion, clearly expressed in the final paragraph, that someone can be called a woman if he was born with a penis and scrotum, and someone can be called a man if she was born with a clitoris, vagina and womb. This contradicts basic biology. Not insignificantly, it also challenges the presumed qualifications of APA members, all of whom have requisite training as physicians. The American Psychiatric Association represents psychiatrists—medical doctors who, after their foundational training in medicine, further specialize in the brain, just as other doctors might specialize in pediatric medicine or gynecology. While a small percentage of psychiatrists do counseling or psychotherapy, most focus on the administration of pharmaceuticals. The hope is that the drugs will somehow eliminate depression and regulate mood, even if it blunts the patient's ability to feel deeply or numbs emotions altogether (not to mention the "side" effects of mood-altering pharmaceuticals). It's therefore not surprising that a professional devoted to corporate medicine would advocate extreme measures of hormone treatments and surgery to address a problem, rather than work with a patient to help him or her break free of limitations that negatively affect quality of life. Nevertheless, it's still shocking that someone trained in medicine—which includes anatomy, physiology and biology—could discount basic scientific reality so easily.[3] A reasonable person might also think it incongruous that male-bodied MtFs who receive chest implants and female-bodied FtMs whose breasts are excised still consider themselves members of the opposite sex if they retain their intact natal genitals. But it's pointless to try to make sense out of something that's inherently irrational. No matter which version of "I am actually a woman in a man's body" or "I am actually a man in a woman's body" you follow, by definition a woman has female genitals and a man has male genitals—and even if those genitals have been removed, no mechanical modification or remodelling can change basic biology.

Unlike the American *Psychiatric* Association, which fails to distinguish between sex (biology) and gender (cultural roles), the American *Psychological* Association does—at least in its official policy. Members of the American Psychological Association include psychologists who received their degrees from accredited institutions and graduate students who are taking courses in psychology. Psychologists are not medical doctors and are not authorized to write prescriptions. Therefore, their focus is not on taking pharmaceuticals or receiving surgeries as the solution to mental issues. Instead, they employ a wide variety of therapeutic modalities that help people understand the source of their problems, learn better ways to cope, and ideally find inner peace through greater self-acceptance. Sometimes, people's authentic behaviors and preferences happen to align with many aspects of sex role stereotypes. But those who are atypical for their prescribed gender role and feel persecuted or limited by it are not as fortunate—unless they can get professional help, the kind that facilitates genuine self-understanding and self-acceptance. If people are to be truly healthy mentally and emotionally, they need to be encouraged to discover who they really are and develop according to their nature, rather than try to conform to social roles in the effort to gain the approval of others.

Walt Heyer was a happily married man who became an unhappy MtF transgender at age 43, and after eight years *detransitioned*, or presented again as his natal self. Having earned a degree in counseling, he eloquently discusses the problems of correct diagnosis and the lack of proper support for people who are labeled transgender.

> Psychological conditions present in almost 70 percent of people with gender dysphoria include anxiety disorders (panic disorder, social anxiety disorder, post-traumatic stress disorder), mood disorders (major depression, bipolar disorder, etc.), eating disorders (anorexia nervosa, bulimia nervosa, etc.), psychotic disorders, dissociative disorders, and substance abuse disorders. Dissociative disorder was found in 29.6 percent of those with gender dysphoria and 45.8 percent had a high prevalence of lifetime major depressive episodes.[4]
>
> Being identified as a transsexual or diagnosed with gender dysphoria often stands in the way of getting a proper diagnosis... [Yet most mental health professionals] don't consider that by pushing patients toward gender change they are preventing them from being diagnosed and treated for another disorder [that's]...

likely to be present in two-thirds of patients. For patients undergoing gender change, this can be a quick trip to suicide. For...the ones who suffer from major depressive disorder, when they are not diagnosed and treated for the depression, suicide is a highly likely outcome.

Suicide among transgenders seems proof enough: 1) that they are suffering from undiagnosed mental disorders and 2) that gender change is not effective treatment for...[a certain class of] disorders present in the majority of patients. A physician who works with transgenders makes some great points: "We have so many reports of so-called co-morbid disorders in transsexuals. We need to now ask, do transsexuals have co-morbid disorders or do transsexuals have one disorder (mental illness) with just a fabricated *co-diagnosis* of gender dysphoria?"[5]

Several papers paralleling Heyer's analysis have recently been released, fortunately without suffering retraction (at least not yet). A journal article surveying young people in their teens and twenties in Germany reported that a full 70 percent were eventually able to trace their gender dysphoria to other, deeper issues.[6] And in January 2023, the *Journal of Sex and Marital Therapy* published "The Myth of 'Reliable Research' in Pediatric Gender Medicine: A critical evaluation of the Dutch Studies—and research that has followed." E. Abbruzzese and two co-authors of this critically important paper explained that the entire industry of cross-sex hormones and genital surgeries for young people is based on two highly flawed Dutch studies that were done in 2011 and 2014, and which supposedly proved that transitioning patients is the only option for treatment. The methodological flaws were serious and many. In both studies, the subjects were preselected so that only successes, and not failures, would be tallied in the results. How was this accomplished? One, the assertion that gender dysphoria was resolved was biased toward a positive outcome due to the way in which questionnaires were worded. Two, although it had been suspected (and subsequently confirmed) that hormone treatments caused adverse effects, these symptoms were not factored into the study. Three, even though puberty blockers were supposed to be administered to children who were age 12, in actuality the average age of the subjects was 15. At that young age, being even three years older makes a huge difference. The more advanced physical and cognitive maturity of the 15-year-olds unquestionably contributed to a better outcome at the end of the trial. Four, because the test subjects were all receiving psychotherapy at the same time they transitioned, it was impossible to separate the beneficial effects of the therapy from the effects of hormones and surgery. Five, the test subjects used for one of the studies were disqualified if they exhibited any signs of mental illness. This biased selection for the most stable subjects was guaranteed to skew results, making the outcome much more favorable than it could possibly be in real life.[7]

In any experiment, the selection process should guarantee that the subjects represent an actual cross-section of the population so the outcome doesn't appear more positive or negative than it actually is. But the Dutch studies were heavily manipulated. In the 2014 study, of 196 initial participants, only 70—already biased to ensure a more positive outcome—were placed in the protocol; and of those, only 55 completed it. The 15 people who were removed and conveniently relabeled "nonparticipants," were subjects with serious health issues. Their concerns included severe diabetes, obesity, and a death due to surgical complications.[8]

The publication of the Dutch studies has had disastrous consequences. Based on just two pieces of horribly designed research, the Endocrine Society—which boasts more than 18,000 practitioner members in over 120 countries—has consistently extolled the benefits of administering puberty blockers and cross-sex hormones to young people. The World Professional Association for Transgender Health (WPATH, discussed in Chapter 7) endorses both hormonal manipulations and surgeries—again, citing those two initial studies. It should be noted that Dr. Daniel Metzger, himself a physician at WPATH, acknowledged in an interview that young adults are not equipped to fully understand or evaluate the long-term effects of the treatments, and many feel regret afterwards.[9]

While the Dutch studies did accurately report that the hormonal and surgical interventions succeeded in changing the appearance of individuals—how could one's appearance *not* be affected by such manipulations?—they failed to prove that such drastic physical alterations promoted any meaningful psychological changes that could justify the risks and adverse outcomes of those interventions. The intention of E. Abbruzzese and colleagues could not be misunderstood:

> The burden of proof—demonstrating that a treatment does more good than harm—is on those promoting the intervention, not on those concerned about the harms. Until gender medicine commits to conducting high quality research capable of reliably demonstrating the preponderance of benefits over harms of these invasive interventions, we must be skeptical of the enthusiasm generated by headlines claiming that yet another "gender study" proved benefits of transitioning youth. This time-honored concern about risk/benefit ratio is a sobering reminder that the history of medicine is replete with examples of "cures" which turned out to be far more harmful than the "disease."...
>
> This highly politicized and fallacious narrative, crafted and promoted by clinician-advocates, has failed to withstand scientific scrutiny internationally...In the U.S., however, medical organizations so far [such as the American Medical Association, in 2022] have chosen to use their eminence to shield the practice of pediatric "gender affirmation" from scrutiny. In response to mounting legal challenges, these organizations have been exerting their considerable influence to insist the science is settled....[T]his stance stifles scientific debate, threatens the integrity and validity of the informed consent process—and ultimately, hurts the very patients it aims to protect.[10]

The mental and emotional problems of youth seeking to escape their problems by becoming someone else are numerous and escalating. The Dutch study critics found that before the boys and girls even began to deal with presumed gender dysphoria, they suffered from various emotional and mental disorders including anxiety, depression, autism, and attention deficit hyperactivity disorder (ADHD).[11] Another research team found that a disproportionately larger number of adopted children were seen at a clinic for gender dysphoria compared to the number of adoptees present in the general population.[12] This is not surprising, considering that many adopted children have backgrounds of neglect and abuse; and those who spend any length of time in institutions are more at risk for behavioral and emotional problems such as aggression, depression, anxiety, and attachment disorders.[13] Finally, of the pubescent girls who claim they are transgender, the overwhelming majority don't fit the typical picture of someone who is truly gender dysphoric; other issues play a key role in their claim. This will be discussed in detail in the next chapter.

In 2022, Project Veritas managed to capture on videotape a revealing conversation at the Vanderbilt University Medical Center. Some of the staff objected to transgender procedures being done on children. "If you don't want to do this kind of work," they were admonished by a doctor, "don't work at Vanderbilt. Saying that you're not going to do something because of your conscience, because of your religious beliefs, is not without consequences. And it *should not be* without consequences." Another doctor said—again, without being aware that she was being filmed—"These surgeries make a lot of money." She cited the figures of 40,000 dollars to provide a "male chest" to females and several thousand dollars to give a patient hormones only a few times a year.[14] Money is a seductive incentive.

Schools for young children and teens, along with colleges and universities, also promote transgenderism as a glamorous solution to the common problems of growing up. Trans activists are invited to speak at these schools, after which record numbers of young people decide that they were born into the wrong body and demand hormones and sexual "reassignment" surgery to correct their problem. Many of the trans-identified adolescent girls whom Abigail Shrier interviewed for her book *Irreversible Damage* had never had a sexual or romantic relationship—not even a kiss—with a boy or girl. Yet they adopted an entire vocabulary of transgender ideology with the full support of educational institutions that encourage young people to open up to who they "truly" are.

In California among other states, the administration and teachers of public and even private schools automatically accept students' declarations of being gender dysphoric because, they claim, to question them will hurt them. The schools are not required to tell parents that the children are being called by opposite-sex pronouns, or that they changed their name—in fact, there are special pre-printed forms on which to record them. Colleges are not obliged, either, to advise parents that students are given ready access to cross-sex hormones so they can get an early start in their transition process. In most cases the parents are not told, especially if the child claims that the parents are not being supportive and are refusing to "affirm" his or her identity. Even if the student has a history of depression, anxiety or other mental health problems, the self-diagnosis of transgender is enough for the school counseling service to ignore any possible psychological issues and immediately dispense hormones—as long as the student signs an "informed consent" document. Small-town colleges and Ivy League universities across the United States counsel children to avoid interacting with their parents, and even consider running away, if the parents don't agree with the child's self-diagnosis. As for the parents, they are told that if they don't "affirm" their son's or daughter's new identity, he or she will commit suicide. Even the child is told this—adding to the power of suggestion and ensuring the possible fulfillment of the prediction.

Many of the social agencies that encourage children to obtain genital surgery don't have a legal obligation to notify parents, either. In fact, the schools and agencies generally view the parents as intrusive adversaries who have no right to guide or take responsibility for their own offspring. Some agencies even help the children leave their homes, providing them with travel tickets and shelter. Parents are now fighting to implement legislation making it mandatory for them to be notified within two or three days that their children are exhibiting symptoms of gender dysphoria. In some locations, they are winning.

An alarmingly large number of therapists have also become complicit in encouraging students to take hormones without addressing underlying emotional disturbances. The few therapists who do speak out against this practice risk not only losing their jobs, but also having their licenses revoked. Although of course not all therapists and doctors acquiesce to the trans-friendly agenda of the medical and political establishments, an internet search in the U.S. is not guaranteed to yield the name of a therapist who has withstood the pressure, or at least who is publicly known as remaining independent.

Trans-friendly algorithms are built in to most search engines. After typing the single keyword "transgender" into a popular and widely used search engine, I viewed helpful definitions, advice on how to spot if you're trans, how to come out as trans, trans dating sites, trans models who made it big, trans news, and even trans gear and apparel for sale. In three web page summaries, not one single article or journal study could be found that questioned why so many people are identifying as trans at this time. Nor were there any articles on how transitioning is harmful to children. To obtain more realistic data, you have to type in exactly what you're looking for—and even then, what you may find is how "transphobic" the object of your search is. Many of the films and video clips appearing in even alternative search engines (which presumably have more algorithm choices) are about the struggles that transgenders of all ages have overcome despite society's bigotry. Some documentaries feature remarkable children who—with the help of supportive parents, hormones, and surgery—have overcome the odds of their birth sex and happily transitioned into their "true" selves, the sex they were supposed to be. Still other films feature well-known actors who have transitioned. A number of searches warn about anti-trans movies. Fortunately, more trans people are now publicly speaking out about botched surgeries. And people who had been pressured into receiving cross-sex hormones and surgeries are now coming forward.

In Europe, medical professionals who question the official position may be more visible than in the U.S. In the 2018 subtitled Dutch documentary *Transgender Regret*, psychiatrist Joost à Campo disclosed that in 2000, he sent a survey to colleagues asking follow-up questions about the mental health of their patients who had transitioned. Eighty-six psychiatrists reported that half of the 586 transgendered individuals had underlying problems that required attention. But in return for his concern, à Campo received hate mail. "I was demonized as a caveman who was blocking modern trends. And that's not true. I want to help the vulnerable."[15]

Joost à Campo was not the only one castigated for asking questions. Clinical psychologist Dorine Sellenraad spoke against what she saw as mass indoctrination of both the subjects and the adults who are supposed to take care of them. Between 2000 and 2001, Sellenraad was part of a team at a branch of the VU Medical Center in Amsterdam, the largest facility in the Netherlands that specializes in gender "reassignment" surgeries. "There was an atmosphere of too much agreeing with the patients....I missed critical judgment about diagnostics and indications." Also, she noted, many patients met with each other to discuss "what was best to say and which psychologists were easy [to convince]...I was known as the difficult psychologist. One patient said, 'It was easier in the past. You're making it complicated.'" Believing that it was irresponsible to capitulate, she explained, "I proposed a better diagnostics protocol with stricter criteria for diagnoses and medical treatment. But they [the administration] said it's too complicated, too hard to set the right criteria. Some who need it might miss treatment. So let's keep it like it is." Not wanting to be a party to this, Sellenraad left her job. à Campo agreed how difficult it was for conscientious professionals. The Dutch psychiatric association, despite being repeatedly asked since 2002 to produce clear guidelines for determining who needs surgeries, has ignored these requests.[16]

The filmmakers also interviewed people who had undergone sexual "reassignment" surgery or were planning to. One very masculinized young woman apparently in her late teens or early twenties who was on testosterone and awaiting FtM surgery, smugly reported that an interview process to determine her suitability, which should have taken four months, was completed in one month. She was able to fast-track her surgery, she boasted, because she had memorized all the "right" things to tell the intake psychiatrists.[17]

One attractive MtF transgender, who had received surgery over 50 years ago in Morocco and seemed genuinely happy and content, said it only worked for a man if you were already very "feminine." However, other clients weren't so fortunate. They suffered from many emotional problems that clinicians ignored while immediately dispensing hormones and surgery. "I'm a homosexual man....I had an identity crisis," acknowledged Patrick, "and joined the forum Travestie.org which was loaded with glorified stories about how great a sex change was. And then I thought, maybe I suffer from the same thing." Patrick detransitioned after he realized that changing his body would not make him happy. His new psychiatrist stated that Patrick had been suffering from PTSD (post-traumatic stress disorder) and borderline personality disorder, but that he didn't have—and never had—gender dysphoria. This was something his VU Medical Center psychiatrist should have known; for when Patrick had told him that walking around as a woman made him anxious rather than happy, the analyst said that wasn't a good reason not to do the surgery. The tragedy is, a different clinic that had treated Patrick much earlier, in 1999, had sent a letter to the VU Medical Center clearly stating that he was not suffering from gender dysphoria. Today, Patrick is in a lot of physical and emotional pain. "I can never be myself again. My belly and bladder are constantly bugging me....[I]t was irreversible and I had to live with it. I had regret. It [the cavity that was surgically carved for him] doesn't belong to me."[18]

Another MtF, Braldt Haak, told the filmmakers that trans people don't want to admit that things don't always turn out the way they had envisioned or desired. "They're not always honest and they only show the bright side....They tell stories about how well surgery went and about how well it functions now. But it's not all good." Haak had to discontinue the hormones because he gained 66 pounds and developed cardiac arrhythmia. "I had to decide if I wanted to live as a man, or be dead as a woman." He added, "The chance to be happy also depends on how well you pass as a woman....I think that if you have other psychiatric problems, you have to deal with them first in order to be able to handle a transition....If you still are struggling with things, it will be very rough. Maybe this is a factor that causes regret or suicide, because transition isn't going to solve your problems."[19]

The VU Medical Center did 5000 sex change surgeries between 1972 and 2015. In 2008, there were 200 new intakes. In 2015, there were 700.[20] It might take a while for effective and honest medicine to prevail. "Trans interventions are big money," says medical doctor Michelle Cretella, who is on the advisory board for the U.S.-based non-profit organization Advocates Protecting Children. "Billionaire elites promote trans ideology over truth across all public institutions and media platforms, and [in the United States] a severe cancel culture results in everything from severe harassment and doxing to ending one's career."[21] *Doxing* is the practice of publicly disclosing personally identifiable information about an individual—such as their full name, address of their home or workplace, phone number, financial status—all without the person's permission. This is now being done regularly to government officials who cast an unpopular vote, authors who write a book that does not support a favored agenda, and public speakers who criticize a behavior or disagree with an act. These kinds of hostile attacks are occurring more frequently, and they are being perpetrated—all in the name of tolerance—by those invested in the trans agenda.

Civil Rights and Violence

Another very disturbing issue raised by the American Psychiatric Association definition (see the passage at the beginning of this chapter) is its declaration that social transitioning must involve "transitioning into the affirmed gender's pronouns and bathrooms."[22] Laws have been passed in many states that give transgenders access to bathrooms to which they would never have been granted access prior to the current climate of sexual "reassignment."

This access has caused several major problems. Not every transgender who has taken cross-sex hormones and undergone surgical alterations looks like a member of the opposite sex. In fact, many do not. Although starting the sexual "reassignment" process before puberty does create a much more realistic-looking imitation of the opposite sex—and the clever use of clothing can help with the disguise—the dissimilarity between the the male and female skeletal structures (including the sway of someone's walk) may be enough to reveal that the person is trans. There may also be an aura or energy about the person that sensitive people (especially children) can detect—an energy indicating that something is slightly odd or off. Therefore, sharing a bathroom with a transgendered individual may feel uncomfortable or unsafe to those who are not trans.

What if the person using that space is a MtF transgender who still has his penis? How "changed" does that person have to be? Even more disturbing—and increasingly common—is a fully equipped male given access to a women's bathroom simply because he says he "identifies" as a woman. What about the right to privacy for women and girls? And what about the very real threat of rape?

The incidences of attempted and actual rapes of women in public bathrooms by men falsely claiming to be transgender are increasing. ASK Academy is a charter school in Rio Rancho, New Mexico, that allows males who self-identify as transgender to use the girls' bathrooms. In October 2021, a 12-year-old female student (calling herself "Ray" to protect her privacy) said she was was raped by an older boy in a school bathroom. In July 2022, the same boy assaulted a 14-year-old female student at a nearby school. Two other girls also said they had been assaulted by that same boy, yet the school did nothing to hold him accountable or protect its female students.

Ray said that she had "felt pressured by teachers and faculty to accept the presence of men in women's spaces, to keep her mouth shut about any feelings of discomfort, and to avoid doing anything that would be construed as 'judging' someone who might identify as transgender." Afraid of reporting the attack for fear of being labeled a "bigot," she was silent about the rape. Her mother, however, noticed that the girl was highly depressed, anxious and grieving, and brought her to therapy. Six months later, Ray's mother learned about the trauma and saw that Ray's medical records confirmed vaginal tears consistent with rape. The mother went to the police and the local Child Protective Services, but they stalled the investigation. When Ray began feeling suicidal, her mother confronted school personnel, who dismissed her concerns. "They treated us like we were a problem when we tried to make them address issues our child was facing in their school," she said. "The school tried to say we must be doing something wrong at home."[23] Since the mother confronted school officials about the attack, four staffers, including two administrators, left. (Did they discover that the mother planned to bring a lawsuit against the school?) Ray's mother wrote to a New Mexico senator, but reported that she was "met with a complete rejection of the notion that he would support anything that goes against gender affirming legislation." Regarding the school, Ray's mom stated:

> We learned that kids were pledging allegiance to the pride flag instead of the American flag. We learned that some teachers were discussing daily, the normalcy of transgender people and gender dysphoria, and that this school had a higher population than anyone would expect for such a small school, of kids saying they were trans and parents not knowing....By them saying the only thing that matters is how they feel and not how I feel, is very selfish of them. If they want their own bathroom, then gladly get your own bathroom. If you want your own sports, get your own sports. If you want to be included, be included in your own way that doesn't cause danger to everyone else.[24]

"Transgender toilet activists," writes Sheila Jeffreys, are sympathetic to MtF individuals' fears about being beaten up if they try to use men's bathrooms— "whereas women's concerns about the egregious violence visited upon them are [considered] spurious....[W]omen's awareness that not all men are violent is no great reassurance against the fact that many are [or might be], and individual women are in no position to work out which ones they need to be particularly vigilant about whilst seeking a safe space in which to urinate."[25]

Females have proportionately smaller urinary bladders than males (probably because they have more organs in the abdominal cavity, which requires the bladder to be smaller to accommodate the crowding). It's not unreasonable to assume that because many girls are unhealthily "holding it in" for fear of being attacked by a male in their own bathroom, urinary tract infections in females will increase.

Allowing biological males to invade spaces that should be keeping females safe is indeed a symptom of mental illness on the part of the invaders and their supporters. Despite the general public's increased disapproval over same-sex bathrooms, trans activists are winning in some of the courts. They are also becoming more vocal in their call for violence. On TikTok, a MtF activist threatened to become dangerous and dared anyone from stopping him from entering a women's bathroom. Then, addressing the trans community, he exhorted, "Go out and buy a gun. Learn how to use it."[26] The inflammatory video was eventually removed from TikTok, but one site captured it and it can still be viewed.

Other women-only spaces—locker rooms, shelters, and even prisons—are also in trouble. In 2019, a bill was approved in the California Senate that allowed men to be inmates in women's prisons if they simply stated that they "identified" as women. MtF transgenders were already being placed into women's prisons to protect them from the violence they would likely have suffered had they been incarcerated in men's prisons. But thanks to this bill, *any* male—even if he was a stalker, wife-beater, sex offender, or rapist—was now given free access to hurt not only vulnerable female inmates, but also female prison guards. Any man could declare an "identification" with women without being required to provide a letter from a doctor or therapist, and without undergoing any hormonal or surgical changes. A woman who opposed this bill stated during the California hearing, "Right now...a trans-identified male is currently housed with female inmates in Corona, even though he is serving time for targeting, raping, and torturing women. Under no circumstances is this morally justifiable."[27] Similarly, many shelters for homeless and abused women have opened their doors not only to MtFs, but also men who simply "identified" as women—courtesy of the Department of Housing and Urban Development (HUD). The HUD secretary, Ben Carson, objected to this policy, which did not even permit the shelter to ask for identification.[28] A change in the law, he pointed out, would "empower shelter providers to set policies that align with their missions, like safeguarding victims of domestic violence or human trafficking."[29] As the law is now, abusers must be allowed in with the abused.

Lawmakers on both sides of the debate are still fighting over this policy. But in some locations, trans-friendly bills have already been passed and men claiming to identify as female have already imposed their wills on women. Attacks are becoming greater in number, and more violent. I will cite just a few examples. In August of 2019, the Vancouver Rape Relief and Women's Shelter (VRRWS) in British Columbia, Canada was defunded for refusing admittance to any man who identified as trans or female. Graffiti with the message "Kill TERFS" was scrawled onto the building. (*TERF* is a new acronym for *trans-exclusionary radical feminist.*) "The women who come to our support groups are rape victims and battered women," said a member of the staff. "One of them said to me, 'Haven't we suffered enough?'"[30] In the U.S. at the largest women's prison in Illinois, a female prisoner filed a lawsuit against a trans inmate for having raped her in 2019.[31] And in 2018 in the UK, a self-described MtF transgender attacked two inmates after being moved to a women's prison. He had already received a life sentence for raping two women and sexually assaulting two other women prior to being incarcerated. All it took to get into the women's prison was a declaration and a costume consisting of a wig, makeup, and false breasts. London mayoral candidate Rory Stewart stated to the press, "When I was Prisons Minister, we had situations of male prisoners self-identifying as females, then raping staff in prison. So I think if somebody is biologically male, particularly in an environment like a prison, we shouldn't allow that to happen....I think the rights of women to feel safe trump the rights of somebody who's biologically male to enter that space."[32]

The infiltration of women's prisons by biological men and trans "women" with penises—and the subsequent escalation of rapes—have become so common that class action suits are now being instigated by female inmates. These women, rightly protesting that they don't feel safe, blame politicians, lawmakers and wardens. The mainstream press loudly protests the diminishing protections of a handful of transgenders—but what about the millions of natal women who require protection? No woman or girl should have to fear for her public safety. Yet the majority is being asked to sacrifice privacy and safety to accommodate the desires and special privileges of a very few.

Politicians are forcing all types of woman-centered businesses to admit men. In June 2023, the Olympus Spa in Seattle, Washington—whose website had stated that "women can relax in this all female environment"[33]—refused to serve a self-proclaimed transgender "woman" with intact male genitals. A judge forced the spa to admit men if they identify as women. "Aside from…nudity [as when employees give patrons exfoliating massages]," she said, "there is simply nothing private about the relationship between Olympus Spa, its employees, and the random strangers who walk in the door seeking a massage."[34] One must question the intentions of the men who will take advantage of this ruling.

Back in the 1970s, feminists were arguing whether men who self-identified as women (and sometimes even as lesbians) should be permitted to attend women-only conferences and music festivals. One woman wrote, "being a woman is a long-term experience, and one that isn't summed up by a collection of female genitalia with some clothes draped over them….[T]he state of mind, the process of becoming—we didn't have any choice about that."[35] As political commentator Brett Cooper has stated in her podcasts, addressing MtF transgenders, "My biology is not your costume."[36]

What about FtM individuals in a public bathroom for males? I asked a man I knew—a former police officer who had routinely been in dangerous situations—how he would feel if a FtM transgender entered a public men's bathroom while he was in it. "Emotionally, it's an invasion of my space," he replied. "A bathroom is for private body functions. Also, in today's climate if a trans person thought I looked at them the 'wrong' way, they could leave the bathroom and falsely accuse me of rape—and there's nothing I'd be able to do about it." Would he feel unsafe? "You'd be surprised at the damage they can do," he responded. "Female bodybuilders who take testosterone are known for being able to put their boyfriends through a wall. Transgenders on testosterone are taking a lot more. Plus, there's potentially a lot of tension and anger. So being attacked feels like a real possibility to me." He was indeed correct about the muscle-enhancing effects of high-dose testosterone, which will be addressed in great detail in Appendix B.

It's important to recognize that only the very vocal radical trans activists are attempting to impose their wills on everyone else. Not all transgender people are activists who want to recruit and harm children. Many, if not most, transgenders regard their transformations as private, personal decisions, and they just want to live their lives in peace. However, as the radical agenda heats up, some trans individuals are being moved to speak up about the need to protect children.

We can have compassion for mentally ill people without humoring transgenderism as normal—and without glamorizing it, turning it into a political movement, or allowing it to oppress others. "Forty years ago," Jeffreys comments, "radical feminist thinkers and activists were very clear in their view that persons who were born biologically male and raised as males, but sought recognition as women" were in fact engaged in an "insulting practice in which men caricatured stereotypes of women for their own amusement or pleasure."[37] Dr. Paul McHugh, Professor of Psychiatry at Johns Hopkins Medical School and Psychiatrist in Chief of Johns Hopkins Hospital, agrees. "Transgendered men do not become women, nor do transgendered women become men....[They] become feminized men or masculinized women, counterfeits or impersonators of the sex with which they 'identify.'"[38] McHugh has also pointed out that to a man, "feeling like a woman" is usually based on sex role stereotypes, "something that women physicians note immediately is a male caricature of women's attitudes and interests....We don't do liposuction on anorexics. Why amputate the genitals of these poor men?"[39] He adds, "I have witnessed a great deal of damage from sex-reassignment...We have wasted scientific and technical resources and damaged our professional credibility by collaborating with madness rather than trying to study, cure, and ultimately prevent it."[40]

Should archeologists of the future unearth documents of 21st century Earth, they might wonder how it was possible for such a tiny minority of bullies to shut down the voices—and so drastically interfere in the lives—of so many.

The Suicide Threat
Falsified Data

Trans activists repeatedly claim that because of society's bigotry and intolerance of trans persons—and attempts to prevent transgenders from finding their "true selves"—the rates of attempted and actual suicide among transgender youth are much higher than those of their non-trans counterparts. According to figures from an American Academy of Pediatrics 2018 study of suicide attempts, FtM adolescents reported the highest rate at 50.8 percent. MtF adolescents reported 29.9 percent. And in "non-binary" adolescents who did not exclusively identify as either male or female, the suicide attempts were 41.8 percent.[41] This contrasts with 2018 figures of adolescents who do not identify as transgender: 17.6 percent of females and 9.8 percent of males.[42] Significantly, a 2015 study conducted by the Harvard School of Public Health found that almost 51 percent of transgender people between the ages of 12 and 29 were diagnosed with depression.[43]

However alarming these statistics are, we must ask: Are the suicidal ideation, alienation and depression a result of the ridicule, violence and rejection that trans people say they endure from family members and society? Or is the desire to become trans a result of feeling depressed, anxious, alienated and rejected? Attributing the cause of psychological problems to society's bigotry might not be accurate, journalist Daniel Payne points out, "when compared to other minority groups who suffer disproportionate...amounts of bigotry and negative discrimination" but don't have similarly high suicide rates. Instead, it seems that "the rate of successful suicide is extremely correlative with conditions of mental illness."[44] Could it be that statistics have been deliberately gathered and interpreted in ways that yield misleading results?

The British organization Transgender Trend explains how certain data suggests higher numbers of suicide in trans youth than what might actually exist. After analyzing two studies that included questionnaires dealing in part with suicidal thoughts and attempts, Transgender Trend described problems with how the research was designed.

> The questionnaire was promoted within the LGBT community and people chose whether or not to fill it in. In total 2078 questionnaires were analysed, however only 120 of these were transgender people, and only 27 of these were under the age of 26 years old. *It is only the results from the 27 young trans people that was reported in relation to suicide.* Of these 27 young trans people 13 of them reported having attempted suicide at some point in the past. This is where the 48% of all trans youth attempt suicide stat[istics] comes from....We don't believe that the suicide history of just 27 self-selected trans people is sufficiently large...[We must also consider that] Participants were not randomly selected. This will mean that trans people who have experienced the most difficulties in life may be more likely to fill in the form. This risks artificially increasing the percentage of participants with a suicide history. [emphasis added][45]

Another anomaly in transgender suicide statistics, which Transgender Trend found in a second survey, was the inclusion of lesbians, gays and bisexuals in the trans category. This yields highly misleading results because members of the non-trans homosexual population have a much higher rate of suicide than the heterosexual population. The misrepresentations are so many and glaring that one must conclude that transgender activists deliberately skewed the statistics to secure sympathy for their cause.

Even if societal bigotry does play a major role in transgender suicides, and the trans population does suffer from abnormally high suicide rates, the truth remains that only people who suffer from self-hatred and have severe emotional problems want to kill themselves. Under such circumstances, writes Payne, "A sane society would be advocating for robust, ameliorative psychological therapy [but]...Instead, we indulge this [mutilation] sickness on an industrial scale."[46] Alan Finch, a British man who received MtF surgery, decided he wasn't trans, and then sought to reverse the process, once remarked, "The fact that someone's suicidal and wanting something, isn't a reason to provide it."[47] Scott Newgent, a FtM who strongly opposes subjecting children to hormones and surgery, emphasizes that transitioning "doesn't fix suicidal ideation....[A] child that's suicidal, you take them to a mental hospital...If you can't handle life now, there's no way in hell you're going to be able to handle it when you medically transition, because it is brutal. So you are the *worst* person to medically transition." Newgent also points out the lack of incentive to conduct psychological follow-ups on those who have medically transitioned—because the goal of getting these people on drugs for life has already been accomplished.[48]

Fortunately, some studies have been conducted that point to emotional disturbance in transgenders independent of their transition. A 2014 article in *Psychiatry Journal* concluded that 62.7 percent of patients with gender dysphoria were diagnosed with at least one emotional disorder.[49] Another seminal article, this one by Cecilia Dhejne and colleagues—"Long-Term Follow-Up of Transsexual Persons Undergoing Sex Reassignment Surgery: Cohort Study in Sweden"—studied two groups. One was "sex-reassigned." The other was "random population controls." Each group was matched by age and other factors. The authors showed that suicidal thoughts and actual suicides *increased* after people transitioned. The overall mortality rate for transgenders was higher—especially death from suicide—than those in the control group. The "sex-reassigned" group also had a higher rate of psychiatric inpatient care. "Persons with transsexualism, *after sex reassignment*, have considerably higher risks for mortality, suicidal behaviour, and psychiatric morbidity than the general population," the authors stated bluntly. "Our findings suggest that sex reassignment...may not suffice as treatment for transsexualism, and should inspire improved psychiatric and somatic care after sex reassignment for this patient group." The study also showed that FtM individuals, as compared to MtFs, had a higher risk for criminal convictions than the non-trans control group.[50] As previously mentioned—and I'll expand on this in Chapter 6—some females on high-dose testosterone report feeling uncontrollable rage. Could increased criminality result from abnormally high testosterone levels that their bodies were never supposed to produce and were not designed to handle?

Dhejne and her colleagues also criticized data presented by psychiatrist Jack Turban, co-author of the often-quoted "Pubertal Suppression for Transgender Youth and Risk of Suicidal Ideation" that appeared in a 2020 issue of *Pediatrics*. Turban and his colleagues believed that efforts made to discourage someone from transitioning worsened mental health and contributed to suicide attempts—and that subjects receiving puberty blockers, compared with those who wanted the drugs but did not receive them, have a lower risk of suicidal ideation for their entire lives.[51] But as Dhejne pointed out, such research failed "to control for the individuals' pre-GICE-exposure mental health status."[52] *GICE* is an acronym for *gender identity conversion efforts*. If the problem was "being in the wrong body," one might reasonably assume that sex "reassignment" would lower the percentage of emotional problems, not raise it. Turban's article showed, once again, the machinations of mental health workers who are complying with the trans agenda. If there's no psychological assessment of someone prior to transition, how can we be sure what has caused the depression, suicidal ideation, and other mental health problems?

More unbiased researchers began to publish. In March 2023, *Archives of Sexual Behavior* released an article on rapid onset gender dysphoria (ROGD). Seventy-five percent of the ROGD children, who were between the ages of 11 and 21, were girls. Pre-existing mental health issues plagued these children, and the more issues they had the more likely they were to socially and medically transition. Their parents reported that clinic personnel demanded that they "affirm" their children's newly-assumed "gender" and support their transition. Significantly, the children's mental health greatly worsened *after* they socially transitioned.[53]

Apparently, someone didn't want data disseminated about pre-existing psychological issues in a group of transitioners. The publisher and editor-in-chief of the journal quickly retracted the article, stating that the authors had not complied with the journal's editorial policies and had violated the privacy of the survey participants.[54] That claim was not only implausible, but ridiculous. The survey was purposely anonymous, and consisted of volunteers—parents who were recruited from the website Parents of ROGD Kids by one of the authors whose own daughter had been seduced by the trans agenda. The authors publicly denied having broken any policies surrounding consent. One of the researchers, Northwestern University Professor J. Michael Bailey, said, "Informed consent means that you're supposed to inform participants what it is that you're studying, and get their consent [which we did]."[55] In fact, Bailey's own Institutional Review Board (IRB), which reviewed the article prior to its publication, had reassured him that it was ethical to publish the results of the survey as long as the identities of the respondents were not revealed—which they weren't. So what made the editorial board change its mind? As it turns out, in May 2023, soon after the article was released, the Center for Applied Transgender Studies had written to the publisher with a threat: "We are informing you that we will no longer submit to the journal, act as peer reviewers, or serve in an editorial capacity until Dr. Zucker [the editor] is replaced with an editor who has a demonstrated record of integrity on LGBTQ+ matters and, especially, trans matters....[The paper] raises serious concerns over research ethics and intellectual integrity."[56] What, exactly was unethical, and how was "intellectual integrity" compromised? The Center for Applied Transgender Studies did not address this.

In 2021, "Rates of Psychiatric Emergencies Before and After Gender Affirming Surgery" published in *The Journal of Urology*, found that among men who had received a vaginoplasty, the attempted suicide rate was twice as high after the surgery compared to before it. The message was clear: Getting a vital part of his body removed—his penis—does not benefit a man's mental health.[57]

The evidence keeps growing that trans activists are deliberately miscategorizing and misinterpreting suicide statistics to elicit sympathy for their agenda. It appears to be working, as more laws keep getting passed to give trans people special privileges over the rights of the majority.

Drug-Induced Death

Another issue that trans proponents avoid making public is the effects of castration chemicals (puberty blockers) themselves. These drugs not only cause severe physical harm (discussed in depth in Chapter 3), but they also encourage the precise emotional state of mind that the act of transgendering is supposed to eliminate: depression, suicidal ideation, and actual suicide. Package inserts and website warnings for Lupron (leuprolide acetate)—the foremost prescribed puberty blocker in the United States—specifically lists "emotional instability" as one of the undesirable "side" effects, along with unstable, wild fluctuations of mood, crying, irritability, impatience, anger, and aggression (not to mention decreased libido). Prescribers are warned to "Monitor for development or worsening of psychiatric symptoms during treatment."[58]

The aforementioned journal article by Jack Turban and his colleagues is often cited as an example of how children on puberty blockers have a lower risk of suicide—which then justifies the administration of such drugs. Statistics can be manipulated or falsely reported to suggest the opposite of the truth, but sloppy science hasn't stopped mainstream headlines from enthusiastically proclaiming, "Puberty blockers reduce suicidal thoughts in trans people."[59] Not only did the press celebrate this presumed good news, so did all the transgender-influenced websites, which advocate the chemical castration of prepubescent teens. But if you examine the original research and look at a table further into the article, statistics indicated that about 50 percent of the trans people being studied reported suicidal thoughts—hardly a success story! Furthermore, of the study participants who had reported not only suicidal ideation, but also *active plans* for suicide and *attempts* at suicide, *more*, rather than fewer, were revealed to have been taking puberty blocking pharmaceuticals.

Oxford University professor Michael Biggs is another researcher who has criticized the flaws in Turban's information-gathering process and conclusions. The study omitted those who had actually committed suicide, Biggs observed. Further distorting test results, the majority of the respondents had reported taking puberty blockers after age 18. This is impossible, because puberty generally occurs six years prior, at around 12 years of age, and certainly no later than ages 13 or 14. Evidently the respondents had mistaken the cross-sex hormones they were taking for puberty blockers. Biggs also pointed out that many of the questions were not answered. Of the 89 respondents who said they took puberty blockers (and probably did not), only 11 answered whether they had been hospitalized in the past 12 months due to a suicide attempt.[60] The data was more than incomplete. It was incorrect, rendering the results of the entire survey fictitious and useless.

Like Cecilia Dhejne and other critics, Biggs explained that pro-trans researchers consistently fail to account for the fact that their surveys eliminate those with psychological issues—which is *not* done in the real world today with most people who ask for puberty blockers. Biggs also stated that prior research omitted people who actually did commit suicide after being on puberty blockers, as well as those who "underwent medical intervention and then subsequently stopped identifying as transgender." Biggs pointed out, too (again) that respondents recruited online for Turban's survey had erroneously reported receiving puberty blockers after age 18.[61] The necessity for Biggs to keep reminding his readers of errors made by other researchers shows how a person's first exposure to information (or misinformation) is difficult to forget. Trans-friendly media still pummel the public with the original incorrect data. "The data," wrote Biggs in yet another paper, "showed no statistically significant difference in psychosocial functioning between the group given [the puberty blocker] GnRHA [gonadotropin-releasing hormone analog] and counseling and the group given only counseling."[62] So how do we know it wasn't the counseling that helped the research subjects?

In case there are any doubts that chemical castration in prepubescent children causes serious negative effects, let's look at a negative outcome in an adult who is using a castration drug for an entirely different purpose. The title of the article is "Acute manic and psychotic symptoms following subcutaneous leuprolide acetate in a male patient without prior psychiatric history: A case report and literature review." The 62-year-old patient was taking the drug for prostate cancer. Severe health problems—the medical establishment likes the phrase "adverse events"—included depression, fatigue, hot flashes, and low or no sex drive. The authors claimed that sudden-onset, intense mental and emotional reactions (including mania) from Lupron injections are uncommon, given the scarcity of documented reports of such reactions. The man had gone through normal puberty, which one might think would have helped prevent some of the more intense psychological symptoms. But he developed mental health problems just two months after his injection (which may be why he eventually quit the protocol).[63]

Other "adverse events" from Lupron affect the central nervous system. This can result in mood swings, insomnia, depression, blurred vision, and listlessness. Although the authors reported these effects occurring in less than 5 percent of patients,[64] that figure is still alarming. Five percent is not a small number. Also, if someone's trying to minimize concern, instead of saying "*close to* five percent," they'll say "*less than* five percent." Keep in mind, too, that 5 percent is *what has been reported*. If a child experienced drug-induced "adverse events," would the distressed parents know enough—or be calm enough—to report these "side" effects of mental instability to the FDA? Would they even know how to do it? You have to search pretty hard for the form on the FDA website. And what about doctors? Medical personnel who make lots of money from these drugs would understandably be reluctant to report "adverse events." Thus the depression due to taking Lupron is very likely much higher than what has been reported. Hormones are extraordinarily powerful. When the body's hormone balance is tampered with, the consequences can be severe and even life-threatening.

As discussed in Chapter 2, the medical industry dishes out misinformation and outright lies. And the press will publish erroneous data, or misquote accurate data, to bolster whatever agenda it wants to promote.

Drugs and Surgeries Versus Psychotherapy

There are basically two protocols for treating gender dysphoria (or the belief that one is gender dysphoric). The first strategy promotes puberty blockers for prepubescent children, cross-sex hormones for everyone, and surgery for as many people as possible. Once a decision has been made to embark on this path, that person is a customer of Big Pharma for life. If surgery is performed, there's rarely only one operation. Often more than one part of the body is cut, excised or reshaped. In addition, too many things can go wrong, ranging from cosmetic and structural damage to more serious mishaps such as injuries and infections. The Big Pharma approach requires considerable finances, along with a high pain tolerance and plenty of painkillers. The second approach, psychotherapy, can also be painful—although in a much different way. It's not easy to face underlying emotions, perceptions, beliefs, and hurtful or traumatic events that could have contributed to or directly caused the desire to escape one's body.

In many ways, the two approaches are polar opposites. Cross-sex hormones and surgeries force the body—biochemically, neurologically and structurally—to appear and express as something that it was never designed to be. Psychotherapy with an ethical and skilled therapist allows the client to express his or her natural and true state. "Reassignment" protocols impose something foreign onto the person. A psychotherapist helps the client discover and uncover what is already present. With sexual "reassignment," the goal—albeit disguised—is to help the individual pass as someone else. With psychotherapy, the goal is to help the client feel comfortable with and accept who he or she truly is.

These two radically different approaches reflect the degree of agency—the ability to master oneself as well as one's environment. If I am at the mercy of being in the "wrong" body, I'll need outside intervention (hormones and surgery) to fix something that's beyond my control. But if I refuse to be a victim of chance of my "wrong" body, with suitable help I can learn to take responsibility for my uncomfortable feelings and meet my genuine needs. Medications and operations, which are administered to victims of chance, signify a psyche that is open to being passive and manipulated. Psychotherapy, which is sought by someone who does not wish to be a victim of their emotional distress, signifies a psyche that is ready to be proactively involved in whatever challenges life may present.

With this comparison, it's also extremely important to distinguish between the intentions of transgender clinic personnel versus the intentions of a qualified therapist. Someone who works at a gender clinic has a fixed agenda: to transition the client. An ethical psychotherapist tailors the treatment to what the individual truly needs. As we have seen, almost without exception people who want to transition suffer from underlying issues that are making them want to be someone else. A therapist who's doing his or her job has no agenda other than to respect the uniqueness, feelings, and *genuine* needs of the client. This requires delving into what lies beneath the surface.

Anyone can pop a pill. But undergoing psychotherapy requires courage, strength, and determination to allow very deep changes into your life. The reward is being captain of your own ship, which includes befriending the body you were born with. It's not surprising, then, that trans activists and psychotherapists—at least those who are doing their jobs—would be at odds with each other. Some highly vocal researchers condemn all psychotherapy as evil manipulation against the poor gender dysphoric client. But now more psychotherapists are stepping forward to criticize the initial flawed studies that had delighted trans activists.

In 2021, *Archives of Sexual Behavior* published a letter to the editor from Roberto D'Angelo, Lisa Marchiano, and other therapists called "One Size Does Not Fit All: In Support of Psychotherapy for Gender Dysphoria." As others had before them, the authors criticized the biased samples and flawed statistical analyses of Turban and his colleagues and the accompanying undeserved positive media support. They also mentioned the lack of scientific credibility for failing to follow subjects over a period of time. Short-term data doesn't provide enough information for a reliable analysis, whereas long-term follow-up yields more, and hence more accurate, data. What distinguished this article from others, however, was their focus on psychotherapy as the main treatment for gender dysphoria. They warned about Turban's simplistic view of psychotherapy. He believed that there were only two types of therapists: those who "affirmed" the client's claim of being the opposite sex and those who tried to "convert" the client. Turban considered it "conversion"—working against the client's best interests—not only if a therapist refuted the client's claim of being the opposite sex, but also if he or she simply asked probing questions. To Turban, the presence of probing questions meant attempts at "conversion." Of course the trans community is happy to promote Turban's view that only "gender-affirmative" therapy is correct, helpful or legitimate. The authors emphasized:

> The notion that all therapy interventions for GD [gender dysphoria] can be categorically classified into this simplistic binary betrays a misunderstanding of the complexity of psychotherapy....Stigmatizing non-"affirmative" psychotherapy for GD as "conversion" will reduce access to treatment alternatives for patients seeking non-biomedical solutions to their distress....We are deeply concerned...[that] unproven claims of the harms of GICE [gender identity conversion efforts] will have a chilling effect on the ethical psychotherapists' willingness to take on complex GD patients, which will make it much harder for GD individuals to access quality mental health care.... [G]iven the potential of agenda-free psychotherapy to ameliorate GD non-invasively among young people with GD, withholding this type of intervention, while promoting "affirmation" approaches that pave the way to medical transition, is ethically questionable. We believe that exploratory psychotherapy that is neither "affirmation" nor "conversion" should be the first-line treatment for all young people with GD, potentially reducing the need for invasive and irreversible medical procedures.[65]

The "One Size Does Not Fit All" article was also clear that many gay and lesbian teens with low self-acceptance are drawn to transgendering in order to freely love and be loved. This is a population that has been very vulnerable to trans indoctrination and could greatly benefit from caring, competent psychotherapy.

Some sources claim that the current percentage of transgenders in the general population is as high as 3.0 percent.[66] But in 2016 the count was 0.328 percent.[67] What inflated the figure so much? Trans activists are now including gays, lesbians and bisexuals, which is a total miscategorization. Sexual orientation designates the sex of the person to whom one is romantically and sexually attracted. Transgenders believe that they themselves are the wrong sex.

The misdiagnosis of traumatized children and teens as "gender dysphoric" is now occurring with alarming frequency. A teenage girl is raped, feels discomfort with her body—who wouldn't, after that?—and then expresses a desire to be male. Instead of addressing her fear and probable PTSD, clinicians eagerly support her new identity. A sensitive boy who's uninterested in sports and prefers to listen to classical music instead, is relentlessly bullied. He concludes that if he were a girl, he'd fit in. So out come the hormones and scalpels. The number of young people who suffer in silence with current or past trauma, feel ashamed of their sexual orientation, and have a difficult time accepting who they are, is rising. Yet clinicians—who should know better—would prefer to see their clients transition than help them deal with their problems. One must seriously question the mental health—not to mention compassion quotient—of anyone who fast-tracks a client.

The lie that transgendering is not only easy, but solves myriad problems, is causing immeasurable harm. Properly conducted psychotherapy could be a wonderful healing tool. But trans activists are deliberately trying to make it impossible for people to receive real help by getting laws passed against "transphobia." Such laws would ensure that ethical psychotherapists lose their jobs and licenses if they try to provide help to those who need it the most. This is why some professionals are refusing to counsel "gender dysphoric" clients.

Despite the obstacles to treatment, trained professionals who provide agenda-free psychotherapy—who want to help alleviate suffering in a non-invasive, non-medical manner—do exist, even if they might be difficult to find. If you know someone who struggles with issues related to sex, gender, and/or sexual orientation, consider psychotherapy. The purpose of a good clinician is to help clients become more self-aware and develop self-acceptance.

Children and teenagers are especially vulnerable to the false promise that they can live worry-free lives without problems or obstacles. But adults can feel coerced too. Chapter 6 contains poignant accounts from both teenagers and mature adults who felt pressured to transition, and then wanted to reverse the process. However, before you get there, please read the next chapter to learn why someone might want to transition. You may see someone you know in those pages.

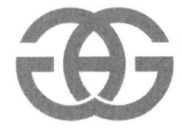

5

WHY SOMEONE MIGHT TRANSITION

What Am I?

There are as many ways to "feel like a boy" (or man) as there are males in the world. And there are as many ways to "feel like a girl" (or woman) as there are females in the world. People who believe that their bodies are not matched with their gender (stereotypes) are following someone else's script of what behaviors, emotions and attitudes are permissible according to what's between their legs. As we have seen in previous chapters, people who feel obligated to follow sex role stereotypes compared to those who are relatively free of them are more limited in their choices—and are thus less well-rounded as people. They also have more restricted emotional lives, may be inadequately fulfilled in their careers, and may even exhibit less intelligence and drive. When they "identify" as the opposite sex—to such an extent that they're willing to mutilate their bodies in order to change their appearance—this indicates that they have lost their sense of self. Decades ago, they would have been considered mentally ill.

Why, then, are so many people today attracted to a movement that—in the name of "gender freedom"—insists that they adhere to the very stereotypes that are enslaving them?

There are many reasons why someone might be attracted to the idea of being trans. I have already touched on some of those reasons, but this chapter will explore them in depth. Depending on which population group the person belongs to, the reasons for transitioning are usually very different. Let's take a detailed look at who transitions, and why he or she might want to do it.

Before the Trend

When the first cases of gender dysphoria were originally diagnosed decades ago (and the subjects were called *transsexuals*), the children who were the most dissatisfied with their bodies and most strongly identified as the opposite sex, didn't merely *wish* that they were the opposite sex—they already believed that they *were*. The ones who believed this were mostly boys. And they were very young when they believed it. Gender dysphoria affected mostly boys age two or three, and such children comprised only about 0.01 percent of the population. In most cases, the issue resolved as the boys reached puberty.[1]

According to the 5th edition of *Diagnostic and Statistical Manual* (commonly known as the *DSM-5*), by 2013 this condition still occurred in a minuscule, although very slightly larger, portion of the population: .005–.014 percent of natal males and .001–.003 percent of natal females. Based on the numbers of people who later sought medical intervention, these figures translate to fewer than 1 in 10,000 people.[2] Contrast this today with what mental health professionals call gender dysphoria: In the U.S., the phenomenon has increased by over 1,000 percent.[3] In Europe alone, girls comprise three-quarters of those referred for gender "reassignment."[4]

Until the last decade or so, parents of young children diagnosed with gender dysphoria were encouraged to help the child feel comfortable with his or her body. They did not indulge a child's wishful thinking, encourage erroneous beliefs and fantasies, or intensify subjective feelings by giving in to the child's demands to wear clothing or hairstyles associated with the opposite sex. (However, if either sex could wear any clothing they wanted, assuming it fit, the act of wearing clothing associated with the opposite sex would very likely lose its charge and hence, appeal. But back to my original point.) The parents certainly did not call the child by an opposite-sex name. They delayed any decisions for cross-sex hormones or sexual "reassignment" surgery until the child was considerably older or became an adult. This humane, commonsense advice was based on what was observed about the far-reaching and powerful effects of hormones on the developing mind and body. No one needed to conduct studies or do fancy tests in laboratories.

Today, parents are advised to allow the child to live as the opposite sex, and even to stop puberty altogether, until the child can make up his or her mind about what sex he or she wants to be—as if people can change their sex as easily as slipping on a garment! Most parents, and their unhappy sons and daughters, are never told that children—whose neural circuits are still forming—are incapable of making rational decisions, and cannot foresee possible future consequences of their behavior. They aren't told, either, that transitioning rarely addresses the source of their misery, which means that attempts to escape their biology will ultimately backfire. Yet young people who cannot legally drink, drive, or vote are actively being encouraged to make decisions that will mutilate them for life.

It's a no-brainer that if children can accept and find peace with the bodies they're born with, this is preferable to becoming dependent for life on expensive hormones and perhaps surgeries as well. As of this writing, close to two dozen US states have banned gender "reassignment" for minors. But the trans agenda, which is everywhere, can be difficult for some people to resist. What makes someone vulnerable? Let's take a look.

Boys

The inability to adhere to a rigidly masculine role is a major reason why boys are encouraged to transition. A boy might be artistic, soft-spoken, shy, and/or not very good at sports. People might assume he's homosexual, even if he's not, and call him a "sissy" or "pansy." If he *is* gay, the more he's perceived to deviate from a stereotypically masculine image, the more he's made to question whether he's a male at all. Sadly, many boys who are homosexual feel pressured into transgendering because they have been taught that loving other boys is unacceptable. A parent may not approve of a son's homosexuality, but which choice is less harmful? Body mutilation, or a loving relationship with another human being?

Boys who are autistic also gravitate to transitioning. One website, Parents with Inconvenient Truths about Trans (PITT), shares that many mothers and fathers of both transitioned and detransitioned teenagers have noticed that their sons fall on the autism spectrum. Emotionally immature for their age, many of the boys also have OCD (obsessive-compulsive disorder). The immaturity and stunted cognitive abilities contribute to "a pattern of black and white thinking that made trans identification appealing. Once 'transitioned,' they felt better, for a time, since all those feelings of anxiety and fear [due to life's shades of gray]… could be reframed as external problems instead of internal ones." However, the relief rarely lasts. In retrospect, most of the young men "felt that their trans identity was a character that took tremendous effort to maintain…the voice, the clothes, the mannerisms…[I]t was all playing a part that began to feel inauthentic (ironic given that trans is promoted as an acceptance of one's authentic self!). It became a chore to put on the character day after day, even for those that 'passed' as female." Of course, the "character that took tremendous effort to maintain" is an unreal caricature. The PITT article describes the futility of the masquerade as the unreality soared to new heights.

> The men we spoke with discussed that the mental illusion was also difficult to maintain, particularly when it came up against hard facts. Increasingly peer groups were fully living in their own delusions, and the detransitioners were seeing the constructed universe that other trans identified men were living in. Discussions of periods in men, and breast-feeding were some of the topics that they believed had gone too far, and they came to believe that they had no basis for understanding the physical realities that actual women faced, like

endometriosis and heavy menstrual bleeding. They also came to feel that transition didn't even serve its original purpose. As one man stated, "It was, in a way, pointless. It was spending a lot of time and money without necessarily making me happy."[5]

The temptation to transition may also be more heightened in males whose testosterone production or utilization are disrupted. This can be the result of a medical condition (see Chapter 1), but products in the environment can also interfere with hormone function. One ubiquitous and dangerous culprit is Bisphenol A (BPA), a common plastic in use since the 1960s. BPA is a major ingredient in bottles and containers for water, food storage, and personal care products. It's used to line tin cans that contain food and is even employed as a coating on cash register receipts. BPA's structure resembles that of natural estrogen, which allows it (and similar plastics) to latch on to the estrogen receptor sites in living bodies. This is what causes the hormone-like effects of plastics. Existing in amounts millions of times more than what a person or animal would normally produce itself, the plastics affect the reproductive systems of both humans and animals, males and females. In some species of fish and frogs, endocrine-induced abnormalities include sex changes. In human males, sex-related abnormalities may include abnormal breast growth, low sperm count or defective sperm leading to infertility, and impotency. In human females, sex-related abnormalities may include premature breast development, early puberty, delayed or suppressed ovulation, and infertility.[6] Reproductive glands of both sexes are more susceptible to cancer. Even the prostate gland in male fetuses can be affected.[7] The DNA of all living things is damaged, influenced by the abnormal rise or fall in hormone levels.[8] Molecules of BPA plastic are unstable, leaching into whatever solid or fluid is in a BPA container. The bodies of over 90 percent of Americans harbor minute particles of these plastics[9] (which is a good reason to store drinking water in glass rather than plastic bottles).

As far back as the 1930s, BPA was considered as a possible medication to treat menopausal women. Therefore, it's astonishing that three decades later, the chemical compound was approved for widespread use in the production of plastics for regular, everyday use. Fetuses, which are extremely sensitive to plastic exposure via the mother, may suffer enough growth disturbances that their gestation period is shortened.[10] But the effects are even more insidious. A 2015 review of previous studies found evidence that BPA interferes with endocrine function in ways that involve the hypothalamus and pituitary gland—and therefore, "The detrimental effects on reproduction may be lifelong and transgenerational."[11] Even experiments with mice show that effects of endocrine disrupters are multi-generational, impacting the structure and function of the brain.[12] While the results of animal studies cannot always be extrapolated to humans, in this case we already know not only that estrogenic plastics affect humans, but also how it affects us. No living thing is immune to these pseudo-estrogens. Nevertheless, even today the FDA claims that the plastic is safe.[13]

Other types of endocrine disrupters can be found in non-stick coatings for cookware and in flame retardants. Because flame retardants are often found on bedding and children's clothing, including pajamas, this is of particular concern.[14] Common chemicals such as parabens and phthalates—present in skincare products, cosmetics, and thousands of ordinary household products—are also highly toxic to the endocrine system. These synthetic chemicals in the environment are inhaled, eaten, and absorbed through the skin.

Exposure to multiple chemicals in their various forms exert exponential effects. This is such a widespread problem that in 2014, the British publication *Lancet Neurology* published a paper on how phthalates (plastics) and similar environmental chemicals disrupt the brain and nervous systems of children. This would affect virtually everything related to cognition, coordination, and perception. Examples of effects include short attention span (attention-deficit disorders) and even impaired social interactions. The changes occur mostly in boys, pointing to endocrine abnormalities in the brain.[15] Pregnant women need to be especially careful about exposure to such plastics because extensive damage can occur to the developing baby at any time during gestation. Once a pregnant woman is exposed to these chemicals, her thyroid hormone levels change. This alone negatively impacts the proper development of the unborn child's brain, and later may cause behavioral problems and learning disabilities.[16]

Although the FDA finally banned BPA due to public pressure, research shows that the plastics now used in its place have similar estrogenic effects. Might BPA be influencing the increase in the numbers of transgendered males by impairing brain function? No fewer than 214 unregulated chemicals, including estrogenic plastics, have been linked to human brain damage.

Pesticides, herbicides and fungicides also affect the molecular structure, and hence function, of hormones. One of the most widely exploited herbicides in the world is atrazine, used for controlling weeds in commercial crops and home gardens. This herbicide is commonly applied to corn, sugar cane, and sorghum, which is fed to lambs and calves raised for us to eat. Atrazine is also mixed into the soil where soy is grown to create a barrier that stops weeds before they even start to grow. And it's sprayed on golf courses and residential lawns. Because of such widespread use, as one scientific paper describes, the herbicide

> is the most commonly detected pesticide contaminant of ground, surface, and drinking water. *Atrazine is also a potent endocrine disruptor that is active at low, ecologically relevant concentrations.*...Atrazine-exposed [amphibian] males were both demasculinized (chemically castrated) and completely feminized as adults. Ten percent of the exposed genetic males developed into functional females that copulated with unexposed males and produced viable eggs. Atrazine-exposed males suffered from depressed testosterone, decreased breeding gland size, demasculinized/feminized laryngeal development, suppressed mating behavior, reduced spermatogenesis, and decreased fertility.

These data are consistent with effects of atrazine observed in other vertebrate classes." [emphasis added][17]

Another possible culprit is soy, an ingredient found in most infant formulas. Compared to endocrine-disrupting plastics and pesticides, soy isoflavones (a major class of phytoestrogens) are weak. However, even low levels can disrupt the endocrine system. Some menopausal women, hoping to benefit from soy's estrogen-like effects, purposely eat it to replace the estrogen that their bodies are no longer naturally producing. Infants reared on soy formulas are exposed to isoflavone plasma concentrations that are about 13,000 to 22,000 times greater than their naturally-occurring estradiol (a form of estrogen) plasma concentrations.[18]

A 2022 study, "Secondary hypogonadism due to excessive ingestion of isoflavone in a man," describes how a 54-year-old man came to develop erectile dysfunction and gynecomastia, or abnormal enlargement of the breast tissue. Every day for three years, he drank about 1.2 liters (a little over one quart) of soy milk—which contains about 310 mg of isoflavones. Blood tests revealed low levels of gonadotropin and testosterone, leading to a diagnosis of hypogonadism—the inability of the gonads (sex glands) to produce sufficient amounts of hormones. Two months after the man stopped drinking the soy milk on his own, he was retested. His gonad function had improved. The authors concluded that the hypogonadism had been caused by the excessive amounts of isoflavones in the soy milk he'd been ingesting. Isoflavones are not as physiologically active as estradiol, but their ability to bind to certain estrogen receptor sites is still enough to produce unwanted changes.[19] Not everyone reacts negatively to soy and soy products, though, especially if the products are organic. The negative endocrine-disrupting effects of soy can be augmented if the conventionally grown soy has been treated with atrazine. Any estrogenic effects can be further reduced or eliminated altogether if the soy is fermented using traditional methods.

Synthetic estrogenic compounds in the environment are creating an entire class of abnormal males. We must ask how many brain cells are being affected by these compounds and what those effects are, which brain cells are being outright destroyed, and if these chemical compounds are depriving the brain of vital nourishment—which can lead to other problems. These estrogenic chemicals are prevalent, but they're not supposed to be in our environment or bodies at all. The question that everyone should be asking is why the chemicals have been created, who developed them, and why they are still permitted to be used, considering that their negative effects are well known by the manufacturers. Eliminating these toxic chemicals from the environment will allow males and females to develop the way they were meant to.[20] A diet high in fresh vegetables and some fruits can help the body excrete BPA.[21]

As stated earlier, those who are most likely to be "genuinely trans" are young boys, although the percentage is still really tiny. What if a very young boy had been allowed by his parents to live as a girl? What if he seemed genuinely happy and well-adjusted? Wouldn't it be better to give him hormones from the earliest age possible to ensure the closest match to the body of a girl? All the research on human development says *no*. Even a "truly trans" boy should be made to wait for cross-sex hormones and gender "reassignment" surgery until he's at least in his mid-20s. The reasons for this were discussed in Chapter 3. You may recall that the brain as well as body is flooded with testosterone during puberty, which can help shape thought processes and emotions. The possibility exists that the boy might later change his mind and decide that he is indeed male—but with an irrevocably altered body, he'd have a very difficult road ahead of him.

The most famous MtF transgender child is probably Jazz Jennings, who captured the attention of the media worldwide with documentaries and a TV series. Even as a young child, Jared (his birth name) proved highly intelligent and articulate, which made for a good interview. "My little penis felt so wrong on me," the teenage Jazz wrote in a *Time* magazine article. "I didn't just like girly clothing—I felt ashamed and humiliated if I had to wear anything else....Whenever my mom or dad would compliment me by saying something like 'Good boy,' I'd immediately correct them. 'No. Good *girl*.'"[22] At what age did it start? It depends on which account you read. According to one report, from the tender age of two or three, the boy said that he "knew" he was actually a girl. His mother later explained that when young Jared asked her whether he was a boy or girl, she asked him what he *felt like*. He said a girl, and that was the end of the conversation. Jared must be a girl, not a boy. Others tell a different tale. Malcolm Clark writes that in 2003, Jazz's mother noticed that her 3-year-old son "kept opening up his onesie [a one-piece garment]. To most parents, this might not have seemed like a big deal, but Jennings became convinced that her son...was trying to make his onesie into a dress."

> Jeanette alleges that her son, at the age of four, told her he wanted God to replace his penis with a vagina. I once asked my dad how I could get laser vision like Superman. He told me to finish my dinner. If only Jeanette Jennings had done the same, her son might still have his genitals. Instead, she sought out the *Diagnostic and Statistical Manual of Mental Disorders*, the bible of mental health, and became convinced her little boy was [actually female]...."I diagnosed her before ever taking her to see a professional and then had it confirmed," she would often say....You'd think a mother would take a lot of advice before telling her son he would be happier once he lost his penis. Not so with Jeanette....
>
> In a 2019 interview, Jazz explained that he loved designing mermaid tails that he could swim in. He liked mermaids, he said, because they have no genitals. If you or I heard that a kid wanted to have no genitals, we might recommend his or her parents seek professional psychiatric help.[23]

Instead, Jeanette sought the counsel of Florida-based sex therapist Marilyn Volker, whom Jeanette asserts was "instrumental in who Jazz is today." On a television show, Volker stated that she knew Jazz "clearly" had a female gender identity. Clark's response is worth noting. "What exactly does Volker mean by 'female gender identity'? Often this just refers to discredited sex stereotypes."[24] Clark—whose observation is astute—may rightly discredit these stereotypes, but many people do not. This includes the late news anchor Barbara Walters, who interviewed Jazz and helped justify his transition by promoting typical myths. "Gender organizes our world into pink or blue," she stated. "As we grow up, most of us naturally fit into our gender roles. Girls wear dresses and play with dolls. For boys it's pants and trucks."[25]

There are so many conflicting reports as to whether Jazz was coached, who coached him, and who said what, that it's difficult to accept Jazz's story at face value—especially considering the psychological state of this transitioned individual now. We do know that after the young boy grew his hair long, played with dolls, and was allowed to wear dresses in public, he appeared to be happy—at least in widely disseminated video clips. Was it because of all the positive attention he received? Jazz's parents and siblings were publicly supportive of the child's transformation to appear feminine, and the public adored him. He was eventually administered puberty blockers. The family allowed a camera crew into their home to chronicle Jazz's presumably successful transition, which resulted in the ongoing series "I Am Jazz," now in its seventh year. However, after passing the age at which a normal male puberty would have occurred, by the time the star was supposed to attend college, physical and emotional problems proliferated. Clearly depressed, Jazz could not stop binge eating and gained 100 pounds. According to Clark, no one on the show ever discussed the connection between Jazz having taken cross-sex hormones and his binge-eating, anxiety, and severe depression. A 2023 episode shows Jazz crying with his mother and saying, "I just want to feel like myself. All I want is to be happy and feel like me, and I don't feel like me, ever."[26]

Why didn't Jazz "feel like me, ever"? At a young age, not only were essential parts of his body removed, but his natural maturation process had been halted and erased—irrevocably disturbing his physical, sexual, and emotional development. In another video clip filmed around the same time, Jeanette remarks that she has to awaken Jazz in the middle of the night to dilate the pseudo-vagina that surgeons had constructed because Jazz doesn't want to do it, and Jeanette is determined to prevent the cavity from closing. Rightly so, the body perceives the cavity as a wound, which is why it closes unless it's actively prevented from doing so.

"If we are to believe the trans lobby," writes Clark, "for whom Jazz is now a prominent advocate, he is walking proof of the importance of early 'affirmation' of transgender identity in children. But like so much of the propaganda churned out by the trans movement, the true story of Jazz is much darker than we have been led to believe."[27] That darkness is now being brought to light as journalists and mental health professionals are asking: When the time came for Jazz's transition, were the young boy and his parents told that he would experience dangerous and irreversible "side" effects from cross-sex hormones? Or intense pain from multiple surgeries during which so many things can go wrong? And they did go wrong. Jazz had to undergo three more "bottom" surgeries to repair the damage after the initial one. Were Jazz and his parents warned about the likely repercussions of using pieces from the colon to construct the pseudo-vagina? Colon tissue had to be used because the little boy's penis was too small. Had the child gone through puberty, there would have been much more penile tissue to use in the construction of the cavern. Were Jazz and his parents informed that he would be infertile, have limited or no sexual sensation, and be unable to sexually climax? Even if the family was told, how could the child have possibly understood enough to give informed consent?

Because Jazz had been dosed with puberty blockers and undergone the complete removal of his penis and testicles, not only will he never experience an orgasm, but he is developmentally stuck as a prepubescent eunuch. The organs that were supposed to exist—for which the body had been biologically, neurologically and energetically prepared—have been permanently severed, and in their place is a gaping wound whose presence is justified and normalized by being called a "vagina." The body's neural pathways that would have deepened through sexual arousal and communion with another human being are withering away. What does being stuck in this sexual limbo do to a person's development—physically, mentally, and emotionally? Or spiritually? Depression is an understandable and predictable outcome, independent of the direct pharmacological effects of the hormones.

Some critics question whether "changing gender" was truly the child's idea. One possibility emerges: The mother always wanted a daughter and killed her son's unwanted maleness, turning him into a girl. It's easy to speculate that because very young children are extremely impressionable and do almost anything to please a parent, the boy adopted his mother's wishes as his own. But the truth appears more complicated. In an interview, when Walters asks Jeanette if she misses her boy before he became Jazz, she breaks down in tears and replies that she does. Also, after viewing available video clips, it does seem that from a very young age Jazz genuinely loved "girly" clothing.[28] We may never know the truth. "If only, years ago, they'd let this child be, Jazz would likely now be a feminine, perhaps gay, boy," writes Dr. Miriam Grossman. "Instead, Jazz's physical, emotional, sexual, and cognitive development were chemically interrupted…[and Jazz] has been led to believe surgery can create female genitalia."[29]

Girls

Despite the fact that historically it has been mostly very young boys who perceive themselves as female, many prepubescent and teenage girls who never expressed any interest in transgenderism are suddenly clamoring for hormones and surgery. Why? Journalist Abigail Shrier—who describes her shock at discovering how many girls are becoming convinced that they are really boys (or should be boys)—shares her research in *Irreversible Damage: The Transgender Craze Seducing Our Daughters*. "Two patterns stood out," she writes. "First, the clear majority

(65 percent) of the adolescent girls who had discovered a transgender identity in adolescence—'out of the blue'—had done so after a period of prolonged social media immersion. Second, the prevalence of transgender identification within some of the girls' friend groups was more than *seventy times* the expected rate." [emphasis added][30]

There are many reasons for this overwhelming influx of girls. Announcing their newly-found "transgender identity" gives the girls a way to rebel against their parents. But more importantly, having a trans identity makes them feel special, because they now belong to a minority club and are accepted by their peers. Dr. Lisa Littman, who coined the term "rapid-onset gender dysphoria," said:

> I became interested in studying gender dysphoria when I observed, in my own community, an unusual pattern whereby teens from the same friend group began announcing transgender identities on social media, one after the other, on a scale that greatly exceeded expected numbers. I searched online and found several narratives of parents describing this type of pattern happening with their teen and young adult kids who had no history of gender dysphoria during their childhoods....Then, I spoke with a clinician who was hearing her clients describe this phenomenon as something happening in their families. The descriptions of multiple friends from the same pre-existing group becoming transgender-identified at the same time were very surprising.[31]

Although social contagion is not "contagion" in the medical sense, it does speak to the power of peer pressure—especially if children start to think and act in ways that are harmful to them. Columnist Chad Felix Greene, who happens to be gay and is self-proclaimed pro-LGBT, posted a thread on Twitter in November 2022 about the effects of this social contagion on his niece. The post was since deleted, but a screen shot was captured. "My 12 year old niece who has very suddenly come out as asexual and trans has been cutting herself," he wrote. "She's broken down crying with her mother that she isn't queer enough to be accepted by her friends. All of her friends have suddenly come out as trans. The most disturbing [thing] is she is thinking of suicide...My niece broke down and told my mom she wishes she could just be a [normal, unencumbered] little girl. She thinks she'll let her mom down if she's not queer."[32]

One woman retrospectively explains her attraction to becoming trans.

> As a child I developed a trans identity as the result of a brutal sexual assault. I decided I was going to be a boy, because I never wanted to have my body violated the way it was when I was a girl. Thankfully, my school psychologist was able to work with me and help me resolve those feelings. Unfortunately now, many states have banned therapy that would help children who have developed a trans identity as a result of a trauma. And even worse, these children have been pushed to medically transition. Thankfully, I wasn't medically transitioned. But a lot of other children have not been so lucky.[33]

The onset of puberty also makes girls extremely susceptible to the trans agenda. Puberty is a time of potentially frightening hormonal changes, which include menstruation and often with it, painful cramps. Estrogen, whether from a high pubertal surge or an externally administered drug, has a reputation for causing moodiness and depression. But the estrogenized body that develops during puberty can itself be a cause for depression in bewildered, distressed girls who have not been mentally or emotionally prepared for maturation.

One change that especially concerns girls is additional fat on the body, which creates a curvy shape. This aspect of maturing conflicts with what a girl sees in the media. Female models weigh at least 23 percent less than the average (not overweight) woman. Compare the typical height and weight for a model at 5'10" and 110 pounds to the average woman at 5'4" and 145 pounds. Unhealthful skinny images constantly bombard teenage girls with an unattainable ideal.[34] Also, the average young person in the United States sees from 13,000 to 30,000 television advertisements per year.[35] Add to this the unrealistic portrayals in films, video games and print, and it's easy to see how girls can grow up to hate their bodies. The authors of a study on body image dissatisfaction and depression in adolescents point out that girls who think their bodies don't measure up to typical cultural standards of beauty are vulnerable to becoming depressed. Despondency about unrelated issues also contributes to a negative body image, as does negative input from others. Depression is highest not only in girls who are genuinely overweight, but also in those who only perceive themselves as too fat, whether or not they actually are.[36] Teenagers of both sexes with body image dissatisfaction are 3.7 times more likely to report symptoms of depression,[37] but twice as many girls as boys are dissatisfied with their body weight and shape. Even girls of an objectively normal weight see themselves as undesirably heavy.[38] In a recent study, almost 38 percent of girls were at least moderately unhappy with their bodies.[39] Based on what I have observed, I believe the percentage is much higher.

Body image dissatisfaction is closely linked to eating disorders. Bulimia and anorexia affect almost 300 million people of all ages, but the majority are girls and young women.[40] Studies show that the pressure on women to be abnormally skinny—and to achieve a "perfection" that cannot exist—comes from all over the world, including in Germany, Spain, Australia and Brazil, as well as the U.S. Females obssess about their appearance no matter where they live. Furthermore, the cultural demand that girls and women be "sexy" has nothing to do with their own enjoyment of their bodies and everything to do with their appearance, how others judge they should look. It's not surprising that girls and women of all ages are especially hard on themselves and might not appreciate being female.

During puberty, sexual desire blossoms. Girls and women are still regarded as sexual objects; so when secondary sex characteristics emerge, along with often intense sexual desire, girls may feel even more vulnerable. In the U.S., the female breast is the quintessential symbol of womanhood and sexiness—again, from an appearance standpoint and not from the perspective of bringing pleasure to its owner. Developing breasts often lead to excessive and unwanted attention from boys, which may contribute to the reason that so many girls want them removed.

Sadly, unwanted sexual attention also corresponds to the use of pornography—which often includes violence, and has become commonplace due to the popularity of the internet. In the United States alone, 20 to 30 percent of children 10 to 12 years of age have reported some exposure to pornography. Pornography use has a clear correlation with objectifying one's sexual partner.[41] *Objectifying* a woman means treating her as a sexual object whose sole purpose is to gratify someone else's desires, rather than respecting her as a human being who has her own needs and wants. Men can be objectified as well, although it doesn't happen as often. Our culture does not consider being a sexual object as a defining trait for masculinity the way it does for femininity. Once someone is taught to objectify others, they lose the ability to be compassionate and it's much easier to inflict sexual violence on them. Sexual violence could include verbal sexual harassment, forcefully touching sexually sensitive areas with or without the threat of violence, and forcing oneself on another sexually—which is rape, whether or not the perpetrator manages to complete the act. Shrier points out that violent pornography now includes choking, which horrifyingly, women in films are portrayed as enjoying. "Violent porn," she writes, "not only terrifies young girls about men and the prospect of sex with them, it is changing the expectations and behavior of boys." One sex researcher "found that nearly a quarter of adult women said they have felt scared during sex." In addition, "13 percent of sexually active girls ages 14 to 17 have already been choked."[42]

A 2019 study linking violent pornography to increased violence among dating teens found that boys who were exposed to violent pornography were two to three times more likely to report victimizing others—and because this figure is based on self-generated reports, it's probable that the incidence of teen dating violence is much higher.[43] How vulnerable a girl must feel when she realizes that as a fully developed women, she could easily be the recipient of sexual violence! If becoming a physically maturing female is so difficult and dangerous, what better way is there to opt out than by being a less vulnerable male? Girls who frequently find themselves subject to ridicule and unwanted sexual attention—not to mention being exposed to violent pornography—may find FtM transitioning especially attractive. Possessing masculine secondary sexual characteristics is a great way to discourage predatory males from perceiving a biological woman as a vulnerable female. Moreover, having a penis isn't even required. According to the 2015 *U.S. Transgender Survey*, only two percent of natal female respondents underwent genital surgery. One percent had phalloplasty, which is the creation of an artificial penis-like structure from existing tissue, usually taken from the forearm. Another one percent had metoidioplasty, which involves cutting ligaments around the erectile tissue to give the shaft of the testosterone-enlarged clitoris greater length.[44]

"The detransitioners I see in my practice," psychotherapist Lisa Marchiano writes, "are all female, and they are all in their early twenties."

> At the time they became trans-identified, many were suffering from complex social and mental health issues. Transition often not only failed to address these issues, but at times exacerbated them or added new issues....
>
> The young women with whom I have worked became trans-identified during adolescence. They frequently did so in the context of significant family dysfunction or complex psycho-social issues. Sexual assault and sexual harassment were common precursors. A majority had an eating disorder at the time they became trans-identified. Since detransitioning, most now understand themselves to be butch lesbians. In our work together, they traced complex histories of coming to terms with their homosexuality. Some faced vicious homophobic bullying before they announced their trans identification.[45]

The experiences of other clinicians and researchers align with Marchiano's. Most of the girls who gravitate toward sexual "reassignment" suffer from emotional problems, especially depression, anxiety, and feelings of self-loathing about their bodies. In addition to eating disorders, some have issues with self-harm such as cutting. It shouldn't be surprising that such girls long to escape the bodies that, in their eyes, are the cause of so much pain and distress. Why be someone with a "front hole" (the new, ugly word for vagina) when you can be a cool FtM? Not only has social media glorified transgenders, but unless a female's appearance lies within a very narrow band of what's considered attractive, she thinks she's not enough of a woman. In a huge anti-female (and anti-feminist) backlash, a girl who excels at math or science, is not particularly "girly," and is good at sports—who is what we call a "tomboy"—is made to question whether she's female at all. If she's attracted to other girls, and *especially* if she's butch or masculine-looking, it's unlikely that she's simply a lesbian—she must be a male! Declaring that one is a FtM transgender bestows great social status compared to coming out as a lesbian, which earns demerits.

During Abigail Shrier's extensive interviews, one girl shared that at her all-girls school of 500, there were 15 trans students. That translates into 3 percent of the school population "born in the wrong body." Compare these numbers to those cited in the *DSM-5*, published less than ten years ago, which listed an expected rate of 0.002–0.003 percent—less than one in 10,000. How many lesbians attend the school? None. This both hides and disappears the gay female population. "Symptoms that some see as evidence of being transgender," Marchiano writes, "can also be an early expression of being lesbian or gay. Given that research indicates that the majority of cross-sex identified kids will desist if left alone, and that most of these will grow up to be gay, lesbian, or bisexual, it seems prudent in many cases to wait and see."[46]

As with boys, girls that are not stereotyped caricatures are branded "gender nonconforming." At a young age, they're expected to declare whether they are "gender-fluid," "gender-queer," "asexual," or "non-binary." What they *don't* want is to be "cis-gender," or ordinary natal, biological females (just as some boys don't want to be regarded as ordinary biological males). Shrier rightly calls this "indoctrination in gender ideology that is both so radical and so pervasive" that it's not surprising that so many students fall for it.[47] "All that's required is the insistence that students display decency, civility, and kindness to their classmates.... But instead 'bullying' is used as an excuse for a thorough indoctrination in gender ideology and the insistence that transgender students must be 'affirmed' or suffer a steep psychological toll."[48] Incredibly, students of all ages are being indoctrinated with the trans agenda: in grammar schools, high schools, colleges, and universities. California leads the trend, but other institutions across the United States—New York, New Jersey, and elsewhere—are quickly following.

The optimistic demeanor conferred by taking testosterone also plays a huge role in FtM transitions, Shrier reports. Many teenage girls post how good they feel from testosterone injections. They feel liberated by testosterone's calming and euphoric effects, not to mention increased energy. Anxiety and depression markedly decrease.[49,50] Excessively high testosterone levels have also been shown to reduce fear, increase risk-taking behaviors, and lower sensitivity to punishment. Compared to patches and pills, the injections are reported to have an addictive quality. For a developing adolescent girl, the promise of relief from not only anxiety (which rises during puberty), but also messy periods and painful cramps, can be too tempting to resist. The act of injecting testosterone is even regarded as a rite of passage, as evidenced by celebratory injection rituals found on the internet. Therapists might claim that the girls feel better because now their bodies are in greater alignment with their brains. But in reality, the enjoyable feelings are due to the effects of a *drug*. Testosterone is a hormone produced in the bodies of females as well as males, but when it's administered in unnaturally large amounts, it's a drug. Many people forget this. Another lasting alteration in girls from testosterone is lowered vocal pitch. Sometimes all it takes is a mere six months on the hormone for permanent changes to occur. So despite her stopping the testosterone, her voice will never revert to its natural range and she may sound like a man for the rest of her life. Other parts of her body will most likely be permanently disfigured in some way, and her options in life will be lessened.

The sad thing is, girls who want to escape their bodies haven't been taught coping skills. As one adolescent female said, "I don't know exactly that I want to be a guy. I just know I don't want to be a girl."[51]

Children Who Have Divergences of Sexual Development

In the first chapter I discussed in detail Divergences of Sexual Development. Due to most people's discomfort with atypical genitals that deviate from an arbitrary norm, infants are routinely subjected to surgery and are often given hormones as well. Children are rarely given a choice. For the rest of their lives, they will have to live with the decisions that others made for them. Fortunately, with the support of the growing intersex movement, which embraces all people with atypical genitals, more people are coming forward to talk about how they were abused by the medical profession. Many of them mourn the loss of their genitals and their inability to experience sexual pleasure.

Dr. Sarah Creighton, author of the 2001 article "Surgery for intersex," reported that not only were adult subjects "dissatisfied" with both the structural and cosmetic outcomes of surgery performed on them when they were children, they were also "unhappy and feel mutilated and damaged by surgery performed... however worthy the clinician's motives." She pointed out that the Intersex Society of North America "regards vaginoplasty and clitoral reduction as cosmetic surgery that should be deferred until the patient can consent. This means leaving even the most virilized female babies without surgery"—despite the fact that this "goes against current practice in the UK." She advocated using surgery "sparingly," as "it is impossible to define who actually 'needs' a clitoral reduction or vaginoplasty in childhood....Clinicians working in this field must step back and review their practice. Surgery may not be necessary."[52] Physicians have yet to heed her advice.

It amazes me that there's still a debate over whether cutting into the genitals of an infant (or grownup) can cause physical and psychological damage.[53]

Men

Some adult men transition relatively late in life, when they're in their 40s or even 50s. Many of them are husbands. A typical candidate has had a satisfying relationship with his wife and children and has enjoyed a successful career, often in a respected white-collar profession. His ability to enjoy sex with his wife and father children, and decades of living in apparent congruence with his body, make his decision to transition even more puzzling. As it turns out, such a man usually declares that he's transgender for one of three reasons: he's a cross-dresser (likes to wear clothing made for women), he experiences sexual excitement when perceiving himself as a woman and masquerading as one, or his desire to transition is underscored by a trauma, possibly decades old.

In today's climate, cross-dressing is often erroneously conflated with transgenderism. Whereas a woman might have occasionally accepted seeing her male partner in a dress, trans-oriented doctors pathologize this behavior to mean that he is in the wrong body and pressure him to accept cross-sex hormones and surgery. Once the medical establishment insinuates itself into a cross-dresser's life, tension may be created where there previously had been none. The cross-dressing man's partner fears that anytime, he might change irreversibly before her very eyes—physically, mentally, and emotionally.

In such relationships, there might be a fundamental clash of values between those who love extreme sex role stereotypes and those who don't. One woman who was married to a cross-dresser said, "I, who had never cared much about clothes and resented the 'Barbie doll' image of women, had a husband who seemed obsessed with clothes and was helpless while his nail polish was drying." Her husband loved the "teenage primping I have never wanted to do."[54]

A man's erotic arousal at dressing up in clothing meant for women is another issue entirely. Back in 1989, psychiatrist and sexologist Ray Blanchard coined the term *autogynephilia* to describe this tendency in some MtFs. The term comes from the Greek words meaning "self," "woman," and "love," which, when combined, translate to "love of oneself as a woman."[55] Several basic autogynephilic fantasies can arouse a man: when he wears or fantasizes wearing women's clothing, when he does something else regarded as feminine, when he fantasizes female-specific body functions, and when he possesses a woman's body or parts of a woman's body. Autoeroticism is quite different from the perception that one actually *is* the opposite sex. The extent of the autoeroticism is illustrated by an observation Blanchard once made of biological males with autogynephilia who had sex with other males as well as females. When such a man fantasizes being penetrated by a man, this is not homosexual attraction, a male's sexual desire for another male. Rather, for an autogynephilic man, the erotic stimulus is the thought of being a woman himself. Having a male sexual partner anchors and strengthens the fantasy that he is a woman.[56]

In 2003, sex researcher and psychology professor J. Michael Bailey published *The Man Who Would Be Queen*. In it he discussed Blanchard's observations. Trans activists tried to discredit Bailey and ruin him, both personally and professionally, by spreading lies of misconduct. "I think," Blanchard commented, referring to the resistance that Bailey had encountered, "the idea of autogynephilia cuts too close to the bone. If the idea had no resonance with them [trans activists], they would simply have ignored it." He explained that online forums are regularly monitored for posts that mention autogynephilia. Anyone who posts is quickly told "that this is wrongthink and that autogynephilia does not exist. It is therefore hard to get any sense of how many autogynephilic gender dysphorics privately think that autogynephilia describes their own experience, because stating that online will produce scorn and other negative reactions."[57] Blanchard was aware that the controversy had nothing to do with science and everything to do with politics.

> I very much doubt that the prevalence of autogynephilia per se, or the prevalence of autogynephilic gender dysphoria, has increased. I think that what has changed is the proportion of autogynephilic trans who have "come out" to their families, friends, and employers, not the total number of autogynephilic trans. Forty years ago, an autogynephile's decision to transition to the female role often had negative consequences in the personal and employment spheres. Now that decision is as likely to get them praised for courage as it is to get them criticized for selfishness and irresponsibility.[58]

Despite pushback from very well-organized trans activists, political pressure has not dissuaded people from investigating the phenomenon. Instances of autogynephilia were observed long before Blanchard. In 1935, British physician Havelock Ellis wrote that while it's natural for a man to identify himself with a woman whom he loves, an exaggerated version of this occurs in those whom we consider transsexual. In 1948, German physician Magnus Hirschfeld observed the autoerotic component of a man who did not feel attracted to a living woman, but to the feminine component inside of himself. Also in Germany, in 1966 Harry Benjamin reported that some MtF transgenders imagine themselves as women being penetrated by male sexual partners.[59] The common denominator of all these descriptions is *the desire to be passive*, which is believed to be an innate quality of women and is then translated into *being* a woman. Yet most real women—on whom passivity is either overtly or covertly enforced as a learned behavior—would not view being passive as sexually exciting. Again, the male transgender's definition of "woman" or "female" is based on *his* idea, *his* construct. What some regard as a transgender issue may be something else entirely: the desire to escape from the pressure of constantly being in the stereotypically dominant male role. The expectation to always be the assertive masculine leader can be a burden.

Some men consider themselves cross-dressers without requiring a transgender label. In "How My Journey in Autogynephilia Began," one man recounts his upbringing of reverse discrimination. His mother wanted a daughter, not a son. When his sister was born a year after him, she "was treated like a princess" and "lived a privileged life." He always felt that he was a "disappointment" to his mother and believed that if he had been a girl, he would have been loved more.

> Girls were provided with pretty, shiny things to adorn themselves. Little girls were even supposed to be smarter than their male counterparts. Sometimes I would play with something pretty, something shiny. I was interested in nail polish, jewels, satin clothing. "You can't do that," I would be told. "That's for girls." I understood that I was just a boy.
>
> I grew up thinking that society preferred girls over boys because girls were pretty, smart, and more virtuous....I believe this overvalued image of females was the glue that hard-wired my brain for its next stage....There was one red velvet dress with a built-in petticoat that was amazing. Just touching it gave me a thrill. I tried it on and I experienced a powerful rush and my whole body was quivering. I couldn't understand what that was all about, but from that moment on I was addicted.[60]

Earlier I stated my hypothesis that if the sex-specific classification for clothing were removed, it would lose its emotional charge and appeal for men who are titillated by what is forbidden. If all clothing was suitable for either sex (assuming it fits), the stigma and unusualness of men wearing dresses would very likely be erased. What gives cross-dressing its power is the assumption that dresses, skirts, makeup, and heels naturally belong in the domain of females.

Not all adult men who decide much later in life to transition do so because they get a sexual charge from wearing dresses. Some of them are suffering from childhood trauma that has been incorrectly diagnosed as gender dysphoria. When Walt Heyer was four years old, he was forced by his grandmother to wear a dress in order to receive her approval. He began his transition in his early 40s. "The reprieve I experienced through surgery was only temporary," Walt writes. "Hidden underneath the makeup and female clothing was the little boy hurt by childhood trauma. I was once again experiencing gender dysphoria, but this time I felt like a male inside a body refashioned to look like a woman....I was deeply suicidal."[61] Heyer eventually went into therapy, got to the root of his dysphoria, and transitioned back to his natal identity and body (minus his genitals). At least he healed emotionally from his trauma. But many men who have been abused don't get the chance to heal at any age.

Women

Even though the transgendering of women and men is treated as the same event, their reasons for transitioning are quite different. A large number of women who take hormones, and most of the small percentage who also undergo surgery, do so to raise their status in a culture that treats men differently than it does women. In one study of FtM transgenders, researchers talked to interviewees before and after their transitions. As it turns out, sexism in the workplace played a huge role in why women decided to look as much like men as possible. They had been sexually fondled, and constantly endured unwanted comments about their appearance. If they were lesbians, they also had to deflect invasive questions about their sex lives. Uniformly, the interviewees reported that after their FtM transition, they earned more—for doing the same job.[62]

FtM transgender James St. James writes, "Quite a bit changed for me over the first couple of years I started testosterone....But just as fascinating as it was to witness my mental and physical changes, it was just as equal of an adjustment to comprehend how other people were responding to me. In short, I was being treated better by everyday America because people were reading me as a young, white, straight (?!) male. And I recognized many new privileges that came my way because of it."[63] Below are the perks. All of the issues underscore what many women experience: disrespect of boundaries, not being taken seriously (either personally or professionally), and diminished earning power compared to that of men. The list is worth reproducing in its entirety because St. James so clearly and thoroughly highlights the issues that so many natal women face.

Appearance:

- I Rarely Look in the Mirror Before Leaving My Home. I've learned that the male me is never appearance policed, so what the hell do I care?
- My Clothing Is More Practical. And better made and longer lasting and cheaper and less judged.
- My Abilities Speak Louder Than My Appearances at Work. When I work on-site gigs, I tend to just wear jeans and a t-shirt. Nobody cares. It's all about the quality of my work.

Fewer Worries for Physical Safety:
- I'm Not Held Accountable for Keeping Rape from Happening. I remember all of the rape prevention education I got, which always focused on how I should behave, where I should walk when, how to appropriately cover my drink, and so on. These days, I'm told nothing. Not even not to rape.
- I'm Very Likely to Arrive Home Safely After Walking Alone at Night. It remains that I walk alone at night far more than I used to purely because I'm a dude. Put up my hoodie, and people have even been known to cross the sidewalk to avoid passing me.
- I Can Be a Gamer Without Worry of Being Threatened, Insulted, or Demeaned. The gaming industry is still very much a man's world. Female characters are frequently sexualized, brutalized, and demeaned when they're represented at all—right along with the female gamers themselves.

Boundaries:
- I'm Not Told by Strangers (Or Anybody Else) to Smile. Not once has it happened since [my transition].
- I Don't Have Strangers Giving Uninvited Opinions About My Body as I Pass By. (Or them expecting me to thank them for it).
- Instructions or Opinions Are Only Given When I Specifically Ask for Them. Apparently I'm seen as somebody who suddenly knows what he's doing.
- People Don't Find It Their Business to Correct Me. Unless it's a person clearly of more authority than me in a working environment and they're telling me about a very specific mistake made on a very specific issue, I never get corrected in life anymore. I'm simply allowed to be, mistakes and all.
- My Facial Expressions Are No Longer Public Property. A bit like the "I'm no longer told to smile" point...but more like, "Why do you look so angry/unhappy/pensive/anything else other than super bubbly happy?" As if any ol' stranger had the right to demand a reason for my surly, surly face because it was—I don't know—offensive to them? Now it's no longer considered my duty to brighten someone else's day.
- I'm Rarely Told to Shut Up Anymore. I used to often be told to stop talking or to be quiet after a few minutes of prattling because I was "annoying people." But now people just sit there and take it. I still haven't figured out if this is because a) they think what I have to say is suddenly more important, or b) if they just don't think it's their place to tell me to shut up.
- I Rarely Get Interrupted. I used to be interrupted so often while presenting as a woman that I in turn started to talk over people as a form of conversational survival.
- It's Okay for Me to Use Negative or Self-Supportive Phrases. People listen and/or respect it when I say things like "no," "I don't want to," or "stop that." And ironically, my need to say these has gone down significantly.

- My Comfort Comes Before Anyone Else's. Nobody expects me to sacrifice a thing for them anymore. Being asked to grab someone their coffee, help decorate for a work party, or help clean up said party is simply a thing of the past.
- I Can Say the Most Ridiculous Things Imaginable. And people will still think I'm right.

Automatic Personal Respect:
- I Repeat a Woman's Suggestion or Comment—And Get All the Credit. I've since made it my policy to say something like, "As So-And-So just said, I think it'd be a great idea to blah blah blah…" If I'm somehow still the only one congratulated, I politely say, "Thank you, but it was So-And-So's idea first." Sometimes even that doesn't work. And then I give up.
- I Get More Eye Contact. Apparently, I'm suddenly worth engaging in conversation with, as opposed to objectifying with a gaze. I feel like they now look at me and think "Oh! You're a person! And of rational thought, no less!"
- Yet I'm Still Taken (More) Seriously. I'm still amazed at the amount of people that now immediately shut their mouths the second I open mine. Believe me, my ideas haven't improved at all. I've even tried to derail serious conversations with ludicrous stuff just to see what would happen—and I'd still be regarded highly.

Work and Professional Life:
- I Have More Money Left at the End of the Week. Because I'm not pressured to spend it on makeup, bras, diet pills, or ridiculously expensive anti-aging treatments that never work.
- People Ask to See My Work. When it comes up in conversation that I'm a writer, people actually want to know more about it and ask for links or unpublished manuscripts to read. Gone are the days where they'd just verbally pat me on the head like I was the most painfully adorable thing ever—me, thinking I was a writer.
- I Get Thanked When I Do More Work on a Job Than Was Necessary. Especially if it was obvious that I helped someone else out, I sometimes even receive some small trinket. It's no longer an expectation that I'll go above and beyond the job description.
- I'm Trusted More. I'm given bigger deals, more important projects, and am otherwise privy to more sensitive information, both personally and professionally.
- I Get Paid More. The proof is in my paychecks. Actual, numerical proof.
- It's Easier for Me to Be Poor. Aside from usually getting paid more, it's been easier to find work when the person doing the hiring is a white guy. It's like helping out a buddy or something.[64, 65]

St. James's experience of being properly compensated after transitioning is not an isolated incident. Earnings may factor significantly in many women's decisions to appear male. In the United States in the year 2020, women earned 81 cents for every dollar earned by men when doing the same job requiring the same skills. The median salary for men was roughly 19 percent higher than the median salary for women. This is a 2 percent improvement from 2019, but the discrepancy shouldn't exist at all.[66] In the U.S. in the year 2022, women earned 82 cents for every dollar earned by men—a one cent increase in two years. This time, the median salary for men was 17 percent higher. In elite industries, the wage gap is astronomical. In the legal field, on average men earn 59 percent more than white women, and white women fare better than women of color.[67]

Trauma is often a compelling reason to transition. If a woman was assaulted —precisely because of her sex—she might try to escape her pain by changing her body. Carey, a young woman in her 20s, recounted how eagerly she began her transition after she was raped. She believed that if she had a masculine body, men wouldn't be able to hurt her anymore. Astoundingly, the therapist she was required to consult before starting cross-sex hormones never explored this issue with her. She should have encouraged Carey to talk about the pain, anger and vulnerability associated with being raped, and then helped her client devise strategies to heal from the trauma. Instead, the therapist prescribed a powerful hormone that would change her body forever. Had Carey received help to deal with her feelings of terror and lack of safety, she would never have taken the medication. Fortunately, she did not have surgery and did not take testosterone for a long period. Although her body did undergo some permanent changes, they were relatively minor compared to the bodies of women who take testosterone long-term. Carey still looks like a woman and sounds like a woman, even though her voice is lower in pitch than it was before she took the testosterone. But now, not only does she need to process the rape, she must also deal with being mistreated by an incompetent therapist.[68]

In 2019, a conference titled "Detransition: The Elephant in the Room. Medical Ethics in the Age of Gender Identity" was organized in Manchester, England by a feminist collective. One detransitioner, Kira, recounted that she had been a "gender nonconformist child"—a tomboy—but had been pressured to act in a stereotypically feminine manner. Kira took cross-sex hormones. At age 20, she had both breasts removed before realizing that those hormones and surgery were not the answer. She needed to accept herself as she truly was.[69] Chapter 6 contains detailed personal accounts of more detransitioners.

I have already mentioned that some homosexual males, especially if they are very effeminate, choose to transition because they believe that being sexually and romantically attracted to men must mean that they're innately women. Similarly, lesbians—especially women who are very masculine or butch—may feel pressured to transition, believing that they have permission to love other women sexually only if they present as men. The transgendering of homosexuals decreases gays and lesbians as a population by exploiting their internalized homophobia.

Earlier I discussed congenital adrenal hyperplasia (CAH), a condition where the female fetus is exposed to abnormally high levels of testosterone *in utero*. Some research (though not all) has shown that CAH women are more likely than their non-CAH counterparts to identify with traits and activities culturally regarded as masculine. If a CAH woman is taught that these characteristics are incongruous for someone with a female body, the only way she believes she'll gain acceptance is by transitioning. Over and over, we are seeing the damaging effects of gender roles. What's considered permissible "masculinity" and "femininity" is narrow indeed.

When examining the reasons why women transition, it's very clear that the overwhelming majority of biological women want to transition not because they believe that they are truly male, but because they want to escape the condition of being female. There's nothing fundamentally wrong with these women's bodies. The problem lies in how others treat them, based on cultural beliefs about females. While psychotherapy devoted to the release of trauma would certainly help—especially in the case of sexual assault and related experiences—women's perceived need to become transgender may more accurately be regarded as rooted in societal, rather than personal, problems.

Setting aside the health dangers of continually taking high doses of testosterone, many biological women benefit from appearing male. However, one issue I have not seen addressed much is the lack of emotional intimacy that FtMs may face. Unlike women, men have been socialized not to talk about their feelings. So how does a natal-born woman—growing up female before acquiring a male-looking body—feel about that? Would heart-to-heart talks about emotions with men or women be common? Would the FtM be afraid of not being seen as a "real man" for wanting to initiate such intimacy? Or would this not matter?

The one account I found that addresses this topic is recent: "I'm a Trans Man. I Didn't Realize How Broken Men Are." James Barnes, who as a young child felt very different than other girls and transitioned at age 26, writes, "The one thing I didn't prepare for [after transitioning] was how lonely it is to be a man….Men started treating me like their guy friends, which was exactly what I wanted. What I didn't know is that male friendships aren't as deep. Before my transition, guys used to open up to me about all sorts of fears, frustrations, and feelings. Now, they would keep it superficial….I realized that it would take years to build a semi-deep friendship." Related to verbal communion is physical closeness. Instead of "deep, long hugs," James now receives "short pat hugs" and handshakes. Barnes is experiencing first-hand the limitations of our culture's beliefs about how men should behave and what attitudes are and are not appropriate for them.

> As a man, you get to feel safe, but you don't get to be a nurturer or nurtured. You can speak up whenever you want, but not about your emotions, fears, or grief. You have the freedom to do whatever

you want whenever you want, as long as that doesn't involve anything feminine, which turns out to be many incredible things, like emotions, intentional parenting, grooming, baking...[F]ind a way to be safe in your skin as a whole person...who cries, feels joy, and can embrace all aspects of themselves....Focus your time on learning how to be vulnerable, build intentional and meaningful friendships, and heal your relationship with what it means to be feminine....I ask you to stretch your idea of masculinity. Hundreds of men reached out to me, saying they try to cry in front of the women in their lives or try to be nurturing, and they [the women] remind them to "man up" or [say] that it makes them uncomfortable.

How sad—not only for Barnes and for men in general, but also for the narrow-minded, judgmental women in this account—that a full range of emotional expression for all human beings is culturally belittled. Everyone should consider Barnes's counsel: "We cannot have a world of healthy, kind, and strong men if we stick to broken stereotypes."[70] Did Barnes need to transition? Perhaps. Or does our society need to change? Most definitely.

Adults Who Have Divergences of Sexual Development

The late Ben Barres was an extraordinary human being and brilliant neuroscientist whose groundbreaking discoveries about the glial cells in the brain provided a foundation for the treatment of many brain disorders, including Parkinson's and dementia. Born Barbara Barres, Ben wrote in an autobiography that "internally I felt strongly that I was a boy. This was evident in everything about my behavior."[71] The "behavior" was apparently the girl's desire to be a scientist, expressed before the age of 5, along with her passion for microscopes and chemistry sets and an aversion to receiving dresses and jewelry as gifts. Barbara Barres received a degree in biology from Massachusetts Institute of Technology (MIT), a medical degree from Dartmouth College, and a Ph.D. from Harvard Medical School. She was also awarded scholarships. Yet even with all her clearly superior brilliance and first-rate education, she still suffered rampant sexism. She transitioned in 1997 and later wrote:

If innate intellectual abilities are not to blame for women's slow advance in science careers, then what is? The foremost factor, I believe, is the societal assumption that women are innately less able than men. Many studies...have demonstrated a substantial degree of bias against women—more than is sufficient to block women's advancement in many professions. Here are a few examples of bias from my own life as a young woman. As an undergrad at the Massachusetts Institute of Technology (MIT), I was the only person in a large class of nearly all men to solve a hard maths problem, only to be told by the professor that my boyfriend must have solved it for me. I was not given any credit. I am still disappointed about the prestigious fellowship competition I later lost to a male contemporary when I was a PhD student, even though the Harvard dean who had read both applications assured me that my application was much stronger (I had published six high-impact papers whereas my male competitor had published only one). Shortly after I changed sex, a faculty member was heard to say "Ben Barres gave a great seminar today, but then his work is much better than his sister's."...

Gender-blinding studies...reveal that in many selection processes, the bar is unconsciously raised so high for women and minority candidates that few emerge as winners. For instance, one study found that women applying for a research grant needed to be 2.5 times more productive than men in order to be considered equally competent. Even for women lucky enough to obtain an academic job, gender biases can influence the relative resources allocated to faculty, as Nancy Hopkins discovered when she and a senior faculty committee studied this problem at MIT. The data were so convincing that MIT president Charles Vest publicly admitted that discrimination was responsible....Despite these studies, very few men or women are willing to admit that discrimination is a serious problem in science. How is that possible? [Author Virginia] Valian suggests that we all have a strong desire to believe that the world is fair....I am suspicious when those who are at an advantage proclaim that a disadvantaged group of people is innately less able.[72]

"As a transgendered person," Dr. Barres also wrote, "no one understands more deeply than I do that there are innate differences between men and women. I suspect that my transgendered identity was caused by fetal exposure to high doses of a testosterone-like drug [which Barres's mother took while pregnant]. But there is no evidence that sexually dimorphic brain wiring is at all relevant to the abilities needed to be successful in a chosen academic career." "Sexually dimorphic brain wiring" refers to presumed innate differences between male and female brains—even though, as discussed in Chapters 1 and 2, the concept has been proven untrue. Barres might not have known about the research disproving the oft-repeated theory. Or perhaps Barres brought up this issue because some colleagues believed that such differences in wiring do exist, and they were using the concept to justify their prejudice against female scientists.

Barres mentioned one effect of testosterone: losing the ability to cry easily. It's true that men on estrogen are apt to cry more readily. But "the main difference that I have noticed," the neuroscientist wrote, "is that people who don't know I am transgendered treat me with much more respect: I can even complete a whole sentence without being interrupted by a man."[73] Gifted, kind, and much loved by students, faculty, friends and colleagues, Dr. Barres never stopped being a vocal and supportive advocate for female scientists. Ben never forgot the problems that Barbara had faced, and obviously still identified with her.

In addition to articles, Barres wrote an autobiography. "From junior high school on, I had increasingly strong feelings of gender dysphoria, difference, and confusion. I felt very embarrassed and ashamed about my gender incongruity but was totally unable to express what I was feeling to anyone....It is difficult to express the degree of continued emotional pain, low self-esteem, and ultimately strong suicidal ideation that my gender discordance caused me while growing up and as a young adult. It was only at the age of forty...that I finally understood that I was transgender and was able to deal effectively with the problem."[74] In 1997 Barres wrote a letter to colleagues, signing it as Barbara but stating that after transitioning her name would be Ben. An especially poignant line read, "whenever I think about changing my gender role, I am flooded with feelings of relief." The letter continued in part:

> I will begin taking testosterone in February. A change in my appearance will not be visible for several months. By summer, I will begin to dress in men's clothes and will change my name to Ben. Throughout this process I will continue to work normally and to conduct myself in all ways as usual (except that I will only use single occupancy bathrooms). Although the idea of my changing sex will take some time for you to get used to, the reality is that I'm not going to change all that much. I'm still going to wear jeans and tee shirts and pretty much be the same person I always have been—it's just that I am going to be a lot happier.
>
> Many transsexuals change jobs after their "sex change" in order to retain anonymity, but anonymity is obviously not an option for me—nor is it one I desire. I am tired of hiding who I am....Sure I knew that sometimes there were male to female transsexuals but I had thought that these people were perverts. I am not a pervert; I don't seek pleasure—only relief from pain.[75]

Dr. Barres chose cross-sex hormones and surgery as a responsible 43-year-old adult, with—I am glad to report—the full support of friends and colleagues. Note how respectful Barres was in choosing single-occupancy bathrooms.

I am sincerely glad that transgendering made the scientist happy. But there is something deeply troubling about Barbara's transformation. The question must be asked whether she would have felt it necessary to undergo such a radical transformation had she been treated fairly by her teachers and colleagues, had she felt comfortable to wear what she truly desired without censure (casual clothing typical of what men wear), and had she been given the respect, recognition, and honors she so richly deserved. Clearly, Barbara felt that in order to advance in her field she had no other option than to transition.

I must also question whether Barbara Barres was genuinely transsexual (to use her own nomenclature). She did have a Divergence of Sexual Development and clearly believed she was male—citing her exposure to a testosterone-like drug *in utero* as the reason for her "maleness." But as I have explained in earlier chapters, having a passion for science and not wanting to wear dresses could hardly be considered proof that someone is inherently male. Significantly, Barbara mentioned "gender incongruity," and "changing my gender *role*" rather than "changing my *biological sex*." It's a bit surprising that Barres—a highly gifted scientist whose success depended on precision—could have confused gender stereotypes with natal sex. But many people in the medical and scientific communities have made, and are still making, the same error. If Barbara indeed conflated gender with sex, it's tragic that she had to transition—especially as Barres died at age 63 from pancreatic cancer, only 20 years after transitioning. Given the abnormally high dose of testosterone that Barres had to keep taking, it's not unreasonable to believe that it contributed to—if not directly caused—the cancer. According to research cited by FtM Scott Newgent, the act of transgendering erases 12 years from a person's life.[76]

Dr. Barres was not the only woman regarded as masculine to encounter blatant sexism and feel pressured to conform to an unfair stereotype. Unfortunately, the beloved scientist is unlikely to be the last.

******

The majority of adults who have Divergences of Sexual Development report having been bullied, mocked, and shunned as children because they were different. If they had an especially androgynous appearance or displayed nonconforming behavior, they would not have fit our culture's ideas of how men and women should look and act. Girls with moderate to severe CAH (congenital adrenal hyperplasia) state that they were often mistaken for boys, and they were derided and rejected—especially if they exhibited typically masculine interests in play and work. Sometimes their genitals were obviously unusual, another source of ridicule and heartache. Boys with an obviously feminine appearance, and who also demonstrated atypical interests, report being the recipients not only of bullying, cruelty and rejection, but also anti-gay violence. If their genitalia are unusual, they suffer even more.

Is surgery the answer for such individuals when they reach adulthood? Is the solution to irreversibly hack off parts of the body that work perfectly well? Perhaps in the long run it's more helpful and enduring—not to mention far less painful—to change society's attitudes than carve up even a single person's body. Individuals make up society, and all of us are individuals. We may not be able to change anyone else's mind, but we can begin by working on ourselves to eliminate our own biases.

If everyone was a little bit more open-minded and kinder, we might be able to help avert suffering—like the kind of agony that the individuals in the next chapter experienced.

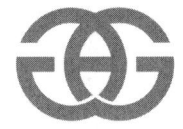

6

TRANS REGRET AND DETRANSITIONERS

Roadblocks to Detransitioning

While a tiny minority of transgenders report feeling freer and happier after their transition, increasing numbers of people are now realizing that they made a mistake and are *detransitioning*—that is, attempting to change back to the body they were born with. If they were solely dressing and living as the opposite sex, returning to their birth identity is less complicated as there's no medical damage. Such individuals who have not taken cross-sex hormones or undergone surgery are known as *desisters*. But they may be few in number, because anyone questioning his or her identity and is seen by "gender-affirming" personnel is immediately given cross-sex hormones and (if they're young enough) puberty blockers. Even in a short time, cross-sex hormones can wreak a great deal of damage. The least fortunate detransitioners are those who have had body parts removed. Girls whose breasts have been hacked off can never get them back. Even if they've retained their reproductive organs and are fertile, they will never be able to breastfeed their children. If females have an artificial penis constructed, they lose their vagina. Men who have their penises and testicles removed will never recover the organ or be able to become biological fathers. And it's highly likely that both sexes will forfeit pleasurable sexual sensation. If puberty blockers are given before Tanner stage two—when high levels of pubescent hormones begin to impart secondary sex characteristics—the ability to have an orgasm is permanently lost.

"The stories from detransitioning young people are strikingly similar," explains a journalist. "As lonely and alienated teenagers, they were exposed to transition on social media and thought it might cure their isolation or unhappiness. They went through a cursory process to acquire 'puberty-blocking' hormones, then testosterone or estrogen, and then surgeries. They realized, horribly, that they had made a grave error. And now they are posting about it on Reddit and Twitter."[1]

Detransitioners typically report that in order to have made the transition, they must have been temporarily crazed. They felt as though they were under a spell, whipped up into a frenzy of emotion. One young man in his 20s who detransitioned, concisely and eloquently summarized the situation:

> For many people, transition is an obsessive quest to compulsively eradicate one's own sexed characteristics. It's born from ideology, self-hatred, trauma, and grooming by online strangers. Gay, autistic, mentally disabled, and gender non-conforming teenagers, as well as victims of sexual violence, are the most affected. Pharmaceuticals and plastic surgery investors are getting rich off of the butchery, mutilation, and mass sterilization of these vulnerable and traumatized populations. Doctors and therapists who assist people in transition aren't providing care, they're enabling self-harm and practicing eugenics.
>
> A transition is never done. There's always more surgeries, new treatments, more work to do. You can never carve away enough pieces of yourself to be satisfied. You can never rid yourself of the fundamental facts of your own biology.[2]

Based on the great numbers of people who tell their stories via email and online support groups, FtM Scott Newgent—who has become an advocate to protect children from trans medical abuse—estimates that 95 percent of people regret "some form, if not all" of medical transition.[3] Obviously this is just one source of information. It's hard to know how many people have detransitioned or regret having become involved in transgendering, because trans activists don't want the public to hear from detransitioners and try to silence them. One trans-friendly website links to statistics from the Charing Cross gender identity clinic in the UK. According to 3,398 patient assessment reports from August 1, 2016 to August 1, 2017, only 16—or 0.47 percent—expressed regret or detransitioned; and of those, 10 detransitioned only temporarily, due to finances, social factors and physical complications.[4] The same website also points to the 2015 *U.S. Transgender Survey* which states that of almost 28,000 people, 8 percent of respondents reported some type of transition—but that 62 percent of that 8 percent did so only "temporarily due to societal, financial, or family pressures."[5] Based on such statistics, one would think that transgendering one's body was a rousing success. But the tremendous backlash by detransitioners indicates the opposite, as evidence by their increased appearance at numerous rallies held throughout the United States. Natal female Luka Hein stated at a 2023 event in Los Angeles, "I was really rushed down a pipeline where my very first medical intervention was a double mastectomy at [age] 16 before anything else. A few months later, I was put on testosterone."[6] Like so many, Hein had been fast-tracked to medications and surgery without anyone investigating her mental health.

Those not connected to clinics or the trans community are finding very different percentages of detransitioners and regretters. Michael Irwig, who published an article in a 2022 issue of *The Journal of Clinical Endocrinology & Metabolism* about detransitioners in the U.S. military, explained the many complex factors involved in detransitioning as well as the difficulty of obtaining data. Not every trans person discusses their problems with their endocrinologist. Sometimes the patients switch doctors. Sometimes the continuity or discontinuity of prescriptions cannot be detected if people fill them at more than one drug store.[7] Other problems in obtaining reliable data include people who volunteer for surveys and then drop out before a trial period is over, those who detransition or have regret but don't talk to researchers, and people such as Scott Newgent (discussed shortly) who are unable to detransition because their bodies have been so damaged by surgeries that they cannot handle any more cutting. It's much easier to find a doctor willing to perform bottom surgery than it is to find a doctor who will try to undo it.

Chopping into one's genitals is not simply stressful, it's unfathomably traumatic and abusive. In order to admit this, though, a person would have to be willing to feel their intense anger at having been misled and betrayed—along with enormous grief over what has been lost. Of those transgenders whose major problems were *not* gender dysphoria, how many have the emotional stamina and support to help them face the horrible truth?

It's difficult to determine how many detransitioners and regretters there are, but common sense indicates that the number is many times higher than what trans activists publicize. In contrast to the aforementioned figures from the Charing Cross gender identity clinic, the 2015 *U.S. Transgender Survey* provides the detransitioner figure as 13.1 percent. But this number was derived solely from those who still identify as members of the trans community and omits anyone who has severed ties to it. Also, the percentage of regretters, as compared to outright detransitioners, is difficult to compute and doesn't factor into those surveys.[8]

A survey conducted by Dr. Lisa Littman of 100 detransitioners—69 natal females and 31 natal males—showed that only 24 out of 100 informed their clinicians that they had returned to their natal sex. This strongly suggests that the actual number of detransitioners is at least four times higher than the highest figures available from trans-related sources. But an even greater percentage of detransitioners may exist, as this number was obtained solely from those who chose to answer Littman's survey.[9] She writes:

> Reasons for detransitioning were varied and included: experiencing discrimination (23.0%); becoming more comfortable identifying as their natal sex (60.0%); having concerns about potential medical complications from transitioning (49.0%); and coming to the view that their gender dysphoria was caused by something specific such

as trauma, abuse, or a mental health condition (38.0%). Homophobia or difficulty accepting themselves as lesbian, gay, or bisexual was expressed by 23.0% as a reason for transition and subsequent detransition. The majority (55.0%) felt that they did not receive an adequate evaluation from a doctor or mental health professional before starting transition.[10]

As already mentioned, a disproportionate number of gay people choose transgendering due to internalized homophobia. Considering the increase in films and TV programs depicting homosexuals and lesbians—along with the prevalence of "out" gays in the entertainment industry—one might assume a greater acceptance of this population in the larger culture. While statistics show that this is indeed the case, it doesn't help the sons and daughters who still suffer intense disapproval and shame from their own families. Results of a 2022 cross-sectional online survey of 237 detransitioners, most of them young women in the 17-to-24 age bracket, show "internalized homophobic and sexist prejudices" among both the males and females who detransitioned.

> A major lack of support was reported by the respondents [to her survey] overall, with a lot of negative experiences coming from medical and mental health systems and from the LGBT+ community....Many expressed a feeling of rejection and loss of support in relation to their decision to detransition, which lead them to step away from LGBT+ groups and communities....Most participants expressed strong difficulties finding the help that they needed during their detransition process."[11]

The study's author, Elie Vandenbussche, also quotes some of the responses from the survey respondents: "The LGBT+ community doesn't support detransitioners and I lost all LGBT+ friends I had because they deemed me transphobic/terfy. Only non-LGBT+ friends supported me." (*TERF* is an acronym for *trans exclusionary radical feminist*, intended to demean those who question the wisdom of body mutilation in the name of gender dysphoria.) "I lost a lot of support and attracted a lot of hostility from trans people when I detransitioned socially." "Telling my trans friends that I'm desisting is nearly impossible. The community is too toxic to allow any kind of discussion about alternatives to transition." "I have several de-trans friends whom [sic] had permanent body alterations they regretted that led to more dysphoria and eventually their suicides. Biggest factors were a lack of medical support and outright rejection from LGBT organisations/communities." "I still have transgender friends who don't want me to talk about detransition. They're okay with me being detransitioned, but they don't want me to criticize transition or discuss the negative side effects of HRT [hormone replacement therapy]." "I've been shunned by most of my trans identifying friends. I had to leave my old doctor, therapist and LGBT group out of shame and embarrassment." And, significantly, "Only lesbians and feminists helped me. The trans and queer community demonized me and ostracized me for my reidentification."[12]

Vandenbussche's respondents made a common error: commingling the LGB (lesbian-gay-bisexual) community with transgenders, resulting in LGBT etc. I want to emphasize that linking the two is a grievous error. Loving a member of your own sex is quite different from believing that you are a member of the opposite sex. But trans activists have been largely successful at commandeering the gay community for their own insidious purposes. Nevertheless, a respondent's comment that only lesbians and feminists were interested in helping her shows a split within the gay community. It's understandable that straight and gay feminist women—who have the most to gain by repudiating sex roles—would be the most horrified by someone mutilating their body to fit a gender stereotype. Not surprisingly, some gay men are not as sympathetic to detransitioners because generally speaking, male homosexuals as a group seem more invested in adhering to gender stereotypes that caricature women.

Medical treatment was difficult for detransitioners to obtain. Some comments from the people in Vandenbussche's survey indicated that "gender affirming" clinicians were outright hostile to detransitioners. They only "affirmed" them as long as the patients didn't want to present as their natal sex: "When I first brought up wanting to stop T [testosterone] to my doctor, they were very dismissive and condescending about it." "I had no medical help from the doctor who prescribed me T, she wanted nothing to do with me." Most medical personnel saw that their only job was to prescribe hormones and administer surgery. If there were unforeseen aftereffects, the patient was simply out of luck: "As soon as I 'detransed' I was discharged from all gender services, despite asking for help in dealing with sex dysphoria should it arise again." Someone else was told, "The team that transitioned you is not willing to help you detransition. You need new doctors." Even a serious medical complication was not addressed: "My hormone blocker implant is several years old and is only barely still functioning but they will not remove it. It's in my arm and I have no contact with the doctor because he shut down his business apparently." And detransitioners had mixed-result experiences with doctors outside the gender-"affirming" business: "I still struggle to find a doctor who has knowledge of detransition and the effects HRT had on me/my best course of action since stopping." Still another: "I needed gender and transition experienced providers to assist with my medical detransition, but none of them seemed to understand or provide the type of care I needed....I got better care from providers outside of the LGBT and transgender specialty clinics."[13]

Obtaining adequate mental health services was difficult as well. "The biggest issue for me was that when I did try to get support from a therapist or psychologist on [dis]entangling the actual reasons behind my dysphoria and how to deal with it, and deal with detransitioning, nobody had any clue or any experience, so they couldn't help me. Which made me even feel more lonely, and made detransitioning so much harder mentally than transitioning was." "Therapists are unprepared to handle the detrans narrative and some that I have seen since detransitioning have pushed the trans narrative," said another, adding, "Some therapists couldn't tell the difference between being transgender and having internalized misogyny and homophobia." With this kind of treatment, no wonder one of the respondents wrote, "My experience with transition left me with greatly diminished faith in medicine and zero faith in the mental health profession."[14]

More websites are springing up to accommodate detransitioners. They contain retrospective analyses from regretful detransitioners, along with reports from a few doctors who have learned that freely dispensing cross-sex hormones, especially to vulnerable youth, is a really bad idea. However, due to the trans infiltration of the medical field, it has been difficult to get researchers to examine the outcome of transitioning for children and adolescents—assuming that journals were even open to publishing their papers. Lisa Marchiano points out that "there are few studies examining adult outcomes for children who present as transgender; and those few studies indicate that the majority of pre-pubescent children who present as transgender eventually drop their trans identity and desist to their natal sex.... Many of the detransitioners I have spoken with...have cut ties completely with the transgender community, and certainly don't identify as trans."[15]

It's amazing how many scientists—or those who call themselves scientists—follow a mechanized paradigm in their approach to transgenderism. Instead of factoring in psychological, social, cultural and political issues, they measure hormone levels before and after death. They also try to find structures in the brain that they believe cause or contribute to transgenderism by doing MRIs on the brains of live subjects and dissecting their brains after they die. But considering the unnaturally massive doses of cross-sex hormones taken by a trans person, the initial "causes" are impossible to find. Also, the person's life experiences have already influenced brain structure and function. It's time to stop doing so much obsessive measuring in an attempt to micromanage every single life process, and let go of the need to control so people can naturally unfold.

Detransitioner Accounts

One of the first and most public detransitioners may be Walt Heyer. For years, he has written and spoken frankly about his unhappy childhood that propelled him to transition. Never having received love and acceptance from his parents, he did gain approval from his grandmother—but on condition that he wore a full-length purple dress that she sewed for him while hearing her say how pretty he was. Walt was taught that wearing clothing typically donned by girls was the equivalent of *being* a girl. "Being a girl," he said, "was where I got...adulation...I felt loved, cared for."[16] However, this mistreatment by his trusted grandmother unfortunately gave Walt's teenage uncle an excuse to sexually abuse him. As with many others who choose cross-sex hormones and surgery, it was a psychological trauma that induced Walt to try to escape his body and his past—his very self—by becoming someone else.

At age 40, Heyer was diagnosed with gender dysphoria. At age 42, he had his genitals removed and received fake breasts. A gender specialist told him it would take time to become accustomed to the changes, but he never did acclimate. After eight years of being "Laura," Walt had the breast implants removed and detransitioned. It was only then that he was diagnosed with psychological issues due to childhood trauma. "Emotionally," Heyer wrote, "I was a mess."

> But with grit and determination, and the love and support of several families and counselors, I pursued healing on a psychological level. With expert guidance, I dared to revisit the emotional trauma of my youth. It wasn't easy, but it was the only way to address the underlying conditions driving my gender dysphoria....
>
> In 1996, at the age of 55, I was finally free from the desire to live as a woman and changed my legal documents back to Walt, my biologically correct male sex. I still have scars on my chest, reminders of the gender detour that cost me 13 years of my life. I am on a hormone regimen to try to regulate a system that is permanently altered....Had I not been misled by media stories of sex change "success" and by medical practitioners who said transitioning was the answer to my problems, I wouldn't have suffered as I have. Genetics can't be changed. Feelings, however, can and do change. Underlying issues often drive the desire to escape one's life into another, and they need to be addressed before taking the radical step of transition.
>
> You will hear the media say, "Regret is rare." But they are not reading my inbox, which is full of messages from transgender individuals who want the life and body back that was taken from them by cross-sex hormones, surgery and living under a new identity.[17]

Heyer says that he still regrets how his poor choices adversely affected his ex-wife and his children. He remarried an understanding woman who didn't care about the changes to his body. Having devoted the rest of his life to helping others sort through their "gender confusion," he encourages them to get the mental health assistance they need.

******

In 2022, a 35-year-old biological male who called himself Tullip R wrote a heartbreaking account of his MtF transition and subsequent detransition:

> I want to tell everyone what they took from us, what irreversible really means, and what that reality looks like for us. No one told me any of what I'm going to tell you now.
>
> I have no sensation in my crotch region at all. You could stab me with a knife and I wouldn't know. The entire area is numb, like it's shell shocked and unable to comprehend what happened, even four years on. Years later, I have what looks like a chunk of missing flesh next to my neo-vagina, it literally looks like someone hacked at me.
>
> No one told me that the base area of your penis is left, it can't be removed—meaning you're left with a literal stump inside that

twitches. When you take testosterone and your libido returns, you wake up with morning wood, without the tree. I wish this was a joke. And if you do take testosterone after being post op, you run the risk of internal hair in the neo-vagina. Imagine dealing with internal hair growth after everything?

What a choice: be healthy on testosterone and a freak, or remain a sexless eunuch.

My sex drive died for about six months on hormone replacement therapy [estrogen flooding] and at the time I was glad to be rid of it, but now 10 years later, I'm realizing what I'm missing out on and what I won't get back. Because even if I had a sex drive, my neo vagina is so narrow and small, I wouldn't even be able to have sex if I wanted to. And when I do use a small dilator—which is like some sort of demonic ceremony where you impale yourself for 20 agonizing minutes to remind you of your own stupidity—I have random pockets of sensation that only seem to pick up pain, rather than pleasure. Any pleasure I do get comes from the prostate that was moved forward and wrapped in glands [he probably means "glans"] from the penis.

Then there's the dreams. I dream often, that I have both sets of genitals, in the dream I'm distressed I have both, why both I think? I tell myself to wake up because I know it's just a dream. And I awaken into a living nightmare. In those moments of amnesia as I would wake, I would reach down to my crotch area expecting something that was there for three decades, and it's not. My heart skips a beat, every single damn time.

Then there's the act of going to the toilet. It takes me about 10 minutes to empty my bladder, it's extremely slow, painful and because it dribbles no matter how much I relax. It will then just go all over that entire area, leaving me soaked. So after cleaning myself up, I will find moments later that my underwear is wet. No matter how much I wiped, it slowly drips out for the best part of an hour. I never knew at 35 [that] I ran the risk like smelling like piss everywhere I went.

During transition, I was obsessive and deeply unwell, I cannot believe they were allowed to do this to me, even after all the red flags. I wasn't even asked if I wanted to freeze sperm or wanted kids. In my obsessive, deeply unwell state they just nodded along and didn't tell me the realities, what life would be like.

Now I get to the point where I'm detransitioned, and the realization that this is permanent is catching up with me. This isn't even the half of it. And this isn't regret either, this is grief and anger. Fuck everyone who let this happen.[18]

******

On social media in 2022, a 24-year-old self-described "detrans male" who called himself Syb described his journey. He explained that the changes caused by testosterone "are upsetting and confusing to many young boys as they enter puberty, but most of them learn to cope with, and even appreciate, the changes that come to their body as they grow into adults. I didn't get that chance, and never will." As with so many young people, Syb made the decision during puberty to radically alter his body. But the original trauma had occurred years earlier. As a child, he had seen his mother being assaulted by a man and "didn't want to be like the man who'd done that to her. The idea of testosterone poisoning made sense to me because maleness itself terrified me."[19] Syb's fear of males increased after he was bullied and sexually abused for years by other boys in school. He was groped and touched in the butt and groin, and endured sexually explicit verbal comments. After that, he concluded that all males were evil and decided that because he was male, he was not acceptable—despite the fact that he himself was a sensitive and kind 14-year-old.

Still a loner at age 15, without friends, and after spending a great deal of time online, Syb was vulnerable to the overtures of trans activists. He described how the transgender community gave him a sense of purpose and belonging. "I wasn't mentally mature enough [to resist]," he posted. "Young boys will want to transition to escape the masculinity they're being told is harmful and toxic." Showing considerable insight and empathy, he continued, "while I can't speak with authority on the subject, I imagine young girls will want to transition to escape the violence they're being told is around every corner, in the eyes of every man who looks at them, and to access the power they're being told they're denied. These hyperbolic, oversimplified distortions of a complicated reality are neither healthy nor empowering, and hurt more than they help."[20] Syb was told what to say to parents and doctors to convince them to allow him to transition. Eventually, armed with transcripts provided by adult transgenders online, he threatened to commit suicide if he did not receive hormones and claimed he would buy them on the black market if no one helped him.

Puberty blockers were begun, and then at age 16 Syb started taking estrogen. At about age 20, he was castrated. "I saw the surgery as a rite of purification," he wrote. "I felt that by removing a part of myself I would become whole. Years of online grooming and ideological brainwashing had made me delusional, but no one pushed back on it." Now Syb must take testosterone for the rest of his life because his own gonads, which would have naturally supplied him with all the hormones he requires, were removed. His doctors never warned him about the phantom pains or intense cramping that he constantly experiences. He was eventually diagnosed with autism and OCD (obsessive-compulsive disorder), which are very different from gender dysphoria. "The end goal of transition isn't self-actualization," he concluded. "It's self-annihilation."[21]

******

Like Walt Heyer, detransitioner Chloe Cole had the courage to tell her story in a very public way because, she said, "I want to create a precedent for other people who have been in my situation to find justice themselves."[22] Cole has been frank about the pressure she'd always felt to be conventionally pretty. "Because my body didn't match beauty ideals, I started to wonder if there was something wrong with me. I thought I wasn't pretty enough to be a girl, so I'd be better off as a boy."[23] Ironically, Chloe looks very pretty in her many online photos and videos. But like most (if not all) girls, she has been bombarded her entire life with stereotypes of "beauty" that are impossible for human beings to live up to.

When Cole was just 13 years old, she was put on puberty blockers and testosterone. Two years later, both breasts were removed. In November 2022, at the age of 18, she notified an endocrinologist, plastic surgeon, psychiatrist, the Permanente Medical Group, Inc., and Kaiser Foundation Health Plan, Inc., of an impending lawsuit for malpractice. Doctors were propagating lies, the lawsuit read. Cole and her parents were "falsely informed" that her "gender dysphoria would not resolve unless Chloe socially and medical [sic] transitioned to appear more like a male." The girl and her parents were also falsely warned "that Chloe was at a high risk for suicide, unless she socially and medically transitioned"—despite the fact that "gender dysphoric individuals who undergo sex reassignment continue to have considerably higher risks for mortality, suicidal behavior, and psychiatric morbidity as compared with the general population. In other words, in a large number of cases, suicidality and psychiatric issues are not resolved by sex reassignment." Neither Cole nor her parents were told that she should receive "non-invasive psychological or psychiatric counseling or treatment" because in the vast majority of cases, gender dysphoria resolves on its own.[24] The "Ninety Day Notice of Intent to Sue," drafted by her lawyers, stated in part:

> This radical, off-label, and inadequately studied course of chemical and surgical "treatment" for Chloe's mental condition amounted to medical experimentation on Chloe. As occurs in most gender dysphoria cases, Chloe's psychological condition resolved on its own when she was close to reaching adulthood, and she no longer desires to identify as a male. Unfortunately, as a result of the so-called transgender "treatment" that Defendants performed on Chloe, she now has deep emotional wounds, severe regrets, and distrust for the medical system. Chloe has suffered physically, socially, neurologically, and psychologically. Among other harms, she has suffered mutilation to her body and lost social development with her peers at milestones that can never be reversed or regained.[25]

Prior to her gender "affirmation" indoctrination, Cole had received mental health diagnoses for ADHD and Disruptive Behavior Disorder. In November 2017, she visited an endocrinologist who advised her not to take cross-sex hormones because she was so young. However, one month later another endocrinologist (the one Cole eventually sued) gave her a prescription for Lupron. The drug caused the girl to develop an abnormally high red blood cell count, which puts people at risk for cardiovascular and coronary heart disease that could result in death.

Perhaps most of all, Chloe Cole mourned the loss of her breasts. "After my breasts were taken away from me, the tissue was incinerated—before I was able to legally drive," she wrote in the *New York Post* in July 2023. "I had a huge part of my future womanhood taken from me. I will never be able to breastfeed....I still struggle to this day with sexual dysfunction. And I have massive scars across my chest and the skin grafts that they used, that they took of my nipples, are weeping fluid today...The resulting menopausal-like hot flashes made focusing on school impossible...After surgery, my grades in school plummeted...I still get joint pains and weird pops in my back....Everything that I went through did nothing to address the underlying mental health issues that I had....I look in the mirror sometimes, and I feel like a monster."[26]

Cole first expressed regret to her doctor about her transition in May of 2021, around the time that she stopped taking testosterone. Now a well-known speaker, the young woman has been interviewed many times by sympathetic journalists. She has also taken part in many events, including "The Rally to End Child Mutilation." On July 27, 2023—her 19th birthday—Chloe Cole testified for Congress. In a passionately delivered speech, she stated in part:

> I used to believe that I was born in the wrong body and the adults in my life, whom I trusted, affirmed my belief; and this caused me lifelong, irreversible harm. I speak to you today as a victim of one of the biggest medical scandals in the history of the United States... I speak to you in the hope that you will have the courage to bring the scandal to an end, and ensure that other vulnerable teenagers, children and young adults don't go through what I went through....
>
> What message do I want to bring to American teenagers and their families? I didn't need to be lied to. I needed compassion. I needed to be loved. I needed to be given therapy to help me work through my issues—not affirming my delusion that by transforming into a boy, it would solve all my problems. We need to stop telling 12-year-olds that they are born wrong, that they are right to reject their own bodies and feel uncomfortable with their own skin. We need to stop telling children that puberty is an option—that they can choose what kind of puberty they will go through, just like they can choose what kind of clothes to wear or music to listen to. Puberty is a rite of passage to adulthood, not a disease to be mitigated. Today, I should be at home with my family, celebrating my 19th birthday. Instead, I am making a desperate plea to my elected representatives: Learn the lessons from other medical scandals like the opioid crisis. Recognize that doctors are human, too, and sometimes they are wrong. My childhood was ruined...[as was the childhood of] thousands of detransitioners that I know through our networks. This needs to stop! You alone can stop it. Enough children have already

been victimized by this barbaric pseudo-science. Please let me be your final warning.[27]

Not surprisingly, Cole has stated that the trans agenda that's so pervasive on social media was a huge influence in convincing her that she had been born the wrong sex. "I saw the unbelievable amounts of praise and attention that they got online," she told the Congressmembers, "and subconsciously, I yearned to have a piece of it. With every milestone of my medical transition, I was given more and more attention and celebration. It was the ultimate high."[28]

One indeed hopes that Chloe Cole will be our "final warning." Even if she's not, she is helping other girls with her willingness to come forward.

******

Layla Jane, diagnosed with social anxiety disorder, entered psychotherapy—but not before she took a puberty blocker and hormones and had her healthy breasts removed at the young age of 13. Shortly after Chloe Cole began preparing her lawsuit, Jane instituted a lawsuit of her own, accusing the medical professionals who had treated her of medical abuse driven by ideology and profit. Like so many girls, Jane had been influenced by the online trans community. Three ethical physicians turned down her request for cross-sex hormones before she found a trans-agenda doctor. Jane was prescribed the drugs after just one 75-minute session with a psychologist. The lawsuit pointed out that the defendants did not even question the girl or try to understand why she mistakenly believed that she was transgender, even though she presented emotional issues that were completely unrelated to her presumed gender dysphoria. Instead, the personnel who treated the 12-year-old were more than happy to dispense a prescription. Her lawyers pointed out that in no other area of medicine would doctors remove a healthy and functioning part of the body at the request of the patient.

"Nobody—none of my doctors—tried anything to make me comfortable in my body, or meaningfully pushed back or asked questions; they only affirmed," Jane said. She suffered nerve damage after the surgery, and says she's been happier since she detransitioned. "The law says children aren't mature enough to make serious decisions that could have long lasting consequences like getting a tattoo, driving with friends, drinking alcohol, smoking cigarettes, or even voting. So why is it acceptable for 13-year-olds to decide to mutilate their body?"[29]

Significantly, the defendants are the Kaiser Foundation Hospitals and the Kaiser Permanente Medical groups—the same facilities that had treated Chloe Cole—along with some of the staff who work there. "Kaiser continues to engage in the quackery of subjecting innocent children to irreversible sex mimicry treatment, including drugs and surgery, without informed consent," said one of the parties representing Jane. "The medical providers responsible for Layla's case, along with countless others, have substituted woke ideology for medically accepted standards of care, including lying to and manipulating vulnerable patients and families....[W]e intend to strongly deter Kaiser's factory-line approach that permanently mutilates an unknown number of American children, subjecting them to a lifetime of harm, regret, and medical consequences."[30]

******

Like so many preadolescent and adolescent girls, Helena Kerschner—who didn't have many friends and suffered from anxiety and depression—was vulnerable to the trans agenda. She especially struggled with body image issues, as her family's business was in the beauty industry. "I was going through a period where I was just really isolated at school, so I turned to the internet," the girl told a reporter after her detransition, confirming the phenomenon known as social contagion. "My dysphoria was definitely triggered by this online community. I never thought about my gender or had a problem with being a girl before going on Tumblr."[31]

In a 2022 interview with Ben Shapiro, Kerschner discussed how her loneliness—which caused her to spend hours on her newly acquired smart phone—exposed her to "gender and leftist woke ideology." Among other things, she was taught that "white people are evil, cis people are evil, straight people are evil." She was reassured that if she felt as though she didn't fit in, if she didn't like her body, or if other girls didn't understand her—typical problems for female teens—she was trans. She was advised that questioning her gender (biological sex) would help her "discover herself." And because she had questions, she was also told, this meant that she was trans, because only trans people ask questions. In order to fit in socially, Kerschner felt pressured to adopt these beliefs. A two-year journey began with changing her pronouns to male, for which she received lots of "positive affirmation."[32] Because Kerschner had a very distant relationship with her parents and they didn't talk to her very much, she was unable to turn to them for guidance or express her concerns to them.

After she turned 18, Kerschner announced to a very shocked mother that she was trans. Her mother, she explained, "shut down" after that, so Helena was on her own. She went to Planned Parenthood, talked to a social worker for about 20 minutes, and then a nurse practitioner for another 20 minutes. There was no medical screening or psychological diagnosis. Kerschner explained to Shapiro that she was diagnosed with an "endocrine disorder" rather than gender dysphoria—and solely on the basis of her having an unspecified "endocrine disorder," she was given a prescription for testosterone. The nurse practitioner suggested beginning with a low dose of testosterone. However, after Kerschner insisted that she needed more because she had large hips, she was given the maximum dose without question. It was five times the starting low dose and twice the amount of a typical dose.

The alarmingly high amount of testosterone affected Helena strongly. She experienced an overwhelmingly strong sex drive and was extremely "irritable." After a year, she was unable to feel most emotions, including sadness. When she did have an emotion, it was usually rage. "I just felt completely out of control of myself. I was spiraling down into...dysfunction," she recounted. "These rage attacks would get so bad that I just felt like I really had to externalize it. It's not that I wanted to hurt anybody, but when I would be overcome with this, I wanted to break something, hit something." Her female body clearly was not equipped to handle that abnormally high level of testosterone. "Completely unprepared for these feelings, I...ended up taking it out on myself....One of those times actually led to me having to go to the hospital...They checked me into a psychiatric unit." After being on testosterone for a year and a half, Kerschner realized that her transitioning was a mistake. "Part of my ability to desist from this ideology was the fact that I had stopped using the internet so much....Because my life was so dysfunctional, I just didn't feel like posting on social media anymore....Being separated from all of these social reinforcements...allowed me to think, and eventually come to the conclusion that I wasn't trans." Fortunately, Helena's light use of the internet shielded her from the disapproval that typically occurs when a member of the trans community detransitions. After she posted just once, so-called friends she had made in the trans community told her how "disgusting" she was and how "disappointed" they were in her. "There's this attitude in the trans community," Helena told Ben, "that if you question your transition, that makes you insane."[33]

When Kerschner was taking testosterone, none of the therapists she saw understood or recognized that some of her "extreme mental health symptoms" were due to the hormone. Fortunately, Kerschner had already gone through puberty. Unlike most other girls who take high doses of testosterone, there were no adverse medical effects that she could see, other than her episodes of rage.

> The trans ideology is a very authoritarian and manipulative ideology. Some describe it as a cult....
>
> I just don't know if there's anything I could say to a 13-year-old [girl to get her to reconsider]; they're just going to call me a fascist....My message usually goes out to parents...If you have a 13-, 14-year-old who's going through this...don't write it off as just...a phase they're going to grow out of...They will when they're in their 20s, but there's a lot of time in between 13 and 20, where there's so much manipulation...[and] dangers...So parents need to become informed, parents need to get in touch with other parents. [She refers parents to www.genspect.org.]
>
> I consider myself very, very, very lucky that I managed to escape this ideology and this medical system relatively unscathed. But many people my age can't say the same.[34]

Helena Kerschner's experience profoundly changed her. "I saw a montage of photos of me," she said to a reporter, "and when I saw how much my face changed and how unhappy I looked, I realized...I shouldn't have done it."[35]

******

Scott Newgent is a fully transitioned FtM transgender man who was born Kellie King. As a child, Kellie was a self-described "alpha," an athletic tomboy. As a woman, Kellie King was a well-functioning, dynamic sales executive. At one point she married and gave birth to three children. After her marriage she was in a lesbian relationship, which Newgent recounted later as being problematic because Kellie's very religious Catholic lover did not want to be identified as gay. The lover kept saying that if Kellie loved a woman, then she must be a man in a woman's body. So at age 42, Kellie became Scott, taking cross-sex hormones and also undergoing multiple surgeries.

Although technically Scott Newgent has not detransitioned—having had far too many surgeries and medical complications to go under the knife again—to say that Newgent has "huge regret" is an understatement.

> I endured medical complication after medical complication due to transgender healthcare. I lost everything I'd ever worked for: home, car, savings, career, wife, medical insurance, and most importantly my faith in myself and God. In a battle to survive, I went from ER [emergency room] to ER, trying to solve a mystery of why my health was failing. I learned firsthand the truth about how dangerous and perilous medical transition really is. I learned the hard way that if you get sick because of transgender health, you will witness physicians throwing their hands up and saying one of two things: 1) "transgender health is experimental, and I don't know what's wrong" or 2) "you need to go back to the physicians who hurt you in the first place."
>
> My medical complications have included seven surgeries, a pulmonary embolism, an induced stress heart attack, sepsis [life-threatening complication of infection], a 17-month recurring infection [because the surgeon used the wrong skin during a failed phalloplasty], 16 rounds of antibiotics, three weeks of daily IV antibiotics, arm reconstructive surgery [only partially successful], lung, heart and bladder damage [both permanent], insomnia, hallucinations [a result of the insomnia], PTSD [which caused Scott to stay indoors for a year], $1 million in medical expenses...All this, and yet I cannot sue the surgeon responsible—in part because there is no structured, tested or widely accepted baseline for transgender health care....[T]he bomb that ignited a fire within me was after I discovered the medical industry was pushing children to transition medically....I was middle-aged and a successful business sales executive. If I was intimidated, children and adolescents don't stand a chance.[36]

The bladder damage resulted from the slip of the surgeon's scalpel during surgery. At some point, all the hair from Scott's head fell out. In addition, Newgent has suffered frequent loss of consciousness due to pain—which resulted from hair on the inside of the urethra (caused by the tissues being moved around during surgery). In an opinion piece in *Newsweek* in 2021, Scott wrote, "Each counseling session and doctor's appointment amounted to one more push convincing me I could be cured of being born in the wrong body. The truth was that I didn't fit in as a dominant, aggressive, assertive lesbian. The dream of finally fitting in dangled like a carrot: The idea that I could fit in catapulted me to a time much like adolescence, with its drive for acceptance, inclusive peers and the fantasy of being normal." In the same *Newsweek* article, Newgent provided a list of "what I could not comprehend before transitioning and what I honestly believe no child is capable of consenting to." On the web where the article is republished, the conditions below are linked to medical papers.

- Decreased life expectancy
- Increased risk of premature death from heart attacks and pulmonary embolisms
- Bone damage
- Possible liver damage
- Increased mental health complications
- Increased chances of mood-syndrome symptoms
- Higher suicide rates than non-trans population
- 12 percent higher chance than non-trans population to develop symptoms of psychosis
- Chance of stunted brain development
- Much reduced chance for lifelong sexual pleasure
- Higher chance of sterility and infertility
- No improved mental health outcomes
- Not completely reversible[37]

Newgent has done a great deal to help people become aware of the dangers of the trans agenda. However, in my opinion, the view that transgendering is "not completely reversible" is unfortunately much too optimistic. I would say, "mostly *not* reversible." In the vast majority of cases, even six months on testosterone can permanently lower a female's voice so that she sounds like a male. Also, the "higher chance of sterility and infertility" that Newgent lists are for someone who transitions *after* puberty. Children who are given puberty blockers and cross-sex hormones before they mature will *never* be able to produce children. Nor will they be able to enjoy any of the sexual pleasure that transitioned adults might. However, Scott's graphic account of the physical and mental damage is correct (although fortunately, not every single trans person has had to endure quite as many botched surgeries and complications). Newgent's website is filled with information to help others make more informed decisions.

A very powerful and eloquent talk, given in November 2022, began with, "My name is Scott Newgent."

> I'm a lesbian, and I'm a trans man. I'm a person who underwent a massive amount of irreversible surgery, and cross sex hormones to create an illusion of a male for comfort. But I am still a woman, and I will always be a woman....
>
> Stop pushing puberty blockers, hormones and surgeries on children and youth. Stop telling kids they were born in the wrong body. They are just different. Different is okay. In fact, different is a superpower. The problem is, being different is not embraced during adolescence. It takes time to accept your differences.
>
> I wish I had embraced my differences earlier. If I had, I would not be standing here today in front of you, as a trans man, with my health destroyed....If the current rate of kids that are being transitioned continues, we're gonna have a whole generation of sterile human beings. And we will have turned a whole generation of children into medically induced lifelong patients without ever having one disease. If I as an adult couldn't resist the allure of the quick fix elixir, do you really think somebody can with an immature frontal lobe? Mental health, love, and compassion are what these children need, not hormones and knives. They need to be told that it is okay to be gay, autistic, mentally gifted, mentally ill, artistically gifted—that it's okay to be weird and different....
>
> Pediatricians, please help. Please don't accept children's invented gender identity. That is not compassionate care. Look at the casualties and why and what else is going on. Don't send kids to get hormone and surgeries. Let them hold on to their childhood and their health....
>
> My discovered purpose in life is to educate people that being unique is not a cause for medical intervention. But these children need people in their lives to help them embrace, accept, and love themselves for who they are, not a delusion of something they will never become.[38]

In addition to public speaking, Newgent works with lawmakers to help them write laws that will protect children from being medically transitioned. Newgent is also committed to helping prevent biological males (whether "transitioned" or not) from participating in sports intended for biological females. In response to accusations from trans activists, Newgent has bluntly stated, "I can't be called transphobic. I am transgender, but medically transitioning children is criminal. There is nothing to debate. It's wrong on every level."[39] A recent photo of Scott Newgent shows a tired, suffering human being with very little head hair and a sad face. There's a good reason that this photo is captioned with the words, "Becoming trans only ruined my life!"[40]

******

Transgenderism has become a highly visible, tantalizing and desirable product, marketed to and consumed by a naïve public. In the mainstream media, trans people are extolled for their courage in finding their "authentic selves." Being trans—or showing oneself to be an accommodating friend or family member of a trans person—garners praise from trans activists and the many media platforms that they control. Of the families who support and encourage the transgendering of their dependent and vulnerable children, I wonder how many have been influenced by the accolades and positive publicity given to them by trans activists and their trans-friendly media allies.

Fortunately, as more people awaken, we will be better able to protect our children. Sheila Jeffreys writes:

> [C]ritical voices do seem to be increasing in number and are likely, at length, to reach the critical mass needed to challenge this harmful practice. As more and more of those who have been transgendered seek help to de-transition and some have the courage to speak out, the quackery of the practice should become more apparent to those who treat them.[41]

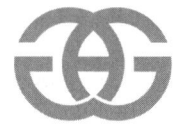

7

WHO'S BEHIND THE TRANS AGENDA

Transgendering is Expensive

Cross-sex hormones and sexual "reassignment" surgery are pricey. The costs of hormones vary, depending on the country in which one lives and whether or not insurance covers some of the debt; but most sources give a similar price range. The average year's supply of hormones is 1,500 dollars, although costs might be as high as 2,400 dollars. Gender "reassignment" genital surgery costs 30,000 dollars or more. Some insurance plans include this type of surgery, but not all do. Most people require more than one operation for the most convincing cosmetic results. Facial reconstruction can range from 25,000 to over 70,000 dollars. Breast augmentation or the removal of breasts can range from 5,000 or 10,000 dollars (the lowest figure) to 40,000 dollars. So-called miscellaneous services for males include laser hair removal and voice coaching. If the two years of psychotherapy before surgery rule is followed (which is rarely the case), there's an additional fee. Without the psychotherapy, in the United States the costs of all procedures are a minimum of 100,000 dollars.[1,2] A transgender person quoted in *Forbes* magazine states that the average price of transition is 150,000 dollars per person. "Multiply that by an estimated population of 1.4 million transgender people, we're taking [sic] about a market in excess of $200B [two hundred billion dollars]. That is significant. That's larger than the entire film industry."[3] FtM transgender Scott Newgent estimates 257,000 dollars for one person.[4] If a child is hooked before reaching puberty, Newgent calculates that over 1.3 billion dollars is spent in pharmaceuticals alone over that person's lifetime.[5]

An estimate for the sex "reassignment" surgery market shows a 24.5 percent compound annual growth rate (CAGR) from 2020 to 2026.[6] While sources vary slightly when discussing costs, they all agree on one thing: Transgendering is a huge, expensive, burgeoning market. And hospitals, clinics, and related facilities are making unimaginable sums of money from it.

The World Professional Association for Transgender Health, or WPATH, holds global dominion over transgender policy. For those who consider themselves transgender, transsexual or gender-nonconforming, its website advises (in 19 languages) what the standard of care should be, based on the most presumably expert medical discoveries and scientific consensus. The organization services and networks medical and mental health professionals, teachers, attorneys, public health officials, pharmacologists, language therapists, academicians, and students in those disciplines. It charges membership fees and accepts donations. "Many, if not most, US hospitals, clinics and private physicians and therapists base their practices on WPATH's SOC [standard of care]," writes psychiatrist Miriam Grossman—even though "its recommendations have been formally rejected by Sweden, Finland, Norway, and Britain and questioned by medical groups in France, Australia, and New Zealand....[W]hile presenting as an unbiased science-based medical group, it is in truth an advocacy organization run by activists who have an unwavering goal of affirmation at all costs."[7] WPATH is apparently funded by politicians, the pharmaceutical industry, and their allies.

The medical establishment has been largely responsible for creating new markets for hormones and surgeries. Originally, hormone replacement therapy (HRT) was intended for older women whose bodies after menopause no longer produce sufficient estrogen (or progesterone or testosterone). But because these drugs caused many unwanted effects—especially because the hormones were not bio-identical (and even then, they can still cause negative effects)—most older women avoided them. The market was shrinking. Then there was more lost income from genital surgeries, which had been performed mostly on children who possessed ambiguous genitalia (see Chapter 1). Doctors tried hard to convince parents that if the child's genitals deviated from their idea of normal, this constituted a "deformity" that would later cause unbearable suffering to the child. The problem was, from the medical establishment's point of view, there weren't enough children who "needed" such surgeries. Who could provide a larger pool of subjects—and give doctors more opportunities to experiment?

Enter the gay community, which was becoming more visible. Not all gay men were effeminate, of course—but those who displayed the most exaggerated female-stereotyped behavior possible made promising targets. Very masculine-behaving lesbians were good targets as well—it was simply not appropriate for women to be strong and assertive; that was a man's department. Feminine men must really be women, just as masculine women must really be men. Individuals who were the least "gender-conforming" were a new, and much larger, market that could benefit from "corrective" surgery. Change the sex—or rather, the *appearance* of sex—of one person in a gay couple, and produce an acceptable heterosexual pair. Surgeons presented themselves as allies who helped fix innate flaws of biology, rather than as members of an industry eager to cash in on the latest fad of compulsory gender stereotyping. Was someone unable to adequately adjust to their stereotype? No problem! He or she could always have their genitals, along with other parts of their body, altered. The drive to radically alter the body through invasive surgery was a logical accompaniment to popping a pill.

Everyone on cross-sex hormones must take them for life (though alas, Big Pharma missed its chance to put anyone older than 13 on puberty blockers). The ones who benefit from this highly profitable scam are the gender "reassignment" clinics, hospitals, surgeons, physicians, nurses, anesthesiologists, trans-influenced psychologists and psychiatrists, and manufacturers of hormones and other drugs. It's quite a nice little racket: *Fix whatever ails you with pills and surgery.*

Drugging children with powerful hormones that permanently alter their minds and bodies is neither assistance nor affirmation—it's child abuse, and a massive human rights violation. Convincing people that they're not acceptable simply because they love members of their own sex is cruel and wrong. Persuading people that they're less worthy because they don't want to be limited by gender stereotypes is also cruel and wrong. Doctors and surgeons who choose to earn a living by operating on misguided individuals are engaging in professional misconduct and should have their licenses revoked. It's time we prosecuted those who benefit from pathologizing normal development and normalizing pathology.

The trans agenda has not just infiltrated medicine. Let's see where else it lurks.

Bombardment from All Sides

Besides the medical industry, many other businesses and individuals are involved in the transgendering business: banks, politicians, even international law firms. Just a few corporations that have contributed financially to bills for transgender "rights" are Apple, Yelp, Microsoft, PayPal, IBM, Salesforce, Box, and Google.[8]

Investments from elite donors, writes investigative journalist Jennifer Bilek, "go toward creating new SSI [synthetic sex identities] using surgeries and drugs, and by instituting rapid language reforms to prop up these new identities and induce institutions and individuals to normalize them…even as it ignores the biological reality of 'male' and 'female' and 'gay' and 'straight.'"[9] Many politicians, educational institutions from grammar schools to universities, and companies that sell food, clothing and other items, are either actively embracing trans indoctrination or allowing themselves to be coerced into accepting it (for fear of not receiving needed business loans from trans-friendly banks). Mainstream media, including television, films, print and internet, are owned by transgender allies. Hence the positive spin to transitioning, no matter who it harms—and an accusation of transphobia if someone simply questions if a gender dysphoria diagnosis applies. Here are just a few ways in which the trans agenda has insinuated itself into our lives.

♦ Social media plays a huge role in convincing young people, especially girls, that transitioning will solve all their problems. Trans people on the internet, known as "influencers," routinely advise adolescents what to say so they'll be given prescriptions. To be trans, Abigail Shrier observes, is no longer a psychological condition; it's "an important social identity, over and above (and even without) the psychiatric condition once thought to undergird it."

> Trans influencers typically promote trans as a lifestyle to celebrate, not the result of a malady they hope to cure....Understood this way, trans is something you might want to become even if you aren't suffering gender dysphoria. Then again, many influencers define "dysphoria" so broadly that nearly every teen would seem to have it....Trans influencers describe symptoms that are vague and ubiquitous: *feeling different, not really fitting in, and not feeling feminine or masculine enough. And this one: ever feeling uncomfortable in your body*....[Influencers say] "So if you're asking the question, 'Am I trans?' the answer is probably yes."[10]

Who *doesn't* feel uncomfortable in their body at some point in their life? And since when does merely asking a question guarantee an affirmative answer? Appropriating the narrative is a common ploy of any totalitarian agenda, and trans activists do it well. It needs to be seen for what it is—a ploy, rather than reality.

In a July 2023 interview, Ash Eskridge told a reporter how, at age 12, she was so depressed that she "leaned on the virtual platform [Tiktok] as an emotional crutch....I saw TikTok videos by influencers saying how...transitioning saved their life....Being transgender is definitely a TikTok trend...I notice that the demographic it most affects is teen girls around 12 to 14, as they're the most vulnerable since they aren't matured yet." Eskridge added that she had always been very "girly" and had never indicated any dislike of being a girl. Nevertheless, she had an appointment with a doctor who didn't deal with her mental and emotional issues, but readily supplied hormones. At age 16, she cut her hair short and began testosterone. This lowered her voice and caused body hair to grow. The drastic changes, rather than helping her feel "affirmed," made her feel "unnatural."Afterwards, Eskridge spiraled into drugs, self-harm, and suicidal ideation. "I assumed this was because I wasn't male enough," she reflected, "but it was really because I wasn't a male at all." In April 2023, Eskridge detransitioned. "After I detransitioned, I lost a lot of friends," she said[11]—which wasn't surprising, considering that those online "friends" consisted of people who are enslaved to ideology that isn't kind to defectors. Eskridge now advocates for better mental health care for teenagers, as well as laws that will prevent children under age 18 from receiving cross-sex hormones.

Thousands of teenagers spend long hours on social media as Eskridge did. When parents take away their phones and computers—or supervise the content watched and the amount of time spent—they're less susceptible to being duped.

♦ Drag queens are being invited by grammar schools, libraries, bookstores, community centers, daycare centers, and other venues to perform and read to young children during "story hour." The Drag Story Hour (DSH) website states, "DSH captures the imagination and play of the gender fluidity of childhood and gives kids glamorous, positive, and unabashedly queer role models....[K]ids are able to see people who defy rigid gender restrictions and imagine a world where everyone can be their authentic selves!"[12]

If *queer* simply meant breaking free of gender stereotypes so we could lead more fulfilling lives, this would be welcomed. But costumes and behaviors in these shows are based on the most extreme stereotypes imaginable. Moreover, as Christopher Rufo discloses, from its inception the drag culture was intended to embrace perversions that include incest and bestiality; and whether people in drag were gay or straight was incidental. Note that drag shows marketed exclusively to adults are considered entertainment, and not all of them embrace perversions. But many drag performers themselves acknowledge their unsuitability for children. In Rufo's article, "The Real Story Behind Drag Queen Story Hour," he writes that the purpose of drag was originally intended *not* solely or even primarily to challenge gender stereotypes, but to undermine

> traditional notions of sexuality, replacing the biological family with the ideological family, and arousing transgressive sexual desires in young children [through graphic depictions that often involve violence and drugs]....The philosophical and political project of queer theory has always been to dethrone traditional heterosexual culture and elevate what [early drag proponent Gayle S.] Rubin called the "sexual caste" at the bottom of the hierarchy: the transsexual, the transvestite, the fetishist, the sadomasochist, the prostitute, the porn star, and the pedophile. Drag Queen Story Hour can attempt to sanitize the routines and run criminal background checks on its performers, but the subculture of queer theory will always attract men who want to follow the ideology to its conclusions....While many of Drag Queen Story Hour's defenders claim that these programs are designed to foster LGBTQ "acceptance" and "inclusion," [drag manifesto writers] Kornstein and Keenan explicitly dismiss those objectives as mere "marketing language" that provides cover for their real agenda.[13]

The "real agenda" is not pretty. As unapologetically admitted by Kornstein and Keenan, "Though DQSH [Drag Queen Story Hour, renamed Drag Story Hour or DSH] publicly positions [itself to]...'help children develop empathy, learn about gender diversity and difference, and tap into their own creativity,' we argue that its contributions can run deeper than morals and role models.... DQSH may be incentivized to recite lines about alignment with curricular standards and social-emotional learning in order to be legible within public education and philanthropic institutions. Drag itself ultimately does not take these utilitarian aims too seriously (but it is quite good at looking the part when necessary)." In other words, Rufo clarifies, "Drag Queen Story Hour has learned the dance of operating a cash-flow-positive activist organization, winning government contracts, and securing access to audiences, while providing a plausible rhetorical defense against parents who might question the wisdom of adult men creating...'queer pleasure' with their children."[14]

In case one still might want to place the same-sex attracted in the same category as drag queens and transgenders, the drag manifesto writers state that "queer and trans pedagogies seek to actively destabilize the normative function of schooling...*This is a fundamentally different orientation than movements towards the inclusion or assimilation of LGBT people into the existing structures of school and society.*" [italics added][15] Put another way, the radical fringe that embraces these "transgressive" drag queens is promoting sexual abuse, not opposite-sex or even same-sex love.

With our understanding of drag's original purpose, it's not difficult to guess the intent of those involved with DSH performances that are designated "family friendly." In Tucson, Arizona, a high school counselor who had organized a drag show was arrested in May 2022 for having a sexual relationship with a 15-year-old girl.[16] Another drag queen who performed in front of children in Pennsylvania was charged with 25 counts of child sexual abuse media possession.[17] At the Houston Public Library in 2019, *two* story hour performers were registered sex offenders. One man was a 32-year-old who had been convicted of assaulting an 8-year-old boy. The other had been convicted of multiple sexual assaults against four children (ages four, five, six and eight) and was registered as "high risk."[18] The Houston Library apologized for not having completed a background check on its story hour performers, but the library has no intention of discontinuing the program.[19]

Even if a background check is done and the individual doesn't have a record, the kind of person who's attracted to this kind of "entertainment" obviously resonates with it—so there's no guarantee that sexual indiscretions won't occur in the future. Some people affiliated with story hour are in political office. Judge Brett Blomme, who presided over Children's Court in Milwaukee, Wisconsin, was also president of Cream City Foundation, which hosted what was then called DQSH. In 2021, Blomme was charged with possession of child pornography depicting the sexual abuse of toddlers and underage boys.[20] (He and his partner had two adopted children, but I could not find information on whether or not the children had been sexually abused.) The judge was eventually arrested, pled guilty to federal charges of distributing child pornography, and was sentenced to prison for nine years, after which he was put on supervised release for two decades.[21]

What happens during such shows? In September 2022, during Pride Youth Day in Chattanooga, Tennessee, the Wanderlinger Brewing Company hosted a drag queen event. As part of the entertainment, young children went up on stage with the performers. A video on Twitter clearly showed a girl about four or five years old stroking the genitals of a man dressed as a mermaid. He stood still and did nothing to stop her. The video clip also shows the men spreading their legs for the children, wearing just thongs beneath their dresses.[22] Another storytelling event in February 2023, held at the Honor Oak Pub in South London, England, was specifically promoted as catering to infants age two and under as well as their parents. One male performer wore bondage gear, tight shorts, and stiletto heels. The show, called Cabababarave, removed its social media pages from public view after it received protests about the controversial footage that someone released.

These shows consist of more than singing and dancing in costume. Their explicitly sexual content is clearly intended to excite children before they are biologically and emotionally ready. Simulating adult-child sex under the guise of entertainment makes inappropriate behavior seem normal. This ensures that children will be more open to being sexually preyed upon later. Such events also cause children to develop a distorted idea of what healthy relationships are about. Yet popular media often puts a positive spin on these spectacles. "The performers," wrote a *Rolling Stone* reporter, "entertain and delight children while introducing them to new types of people and teaching them acceptance and inclusion through storybooks." The article claimed that the political right wing, by targeting the drag community, was not only demonstrating "transphobia" but also "homophobia…[about] all things LGBTQ."[23] But the reporter who associated these drag queens and shows with the gay community might be surprised to learn that most homosexuals and lesbians want nothing to do with them. Drag queens, pornography, and sexual perversions are totally unrelated to sexual orientation, which simply means the sex to whom one is attracted. Committed to having loving relationships and families, most gays are against the sexualization of children, which is also known as grooming.

Simply put, *grooming*—when used in a sexual context—is a strategically employed set of behaviors to establish an emotional connection with a child, and sometimes the child's family, to prepare the child for eventual sexual abuse. A typical child molester identifies a vulnerable child, someone who feels lonely or misunderstood. Rather than making threats or stalking, the groomer is friendly to the child and makes him or her feel special. Sometimes activities are planned so they are alone together. Buying food and presents and playing games is also part of the grooming process. If the child feels disappointed or hurt by parents or friends, the predator is always willing to listen and provide comfort. That "comfort" leads to touching, which the predator tells the child is "our little secret." By this time the child may be confused and frightened, but usually doesn't tell parents or another authority figure due to guilt, shame, or some other feeling.[24] Drag shows with children in the audience are a relatively new phenomenon, and the grooming process is somewhat different, couched in a spectacle of public entertainment. But the goal of all grooming is similar: to acclimate the child to being sexually abused through the normalization of behavior that is sexually manipulative. Drag grooming sexualizes not only children but also their parents—adults who either don't want to be viewed as intolerant, or who themselves are so sexually titillated by such events that they lack the ability to protect their children. If parents believe that drag shows are innocent childhood entertainment, this makes it much easier to train their children to become sexual objects in the future—all in the name of "tolerance" and "gender affirmation."

The "about" page of the Gays Against Groomers website states clearly and emphatically that they are *not* aligned with "all things LGBTQ."

> Gays Against Groomers is a 501(c)4 organization of gay people who oppose the recent trend of indoctrinating, sexualizing and… transitioning and medicalization of minors…under the guise of "LGBTQIA+."…[We also oppose] drag queen story hours, drag shows involving children…and gender [radical queer] theory being taught in the classroom….Our community that once preached love and acceptance of others has been hijacked by radical activists who are now pushing extreme concepts onto society, specifically targeting children in recent years.
>
> The overwhelming majority of gay people are against what the community has transformed into, and we do not accept the political movement pushing their agenda in our name….
>
> The activists, backed by school boards, government, woke media, and corporations, have been speaking on our behalf for too long. When fighting for equality, our goal was to successfully integrate ourselves into society, but now these radicals aim to restructure it entirely in order to accommodate a fringe minority [and]…indoctrinate children into their ideology.
>
> We're saying *no*.[25]

♦ Some branches of the United States military are periodically embracing drag queens. The Navy, according to Yeoman 2nd Class Joshua Kelley, invited him to become the first "Navy Digital Ambassador." In a social media post, he described his journey that began in 2018 when he performed on deck. He was now becoming a "leader" and "advocate" of people who "were oppressed for years in the service," he declared. Matthew Lohmeier, former commander of the 11th Space Warning Squadron in Colorado, commented, "I have to wonder who it is that our senior military leaders…think they're appealing to in the recruiting process by hiring a drag queen as their digital ambassador…What's surprising is that senior military leaders continue to push an agenda like this despite the fact that it's hurting our recruiting efforts and it's hurting our retention"[26]—not to mention the ability to actually do their jobs, which is to defend the United States in case of attack. A strong military presence is critical, especially when faced with international tensions. One must question the motives of those in charge who are promoting trans and drag visibility in the U.S. armed forces.

- Companies and stores are featuring ads, displays, and products that cater to the trans and drag queen communities. In spring of 2023, in honor of gay pride, the box store Target featured displays that included clothing with slogans aimed at children and adults. Corporate management donated 100,000 dollars to the Gay, Lesbian, Straight Education Network (GLSEN), which offers lesson plans on "gender-neutral pronouns" for elementary school children as well as gender ideology lessons aimed at third graders.[27] Another questionable marketing decision involved North Face, which sells camping and other outdoor gear. It released a TV ad with a drag queen telling children to just "come out!"[28] And in the spring of 2023 Anheuser-Busch, which manufactures Budweiser beer, made a huge mistake by hiring flamboyant MtF Dylan Mulvaney to be the spokesperson for Bud Light. Within weeks Bud Light beer dropped in sales by 28%, and the stock of what had been one of Budweiser's best sellers fell dramatically by 17%. During that same time period, the sales of rival beers rose.[29] Unfortunately, an unforeseen consequence resulted from the boycott: An estimated 645 employees at the Ardagh Group—a glass container manufacturer that had been supplying Anheuser-Busch with bottles for Bud Lite and Budweiser—lost their jobs when two plants in North Carolina and Louisiana had to close due to the decline in Budweiser beer sales.[30]

These are only several examples of how the trans agenda has influenced our lives. The influx of trans athletes in sports, particulary women's sports, is discussed in detail in Appendix B. In the meantime, let's take a look at some individuals and organizations that are funding this agenda.

Politics in Our Pants

Many transgender people simply want to live their lives and be left alone. After all, who wants to be constantly scrutinized as "that person who used to be in the wrong body," and have people wonder what they looked like before their transition? Transgender *activists*, on the other hand, do their best to be as newsworthily aggressive as possible. This supports their practice of sexualizing young children at an early age and grooming them for continued abuse later.

It took at least a century for lesbians and gay men to become accepted in mainstream culture and receive legal protections. So why has it taken less than one decade for transgenders to be so enthusiastically embraced and promoted? Someone must be providing financial and other support to this small but in-your-face minority. How else could such a minority population commandeer the country at such speed?

One billionaire who has funneled vast sums of money to the transgender cause, through the Open Society Foundations (OSF) he set up, is George Soros. According to "An Essential Legal Right for Trans People" on the OSF website, "Trans people use many labels to identify their experience with gender, embracing the diverse nature of identity. Trans people can therefore be male, female, nonbinary (gender identities that are not exclusively masculine or feminine), gender nonconforming (expressing and/or behaving outside of existing gender norms), or they may choose to reject any of these labels."[31] Oxford University sociology professor Michael Biggs writes that as far back as 2011, over a period of two years the OSF donated 3.19 million dollars to trans-influenced organizations. Moreover, "Three million dollars on trans issues is a tiny fraction of OSF's total expenditure, merely 0.3%."[32] Jon Stryker, who inherited his family's fortune from the sale of medical devices, set up the Arcus Foundation to disseminate huge amounts to the trans cause as well.[33]

One unexpected donor to the trans cause is the Black Lives Matter Global Network Foundation, Inc. In the recent documentary *The Greatest Lie Ever Sold*, political commentator Candace Owens confirmed that the organization had collected 80 million dollars, according to its filing with the Internal Revenue Service (the public document was shown onscreen). The money had not been given to or invested in black communities. Instead, 2.6 million dollars were donated to transgender organizations, just a few of which are the Trans Justice Funding Project, Transgender Law Center, Black Trans Media, Trans United Fund, and Transgender Advocates Knowledgeable Empowering (TAKE). A Gays Against Groomers journalist, reviewing the documentary, writes, "As Owens takes viewers through the extensive list, she wonders how these donations are meant to contribute to the advancement of Black America. We were also interested in asking whether these organizations promote childhood transition—and they do. Every single one."[34] In the documentary, Owens informs us that an additional 200,000 dollars "went to escorts, BDSM [bondage and discipline, sadism and masochism] workers, strippers, peep show workers, phone sex operators, and webcam performers."[35] Lest Owens be accused of racism, note that she is black.

Other well-known donors funding the trans movement are members of the Pritzker family, who made their fortune in the Hyatt hotel chain and insinuated themselves into powerful political positions in the U.S. One Pritzker is a former U.S. Secretary of Commerce. Another is currently the highly influential governor of Illinois. The driving force behind the sex "reassignment" mutilations could only be Jennifer Pritzker, born James, who had been a lieutenant colonel in the Illinois Army National Guard and fathered three children before transitioning. It's no coincidence that at the time gender ideology exploded in mainstream culture's consciousness, James became Jennifer. Clan members "appear to have used a family philanthropic apparatus to drive an ideology and practice of disembodiment into our medical, legal, cultural, and educational institutions," writes Jennifer Bilek. Recipients of Pritzker money constitute a very long list. They include Howard Brown Health and Rush Memorial Medical Center in Chicago, the University of Minnesota's Institute for Sexual and Gender Health, the University of Arkansas for Medical Sciences Foundation Fund, the Human Rights Campaign Foundation, the Williams Institute UCLA School of Law, the National Center for Transgender Equality, the Transgender Legal Defense and Education Fund, the Gender & Sex

Development Program at Lurie Children's Hospital in Chicago, the American Civil Liberties Union, the Palm Military Center, the University of Minnesota National Center for Gender Spectrum Health, University of Toronto's Bonham Centre for Sexual Diversity Studies, the radical trans activist group WPATH (World Professional Association for Transgender Health), and the Los Angeles-based Ronald Reagan Medical Center at the University of California, whose Department of Obstetrics and Gynecology pitches "gender-affirming care"—in other words, breast removal—to females "who think they can be men."[36]

The amounts of money given to support the trans agenda are almost unimaginable. Back in 1968, in Illinois alone—a state that heavily promotes "gender-affirming care"—the Pritzkers donated 12 million dollars to the University of Chicago School of Medicine. In June 2002, an additional gift of 30 million was given to the University of Chicago's Biological Sciences Division and School of Medicine. According to Bilek, there is also ongoing "research on developments in the field of early childhood education, to which the [Pritzker Family] foundation committed $25 million."[37]

Rarely is a donation (which we call "philanthropy") given without something expected in return—be it a name on a building or a dividend from what's really a business investment. The Pritzker family is no exception to this practice. "Tawani Enterprises," Bilek informs us, "the private investment counterpart to the philanthropic foundation, invests in and partners with Squadron Capital LLC, a Chicago-based private investment vehicle that acquires a number of medical device companies that manufacture instruments, implants, cutting tools, and injection molded plastic products for use in surgeries....it is hard to avoid the impression of complementarity between Jennifer Pritzker's for-profit medical investments and philanthropic support for SSI [synthetic sex identities]."[38]

The marriage of politics and education is likewise entangled. In August 2021, Governor Pritzker of Illinois signed a sex education bill for all public schools in the state. The sex education course was designed to align with the second edition of the *National Sex Education Standards* or *NES*, which is used in all sex ed classes for children up to grade twelve. By the end of fifth grade, 10- and 11-year-olds will have been taught about sexual orientation and gender. By the end of eighth grade, students will have learned about anal sex as well as "a range of identities related to sexual orientation," including "two-spirit, asexual, [and] pansexual."[39] The manual does contain some helpful information in the lesson plan for teachers—such as (this is for tenth-graders) "Explain why a victim/survivor in interpersonal violence, including sexual violence, is never to blame for the actions of the perpetrator" and "Explain sex trafficking, including recruitment tactics that sex traffickers/exploiters use to exploit vulnerabilities and recruit youth."[40] However, in view of the manual's agenda—which is heavily exploitive of children—the tips that seem designed to help protect them from that very exploitation seem to be included only to deliberately mislead. By Bilek's count, in the 72-page manual the phrase "anal sex" appears 10 times, the word "gender" 270 times, and the word "intimacy" a mere five times. "The *NES* manual," writes Bilek, "was crafted by The Future of Sex Education Initiative (FoSE)...[whose] credo is that 'not only are younger children able to discuss sexuality-related issues but that the early grades may, in fact, be the best time to introduce topics related to sexual orientation, gender identity and expression, gender equality, and social justice related to the LGBTQ community before hetero- and cisnormative [biological sex] values and assumptions become more deeply ingrained and less mutable.'"[41]

The *NES* manual was funded by the Grove Foundation, Bilek discloses, which has worked with David and Lucile Packard Foundation (of the Hewlett-Packard fortune)—which, in turn, hired the same Bridgespan Group that in 2012 helped the Pritzkers disseminate their funds. The web gets even more tangled. UCLA training psychologist Jeanne Pritzker and her husband established a scholarship fund for medical students at the David Geffen School of Medicine, which is affiliated with a children's hospital named after the toy company Mattel. In 2022, Mattel introduced the first transgender Barbie, modeled after MtF trans actor Laverne Cox. (Cox has an identical twin brother who is gay and did not transition.) Jennifer Pritzker gave money to the University of Toronto's Bonham Centre for Sexual Diversity Studies. Transgender studies professor Nicholas Matte, an instructor at the Bonham Centre, is also the curator of its Sexual Representation Collection which houses a massive number of pornographic books, magazines, and films.

The arenas into which the trans agenda has insinuated itself seem unlimited. Yet the connections listed here between politicians, businesses, medical facilities, educational institutions, and media outlets, are just the tip of the iceberg. It's difficult to say where this agenda is *not*.

Transhumanism, a Step Up

There's one more important piece of the transgender scheme: a different kind of trans, known as *transhumanism*. The stated philosophy of transhumanists is to triumph over disease, ostensible biological imperfections, and even death. These victories will be accomplished, it is claimed, by enhancing human intellect and physiology. To provide such enhancements, transhumanists suggest implanting artificial intelligence and other technologies into living biological tissue—*us*. Various human-technology interfaces, meant to be widely available, involve implantable computer chips to simulate neurological functions, injectable nanotechnology to manipulate organs and other tissues including the brain, gene splicing to weed out so-called undesirable traits, and drugs that would not only regulate mood but also modify personality. One transhumanist idea to prolong an individual's lifespan is to upload that person's consciousness—or what is believed to be someone's consciousness—into a computerized robot. While this latter task sounds very much like science fiction, some scientists are actually working now to make it happen. As for the other technologies, they already exist.

Cloning is also on the transhumanist agenda. "It is often right to tamper with nature...[and] it doesn't matter whether human clones are natural or not," states a website devoted to transhumanism. It extols using "technological means that will eventually enable us to move beyond what some would think of as 'human.'...Some of the prospects that used to be the exclusive thunder of the religious institutions, such as very long lifespan, unfading bliss, and godlike intelligence, are being discussed by transhumanists as hypothetical future engineering achievements."[42] And, in a particularly sneaky language manipulation, "The important thing is not to be human but to be humane."[43] *The Guardian* reports that "adherents of transhumanism envisage a day when humans will free themselves of all corporeal restraints....when biotechnology will enable a union between humans and genuinely intelligent computers and AI [artificial intelligence] systems."[44] With this kind of engineering available—which, by the way, sounds ominously like the Borg in Star Trek—the soulful, evolving, autonomous human that many of us are still striving to become would be a thing of the past. The power involved in being able to control and transform human beings to this extent is mind-blowing.

Despite claims that transhumanists are technologizing humanity for its betterment and happiness, the intense amount of manipulation required to create, install, and integrate all that technology belies those claims. So does the word "transhumanism" itself. *Trans* is derived from Latin and means "across," "beyond," "through," "on the other side of," "to go beyond."[45] *Humanism* is a philosophy of life that "affirms our ability and responsibility to lead ethical lives of personal fulfillment that aspire to the greater good," and which "considers the welfare of humankind...to be of paramount importance." Therefore, a *humanist* is someone who's devoted to "the welfare of humankind."[46] When the two concepts are cobbled together, the word "*trans*humanist" designates someone whose intention is "beyond the welfare of humankind" or "through the welfare of humankind"—in other words, *bypassing* the welfare of humans! The philosophy of humanism also excludes any form of spirituality and it specifically disavows God. To some, it also suggests socialism.

Transhumanism is similar to its crude bioengineering precursor, the surgical act of transgendering—only on a much more high-tech scale. The difference is really only one of degree. Both use similar linguistics, share the same personnel, and—this is really important—*transhumanists are telling us clearly what their intentions are.* Jennifer Pritzker had created the first chair in transgender studies at the University of Victoria in British Columbia, Canada. The current chair established an annual conference, Moving Trans History Forward. Thanks to Jennifer Bilek's efforts to connect the dots, we know that in 2016, the keynote speaker was transhumanist Martine Rothblatt. Rothblatt, who is also a MtF transgender, was mentored by fellow transhumanist Ray Kurzweil. Kurzweil (known for inventing early electronic keyboard instruments beloved by musicians) is also an expert in computers. When he was working for Google he studied artificial intelligence, including how to interface AI with humans. At that

2016 conference, Bilek informs us, Rothblatt, who "is an integral presence at Out Leadership, a business networking arm of the LGBTQ+ movement...lectured on the value of creating an organization such as WPATH to serve 'tech transgenders' *in the cultivation of 'tech transhumanists.'*" [italics added][47]

Elon Musk, the controversial owner of the social media site Twitter (recently renamed X), also loves AI. He has stated his desire "to achieve a symbiosis [intimate, prolonged association] with artificial intelligence" to such an extent that technology will allow for the "merging" of AI with humans. Musk's company Neuralink has already invented flexible threads, thinner than a human hair, that once implanted into a human brain will allow the person to control their phone or computer with their thoughts.[48] In January 2024, Musk announced that a chip was installed in a human being for the first time. The noble rationale for such technology—to help people "who have lost the use of their limbs"[49]—is belied by a much more sinister agenda.

In an interview, Rothblatt once said, "For us God is in-the-making by our collective efforts to make technology ever more omnipresent, omnipotent and ethical. When we can joyfully all experience techno immortality, then God is complete."[50] When transhumanists mention God at all, it's only in association with technology and the power we can wield by using it. Transcendence, spiritual connection, or even earthly love are never mentioned. Yet another article states, "We are making God as we are implementing technology that is ever more all-knowing, ever-present, all-powerful and beneficent. Geoethical nanotechnology will ultimately connect all consciousness and control the cosmos."[51] The desire, not to mention the ability, to completely transform the human body in such a drastic way reveals an eerie pathological hunger for power. Transhumanists not only want to play God, they want to *be* God—by creating and employing the most unnatural of technologies. What does that indicate about their desire to totally control the rest of us?

Laura Aboli, an expert in finance and interior design, was happy to stay at home with her children but became a public speaker after seeing how people's livelihoods, civil rights, and mental health were being affected by worldwide lockdowns blamed solely on a virus. In May 2020, she founded the United Democratic international Movement for Awareness and Freedom (UDIMAF). During one of her lectures, she stated in part:

> The final goal [of those in power] is to eradicate humanity as we know it. Once you understand the final destination, it becomes much easier to look back and identify the psychological conditioning, the biological tampering, the cultural grooming and the educational prepping that we have been subjected to for decades in preparation to making us accept a post-human future. For this, they first needed to destabilize, dehumanize, and demoralize humanity through every means possible. The destruction of the nuclear family; children being indoctrinated by the state; abortion; the eradication

of God and spirituality from education; life in megacities and away from nature; toxic food, air and water; social media replacing real human connection and interaction; engineered financial crisis and taxation; endless wars and massive migration; stress, anxiety [and] depression; drugs and alcohol; constant fear-mongering; moral relativism as the new religion.

A weak, immoral, disconnected, ignorant, and unhealthy population is an easy target...Masculinity is under attack, psychological, culturally and biologically. Women are being replaced in sports, entertainment, and politics by men pretending to be women. And children are being indoctrinated at school to think that gender [biological sex] is a choice.

The transgender movement is not a grassroots movement. It comes from the top. It has nothing to do with people's freedom of expression, sexuality, or civil rights. It's an evil psyop [military techniques to influence the beliefs, emotions, and behavior of citizens] with a clear agenda: to get us closer to transhumanism by making us question the most fundamental notion of human identity—our gender [sex]. If you don't know who you are, if you already identify as a hybrid between a man and a woman, you will be easily convinced to become a hybrid between a human and machine.

It's the final test to see whether we will follow the most absurd party line towards our own extinction....In the gaslighting process to get us closer to a post-human future, they have mentally and physically harmed an increasing number of children and young people. And it's only getting worse. This must be stopped.[52]

The craving to supplant God and outwit nature is a common denominator of both "trans" movements. Feeling visceral horror at the prospect of both is a sign of sanity and balanced mental health. As unpleasant as it may be to feel that horror, the fact that we experience it at all is a good sign. It indicates the instinctive recognition that disembodiment—features of both transgendering and transhumanism—severs us from our humanity.

Trans activists, along with the institutions behind them, don't want acceptance and tolerance. They want compliance. In the next chapter, I describe in detail some of what is being done to ensure that this is enforced.

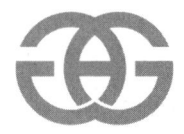

8

STIFLING DISSENT

The Adulteration of Language and Use of Reversals

Language as Propaganda

Language is the auditory, written, or visual communication of ideas, thoughts, and feelings in a systematized way so that others can understand us. When we think of an idea or thing, we communicate it to others. But the converse is also true: The act of naming something gives it substance and clarity in our own minds, thus making it real. That is why public relations and marketing people pay so much attention to words. Words not only express what's already in our minds, words can also *cause something to appear* in our minds. Language is more than a means of communication. It's an incredibly powerful tool for shaping consciousness.

Propaganda is the deliberate attempt to convince others of a certain viewpoint through the use of misleading or falsified information—perhaps with the inclusion of partial truths to make the position sound more credible. A good example is the American Tobacco Company campaign of the late 1920s, which was managed by Edward Bernays (Sigmund Freud's nephew). Americans were exposed to the mindset that smoking would help people lose weight because it was done in lieu of eating candy and desserts. Thus, it was rationalized, smoking was both desirable and safe. Cigarettes also represented freedom, which understandably attracted female customers. After young women were recruited to smoke cigarettes while marching in the annual Easter Sunday parade on Fifth Avenue in New York City, tobacco sales skyrocketed. The strategy today has not changed: Make something so desirable and enticing that people will buy it, even if it's bad for them.

All ideologies that use subterfuge—including the organized transgender movement—require the clever use of language to frame their goals. When trans activists assert that transitioners are brave, unique and special, they are employing an irresistible marketing tool. Young people, who nowadays tend not to feel good about themselves and are besieged by the difficulties of growing up, have found an entire community that seems to validate and care about them. This makes it easier to be convinced that their problems will disappear if they take cross-sex hormones and get surgery. Of course, this so-called solution is a lie. "I didn't need estrogen," a young gay detransitioner told me. "I needed counseling so I could accept myself as I am. But they made it sound like it was the answer!"

Being "Affirmed"

Earlier in this book I mentioned a trick with language: calling the radical reshaping or removal of genitals sexual "reassignment" surgery. Sex isn't "assigned." *Gender roles* are assigned. Sex is a biological fact. Gender denotes stereotypes of behavior, aptitude, and dress based on how masculine- or feminine-appearing someone is and what we believe (or imagine) is between their legs.

"Assignment" is only one of many language mind games that trans activists and their allies have concocted to convince everyone to embrace their agenda. As with any advertising, the agenda's effectiveness is partly based on repetition. Say it often enough and it becomes firmly entrenched in one's memory. The problem is, what's persistent is eventually routine, what's routine is perceived as natural, what's natural is seen as right, and what's considered right or correct soon becomes the only path. There are many ways in which the English language has been adulterated by trans activists. Let's take a closer look at some more of the terminology.

One phrase riddled with reversals is "gender-affirming care." On the surface it sounds compassionate, desirable even. Who could argue with being "affirmed"? Yet with a careful analysis, a completely different picture emerges. Children and teenagers have been brainwashed into confusing gender (gender roles, sex role stereotypes) with biological sex. Take the example of a 13-year-old male. If he has effeminate mannerisms, and if he enjoys pursuits typically allocated to the realm of females, such as sewing or fashion, he believes that this means he's a girl—even if he has a penis and scrotum. This erroneous belief is further amplified if he's homosexual. In the trans activist paradigm, a male who gravitates toward opposite-sex gender roles is assumed to be trans, and the trans establishment quickly steers him to hormones and eventually (it is hoped) surgery. The irony is that if this boy were *truly* being "affirmed," he'd be reassured that *he's perfectly acceptable as he is*—that he's a male, no matter what his interests or inclinations—and furthermore, even if he has atypical interests, that's perfectly fine. Similarly, if a masculine-appearing 15-year-old girl wears her hair very short and enjoys tinkering with car engines and driving trucks—that is, if she enjoys pursuits allocated to the realm of males—the trans agenda tries to make her feel that she's really a boy, and requires cross-sex hormones and surgery to make her body align with her interests. This message becomes even more intensified if she's attracted to other girls. The cruel linguistic trick of making people think that gender roles and biological sex are the same has caused misery for countless numbers of people, especially children and young adults. The trans agenda actually *reinforces* sex role stereotypes instead of helping people to break free of them.

What Member of the Alphabet Are You?

Nowadays, a huge number of college campuses make a point of discussing "gender identity" along with sexual orientation. There are plenty of words to choose from to describe the nuances and varieties of each. One major mind game, courtesy of the trans agenda, is the use of the acronym LGBTQ—or its variations, such as LGBTQIA+—to designate anyone whose sexual orientation is not heterosexual and/or who chooses to discount the biological reality of sex. Someone who identifies as being under the LGBTQIA+ etc. umbrella is special and perhaps even oppressed, because he or she is separate from the ordinary, and presumably privileged, majority. Someone might be "gender-fluid," "gender-queer," or "non-binary." Still others call themselves "asexual," another cool label—although technically, *asexual* is an older term that designates a biological reality, the state of feeling no sexual attraction towards anyone.

On admissions forms, universities have begun asking applicants to disclose details about their sex "assigned" at birth as well as their so-called sexual orientation. The first educational institution to establish this policy may have been Elmhurst College in Illinois in 2011; but other colleges quickly followed, including the University of Iowa, Boston University, the University of Pennsylvania, Duke University, all University of California campuses, and Massachusetts Institute of Technology (MIT). Choices for sex "assigned" at birth are the only two possible, male or female. But "sexual orientation"—which in most cases is erroneously conflated with "how you identify"—offers a much wider selection. Choices include straight, gay, lesbian, bisexual, trans male/man, trans female/woman, queer, gender non-conforming, different, and more. Everything is lumped under "gender role nonconforming," which trans activists have designated as LGBTQIA+. But *transgenders by definition are heavily invested in conforming to sex role stereotypes*. If they weren't, it wouldn't matter what kind of body was expressing "masculine" or "feminine" behavior. Furthermore, to equate gender nonconformity with being gay is deceitful. Although some gays do subscribe to sex roles—and lesbians might be less inclined to adhere to sex roles than gay men—sex *roles* are not sexual *orientation*. As Gays Against Groomers states, "Being gay is not the same as being transgender, or transsexual. Who you love is not the same as how you choose to present yourself."[1]

The MIT website assures students that answering its question about "sexual orientation" will not negatively impact admission. "We know," the website reads, "that people are more than just a set of grades and scores on a screen. So we use a holistic admissions process which entails understanding as much about you as we can, and the context from which you have been shaped, both as a person and a student. The information from the application provides the pieces that help us to create a picture of you."[2] But considering how long gay people were vilified, beaten and murdered before being granted basic human rights—and that now, internalized homophobia is being exploited to transition as many gays as possible—this sudden interest in students' sexual orientation hardly seems benign.

Interestingly, Ivy League schools are now claiming a much larger proportion of LGBTQ+ students than what actually exists in the general population—or even at most other schools. Brown University boasts 38 percent, and Princeton over 33 percent. At Yale and Harvard Universities, more than 25 percent of students say they identify with a minority, or something besides heterosexual. One former undergraduate mused, "Queer is as much politics as it is a sexual identity....The Ivies have a lot of really privileged kids. I'm sure many are motivated to identify into a so-called marginalized community in order to earn some social cache....The 'trans' and 'queer' umbrellas have expanded to include gender-nonconforming people and even people who would normally be considered straight."[3]

Some colleges freely admit that the information allows the institutions to "collect demographic data."[4] But for what purposes? Thanks to educational institutions and especially social media, young people are being trained to volunteer private, intimate data that their grandparents and even parents would never have willingly relinquished.

"Cis" Terminology

A new term that cropped up a few decades ago and is now being used a great deal by trans activists is *cisgender* (or *ciswoman* and *cisman*, or just plain *cis*). *Cis* is Latin, which means "on this side."[5] Its opposite is *trans*, which means "on the other side of" or "beyond."[6] The term *cisgender*, as an antonym for transgender, was first published in an article about transsexuals that appeared in a 1991 volume of the German-language *Journal for Sex Research (Stuttgart)*.[7] The author reasoned that the counterpart of transsexuals should be cissexuals.[8] In English, the term *cissexual* was replaced with *cisgender*, just as *transsexual* was replaced with *transgender*.

Superficially, "cisgender" applies to anyone who is content with their biological sex (or "gender," as it's called in this paradigm). But the term "cis," popular with trans activists, is meant to be disparaging. How *dare* someone be comfortable with who they are, the sex "assigned" to them at birth? They clearly don't need to transition; so therefore, "cis" persons are privileged. Also, reading between the lines, a "cis" person is ordinary, unexciting and predictable—probably because he or she isn't aware (or rebellious) enough to climb out of the "gender" rut into which he or she was born. Being content with one's genitals (and of course being a mundane heterosexual, should that apply) is no longer adequate. "Cis" people are correct in sensing that the intent behind the term is deliberately insulting.

Language can impart knowledge, but it can also be used to erode awareness. Sheila Jeffreys points out that for MtF individuals, the word "cis":

> creates two kinds of women, those with female bodies who are labeled "cisgender," and those with male bodies who are "transwomen." Women, those born female and raised as women, thus suffer a loss of status as they are relegated to being just one kind of woman and their voices will have to compete on a level playing field with the other variety, men who transgender. In this ideology... those who have a "gender" that fits their "biological bodies" have "cisprivilege," which [gives them] advantages...over transgenders.... [Many trans activists claim to be] oppressed by ciswomen, who do not recognize their privilege and do not seek to work off their guilt by supporting the demands and needs of oppressed [MtF] transgender people who are more oppressed than women.[9]

All of the language manipulation by trans activists has the goal of categorizing transgenders as an oppressed class. The prevailing myth is that MtFs are victims of privileged ciswomen whose only crime is being comfortable with (and presumably enjoying) the bodies they were born with. "Cissexism" is displayed by anyone who, purposely or not, uses the "wrong" pronoun for a transgendered person, or insists that a trans person use the "wrong" public bathroom. Bullied into trying to fix what is not their fault or responsibility, too many people are accepting that it's their duty to accommodate the escalating and unreasonable demands of transgender "rights" groups. To coerce the majority into making concessions that are not in their own self-interest—and in fact actively hurt them—the minority gives them an unflattering name. Those susceptible to being shamed are more easily manipulated into giving the demanding minority what they want.[10]

"The concept of cissexism," comments Jeffreys, "is employed by transgender activists [she is referring to MtFs here] to guilt-trip women into silence or support for their cause...The term misogyny is also redefined by transgender activists so that it means disparagement of the femininity that is attractive to cross-dressers... Transgender ideology is full of such reversals, in which the material reality of biological and existential womanhood is usurped by men who fantasise about being women." Biological women have also been instructed by trans activists to refer to themselves as "cis"—even when no "transwomen" are present.[11]

The foundational language of transgenderism itself has been cleverly manipulated through the use of "MtF" and "FtM." These designations give the impression that with the addition of some hormones and maybe a bit of surgery—or even just with different clothing or a simple declaration—a natal man can be transformed into a woman and a natal woman can be transformed into a man. Biology is not only minimized, it's erased. However, Sheila Jeffreys's use of the phrases *male-bodied transgenders* and *female-bodied transgenders* focuses our attention on biological reality, the actual person beneath the drug-induced (hormonal) and mechanical (surgical) transformation.

Words That Eliminate Women

To further entrench the transgender mindset and erase biology, more language keeps being created. *Women* no longer become pregnant or give birth; "people" do. For adoptees it's birth "parent," not birth *mother*. Also, it's "menstruators," "people who menstruate" or "bleeders," rather than *menstruating women* or just plain *women*. All of this is done under the guise of being more "inclusive" and committed to "gender neutral language"—because one should try to avoid offending the delicate sensibilities of "transwomen." It's also considered "cissexist" to say *mother*; an acceptable replacement is "birthing person." One MtF activist referred to himself as an "infertile woman" and found "contraception-focused" feminism "alienating."[12] "Issues related to reproduction are of great importance to women, of course, but may be boring for men who want 'feminism' to concentrate on their interest in impersonating women," Jeffreys remarks.[13] The trans agenda further shows its devaluation of natal women by calling them "egg producers" or "egg carriers"—terms that a U.S. government official was heard using, and which sparked outrage.[14] Other terms are "womb carriers" and "uterus havers."

Even the natural healthy practice of breastfeeding is suspect. Some circles now require the terms "chestfeeding," "milkfeeding," or "human milkfeeding" to avoid offending those whose biology makes it impossible for them to do it. The Academy of Breastfeeding Medicine (ABM) published a position paper in 2021 subtitled "Infant Feeding and Lactation-Related Language and Gender." Reassuring readers of the organization's commitment to respect the human rights of lesbian, gay, bisexual, transgender, and intersex people—note that they were all injudiciously grouped together—the author stated that not everyone who identifies as female can give birth or lactate, and some people identify as neither male nor female. Therefore, in the effort to be "gender-inclusive," language would be adjusted so that instead of the word *mother*—which might offend someone who identifies as a woman but lacks female reproductive organs—"lactating person" would be employed. In addition, every effort would be made to use the pronouns that individuals prefer. Moreover, the words "milkfeeding" and "chestfeeding" would be honored as much as possible, despite the organization's name—which is centered around and contains the word *breastfeeding*. The author conceded that because not every country consents to "asexual" language, "gendered" words would continue to be used. However, she assured readers, the ABM was sincerely on board with "inclusivity"—the trans agenda.[15] The sad thing is, the ABM states that it strives to "serve the broader purpose of promoting, protecting, and supporting the importance of breastfeeding worldwide."[16] This is a noble goal, as mother's milk contains antibodies and nutrients for the growing infant that cannot be found in commercial formulas. In addition, as the ABM points out, infants who are breastfed are healthier than their non-breastfed counterparts, and breastfeeding provides a great opportunity for the mother to bond with her baby. In fact, the organization states, "Breastfeeding is a human rights issue."[17] What tactics did trans activists use to get the ABM board members on their side?

In another remarkable and frankly unbelievable denial of basic biology, educators and students are now being instructed to avoid so-called gender-specific language such as *boys* and *girls*. And a euphemism that would be laughable if it wasn't so egregious, is the newly minted phrase "lady stick." This designates the intact penis of an individual who calls himself MtF. But saying that a "lady stick" belongs to a woman does not change the essence of the organ. By definition, a penis belongs to a male.

Vagina has not escaped modification either. The term is increasingly being replaced with the imprecise and ugly phrase "front hole"—again, so named in order to avoid offending MtF transgenders. Forget about the much higher percentage of women who might be offended, because they don't count. Females, with their distinct biology and anatomy, are being obliterated. "If 'women' can no longer be defined according to physical characteristics or biology," asks Abigail Shrier, "how are we to define them?"

> Prominent transgender author Andrea Long Chu has an answer: "female is a 'universal existential condition' defined by submitting to someone else's desires."
>
> A more offensive or insipid definition of womanhood could hardly be imagined. But in order to redefine womanhood to include trans women, this sort of "solution" has become typical. Bereft of biological markers to explain who counts as a woman, trans activists rely on social stereotypes, many of them archaic or insulting.
>
> In this way, women's biological uniqueness is denied outright... Those who use the terminology claim it offers a more sensitive way of referring to biological women, so that trans women do not feel excluded. But what does it offer actual girls, except membership in a group so grotesquely described that they could hardly wish to belong to it?[18]

If girls no longer desire membership in the group called "women," this may eventually become a non-issue for them if the trans agenda isn't stopped. In the spring of 2023, 20-year-old University of Cincinnati student Olivia Krolczyk posted on the social media platform TikTok that the professor who taught the Women's Gender Studies in Pop Culture course gave her a zero on a paper because she used the term "biological women." The paper was about how unfair it was for male-bodied trans athletes to compete in women's sports. "I 100% know this is the most biased grade ever because my project is about transgenders competing in biological women's sports," Krilczyk wrote. "How am I supposed to do my project if I can't use the phrase 'biological women'?"[19] The student also provided a copy of the professor's comment: "Olivia, this is a solid proposal. However, the terms 'biological women' are exclusionary and are not allowed in this course as they further reinforce heteronormativity [the idea that heterosexuality is the preferred or normal mode of sexual orientation]. Please reassess your topic and edit it to focus on women's rights (not just 'females') and I'll re-grade."[20]

One might have a hard time believing such a tale, but in subsequent news articles the name of the adjunct professor who had graded Krolczyk's paper, Melanie Rose Nipper, became known because she had to surface to defend her actions. Nipper was forced into the public eye after Krolczyk submitted a Freedom of Speech complaint to the University of Cincinnati. Nipper is quoted as saying that debate and discussion end when "you are, intentionally or unintentionally, participating in a systemic harm of some kind....This is unacceptable based on the community, the marginalized individuals that are at stake, and also the foundations of the course."[21] The University of Cincinnati (UC) formally reprimanded Nipper on June 14, but rescinded that reprimand in July after Nipper filed an appeal with school administrators. A frustrated Krolczyk told a reporter, "UC is affirming that professors will have no consequences for failing students with dissenting opinions...[T]hey will not uphold a student's rights to free speech and will take no action to ensure that the educators hired are acting in a professional manner."[22]

If there's no such thing as a biological woman, then there's no reason to use the pronouns *she* or *her*—is there? Pronouns, which make communication in English easy, are in danger of being obliterated too. The pronouns "ze" and "hirs"—which are intended to be neutral, and are also known as "non-binary" or "non-gendered"—were invented to be used regularly, even though the common *they* and *theirs* has been acceptable and in use since the 14th century to refer to an unspecified sex, singular.[23]

Jeffreys comments on a MtF's use of feminine pronouns.

> Women's experience does not resemble...in any respect...that of men who adopt the "gender identity" of being female or being women. The idea of "gender identity" disappears biology and all the experiences that those with female biology have of being reared in a caste system based on sex....Use by men of feminine pronouns conceals the masculine privilege bestowed upon them by virtue of having been placed in and brought up in the male sex caste. If men are addressed as "she," then all this privilege... is disappeared....Transgenderism on the part of men can be seen as a ruthless appropriation of women's experience and existence. The men who claim womanhood do not have any experience of being women, and thus should not have the right to speak as "women."[24]

Journalist, media personality, and former corporate defense attorney Megyn Kelly has strong opinions about pronouns. On one of her podcasts, she explained how she had capitulated to using the "proper" pronouns—"she" and "her"—to indicate MtFs when working at NBC and Fox News. "I figured what's the harm," she said. "It's such a tiny number [of transgenders]. Why be rude, we all know it's really a dude but okay, he wants to call himself a 'she'—whatever, I don't want to hurt your feelings." But Kelly changed her mind.

> Now we see the harm everywhere....It's not about their feelings anymore, it's about the safety of our daughters, it's about our spaces,

it's about the integrity of the word 'woman' and what it actually means....One of the ways we're clear [about women being women and men being men] is by using the proper pronouns. How can I keep you out of my locker room if I'm referring to a man as a she? [If you say] "She can't come into my locker room, she can't come into my bathroom," you've already lost the argument....The reason *he* cannot come in is *because* he's a he. So if I'm required to refer to him as a "she," I've already lost. That's why they [trans activists] are so insistent that we use their terms. And over and over and over again, what we see is biological girls and women getting hurt...in fights with biological men....The more I engage in taking that... pronoun drug, that gateway drug, the less powerful my argument is, the less safe my daughter is, and I am, and my fellow women are. And until we find our strength and our willingness to speak out on this, we're going to keep losing.[25]

Alan Finch, a MtF who detransitioned back to being a male, told a reporter back in 2004, "Their language is illusory. You fundamentally can't change sex. The surgery doesn't alter you genetically. It's genital mutilation. My 'vagina' was just the bag of my scrotum. It's a pouch, like [what] a kangaroo [has]. What's scary is you still feel like you have a penis when you're sexually aroused. It's like phantom limb syndrome. It's all been a terrible misadventure. I've never been a woman, just Alan."[26]

"While all this sexual identity politics marches through the front door," writes Abigail Shrier, "a large-scale robbery is taking place: the theft of women's achievement. The more incredible a woman is, the more barriers she busts through, the more 'gender nonconforming' she is deemed to be. In this perverse schema, by definition, the more amazing a woman is, the less she counts as a woman."[27]

Often, images can convey concepts more efficiently than verbal or written language because they reach the subconscious instantly. Their effects can be compelling even if the person is unaware of having received a suggestion. The ways in which women perceive themselves are being appropriated with increasing regularity as MtF transgenders—*male-bodied individuals*—appear on the covers of women's magazines. *Glamour* magazine even named biological men Woman of the Year in both 2014 and 2015. And MtF transgenders are entering and winning women's beauty pageants. In July 2023, 22-year-old Rikkie Valerie Kollé, a man who says he identifies as a woman, was named Miss Netherlands, which makes him eligible to participate in the Miss Universe pageant.

Negative ramifications of beauty pageants aside, awarding a prize to a male-bodied MtF is sending extremely dangerous messages to young women. If someone with an inherently different bone structure is endorsed as a female role model—even if the body has been padded with a little more (estrogen-induced) fat—how can a teen girl who's entering curvy womanhood hope to achieve such a fictitious ideal? And feel good about herself? A good example is Lesley

Lawson (nicknamed Twiggy), a natal female British model, who in the 1960s was known throughout the world for her thin, androgynous body and pixie-like appearance. "I was very skinny, but that was just my natural build," she stated to the press. "Being thin was in my genes."[28] Nevertheless, Twiggy was criticized for promoting negative body image ideals to females, especially teenage girls—the majority of whom do not have a thin boyish figure. To be fair, the unhealthy expectations of women can hardly be blamed on a single fashion celebrity; the entire modeling industry was promoting unrealistic messages about female body size and weight. In fact, in order to keep their jobs, models were required to be so unhealthily skinny that some women lost the ability to menstruate. Fat cells produce and store almost one-third of the estrogen in a woman's body, so too few fat cells means not enough estrogen, and menstruation ceases. But because all the girls wanted to look like Twiggy, cases of anorexia and bulimia in young females rose dramatically. After enough pressure, normal size women, and then plus size women, started appearing in advertisements. This was good business as well as respectful of women as a group, because the majority of American women are overweight. But now that being transgender has become popular and MtF fashion models are taking the place of actual women, we are back again to unattainable bodies for females. This time, the stakes are much higher because girls and women will never, ever be able to possess the wide-shouldered, thin-hipped, low-waist "skinny" frame of a male, no matter how hard they try.

Language confusion and image confusion equal "gender" confusion. This is no accident. Another linguistic trick is that many concepts and terms have been co-opted so that their meanings are now completely the opposite of what they used to be. I'll discuss an especially nasty reversal on the next page.

Punishing the Non-Believers

Some people have rightly compared transgender activists and their allies to a cult. Psychiatrist Paul McHugh states:

> The idea that one's sex is fluid and a matter open to choice runs unquestioned through our culture and is reflected everywhere in the media, the theater, the classroom, and in many medical clinics. It has taken on cult-like features: its own special lingo, internet chat rooms providing slick answers to new recruits, and clubs for easy access to dresses and styles supporting the sex change. It is doing much damage to families, adolescents, and children and should be confronted as an opinion without biological foundation wherever it emerges.[29]

All cults—whether they're based on religion, politics, or some other ideology, and no matter how they're packaged—share similar traits. The methods used to weaken the will and discernment of devotees uniformly include the repetition of propaganda, the control of people's sexual expression, and sleep deprivation (which can occur if one is constantly online). The following claims are typical.

- *Only the cult has answers.* It doesn't matter what facts, opinions, or experiences others have; their point of view is always wrong, whereas the doctrine of the group is always right. This position is reinforced with confusing language and deceptions, all designed to psychologically manipulate.

- *All outsiders are adversaries.* They don't care about you; only the cult has the disciple's best interests at heart. The devotee must depend on the cult for information, social connections, and validation of self-worth. That is why separation from friends and family is strongly encouraged, if not mandatory.

- *Anyone who leaves the cult is devalued.* She or he is disapproved of, rejected, and in some cases publicly humiliated. Sometimes the defector's property is destroyed and the person is physically threatened.

Immense efforts are made to intimidate and silence those who disagree with trans ideology. On college campuses in the U.S., students are reprimanded and sometimes suspended for using the "wrong" pronoun for trans people. They are told that using the "wrong" pronoun is a violation of trans people's civil rights—not to mention it hurts their feelings. But since when were hurt feelings a crime? And what about the civil rights of those who speak? Health professionals who disagree with the trans agenda are also highly vulnerable. As of 2019, eighteen states and the District of Columbia regarded even simple *questions* about a child's gender identity as the equivalent of so-called conversion therapy, punishable by making therapists forfeit not only their jobs, but also their professional licenses. In this paradigm, "conversion therapy" means anything that appears to discourage a prospective trans candidate from self-identifying as a member of the opposite sex, taking drugs, and undergoing surgery.

Accusing mental health professionals of conversion therapy is such a sinister mind game of the trans movement that the history and origins of the practice are worth noting. *Conversion therapy* has a very different meaning today than it did when it was first introduced almost a century ago. A major component of this practice was electroconvulsive therapy or ECT, also known as electroshock. ECT was first used in the U.S. in 1940 after being developed in Europe.[30] To administer ECT, an electrical current is introduced into the brain. This elicits an epileptic seizure for the presumably therapeutic purpose of "rebooting" the brain. While some medical professionals tout its success, others rightly call it torture. The "therapy" in the phrase "electroconvulsive therapy" is anything *but* that. The website for the Citizens Commission on Human Rights explains:

> The human brain is a highly intricate organ, controlling the body with more than five trillion signals every second....It operates on 0.2 volts, nearly eight times less than the power of a watch battery [which is 1.5 volts]...[Yet] up to 460 volts [are] put through the brain in a single shock treatment, 2,300 times the electricity that the brain uses to function....There is considerable evidence that ECT causes significant and irreversible brain damage.[31]

The "side" effects of ECT include headaches, nausea, first- and second- degree burns (due to overload from the electrodes that are placed on the skin), confusion and disorientation, substantial and permanent memory loss, lowered intellectual function (there may be an IQ drop of between 20 and 40 points), loss of interest in oneself and one's surroundings, and death.[32] After ECT sessions, it's not uncommon for people to lose some of the essence that had made them who they were. Despite claims that ECT lowers the suicide rate, statistics show otherwise. Patients who receive ECT are 13 times more likely to commit suicide than those who do not—undoubtedly due to their loss of a sense of self.[33] No clinical trials have ever proven that this practice is safe, but the FDA has allowed ECT units to remain on the market.[34] ECT is still legal in some U.S. states.

Brain surgery is sometimes used in conjunction with ECT. Candidates for either include people who are depressed (and sometimes catatonic) or schizophrenic, women who are unmanageable (due to their unwillingness to remain passive and acquiesce to their assigned gender role stereotype), and patients unresponsive to other methods. Another group of people administered ECT, especially some decades ago, was homosexuals (mostly male). This population was considered ideal for conversion therapy because, according to the prevailing medical opinion, they needed to be "cured" of their same-sex attraction. Besides receiving ECT, homosexuals were often chemically castrated with drugs similar to what today we call *puberty blockers*. Homosexuals were also sometimes surgically castrated, only today we call it *gender-affirming surgery*.

How insidious that transgender advocates accuse psychotherapists and doctors of employing conversion therapy when they simply *talk* to their patients—when historically, the original attempts to "convert" were made on homosexuals, and the tools that were used were hormone disruptors and genital castration! In the most ironic reversal possible, transgender clinics today actually *are* attempting to convert male and female homosexuals by chemically and surgically altering them—only this time, into an approximation of the opposite sex. Distorting words and concepts so that they mean the exact opposite of what they actually are is a brilliant, albeit twisted, line of attack—a classic gaslighting technique. The "hide it in plain sight" strategy also indicates immense arrogance.

Some scientists and researchers as well as physicians have voiced their concerns that diagnoses of gender dysphoria and gender "affirming" regimens are being made much too readily. They, like detransitioners, aren't exempt from trans wrath. Sexual physiology researcher Alice Dreger, known for her advocacy work to protect children from being mutilated with hormones and surgery, has been a high-profile target. After Dreger was accused of not being "inclusive" enough in one of her articles, another, unrelated article—which was acknowledged to be helpful—was removed from a website. "A number of my fellow feminists," Dreger responded, "have pointed out that today, women like me can be subject to silencing simply on the basis that they have supposedly said something that is anti-trans rights, *even if they have not*....As soon as you assert anything that someone with the trans identity card claims is anti-trans, you are stripped of your rights."[35] Sheila Jeffreys, well known for her stance against transgenderism, reported that on more than one occasion, invitations to speak at feminist conferences were rescinded after trans activists discovered that she'd been asked, and pressured the symposium organizers to change their minds.

Dr. Lisa Littman summarizes trans activist tactics.

> Activists appear to follow a very conscious strategy of harassment and intimidation, which I'm sure they feel is justified. They go after the reputations of the people they wish to silence, and they also attack the organizations those people are affiliated with, offering to back off if only those organizations take swift and decisive disciplinary action.
>
> The decision to make a medical transition is a difficult one and people need accurate information about risks, benefits and alternatives to assess whether, in their individual case, it will be beneficial—that is the essence of informed consent. When activists shut down gender dysphoria research about potential risks and contraindications of transition, they are depriving the transgender community of their right to receive accurate information.[36]

Earlier I mentioned the phrase "lady stick" to designate the intact penis of a MtF—who no doubt hopes that using such a euphemism will make him more desirable to lesbians. But no figure of speech can obscure the fact that he's a biological male pretending to be a woman. Therefore, it shouldn't be a surprise if gay women don't want anything to do with him, sexually or otherwise. Nevertheless, lesbians and heterosexual men who refuse to date trans people are publicly accused of being narrow-minded, bigoted, and transphobic. Yet only someone who's arrogant, self-centered, and narcissistic would insist that people should be attracted to him (or her), and attack them if they're not.

Anyone is fair game for trans censure. In June 2023, Professor Michael Joyner, an anesthesiologist who teaches at the Mayo Clinic College of Medicine, was suspended by the administration for one week without pay. He was also told not to speak to the media without permission. His offense? In June 2022, he told a *New York Times* reporter that biological males, and those who claim to be transgender, have a competitive edge when playing against natal women in sports. "You see the divergence immediately as the testosterone surges into the boys. There are dramatic differences in performances."[37] But there's also another reason why Joyner was silenced. In a memo to Joyner dated March 5, 2023, the department chair referred disparagingly to a later interview, this one between Dr. Joyner and a CNN reporter on January 12, 2023. During the interview, Joyner had expressed frustration with the "bureaucratic rope-a-dope" behavior of the National Institute of Health (NIH), calling the agency's guidelines a "wet blanket" because it was discouraging doctors from trying convalescent plasma on immune-compromised patients with Covid.[38]

To explain Joyner's comment: The normal immune response to an infection is to produce *antibodies* against the pathogen, which help neutralize it. *Convalescent plasma* is blood plasma that contains antibodies to a specific pathogen that has caused an illness. Produced by someone who has recovered from that illness, it's donated to another person who currently has the illness but whose lowered immunity and overall weakness make it difficult for them to produce enough antibodies to defend against the disease. Convalescent plasma therapy has proven effective in many rapid-onset illnesses whose human hosts have not had the time, or lack the ability, to mount an effective defense.[39] In fact, Joyner had co-authored a journal article on the benefits of such treatments. The article read in part, "These findings suggest that transfusion of COVID-19 convalescent plasma may be associated with a mortality benefit for patients who are immunocompromised who are susceptible to refractory infection." Patients so treated were 37% less likely to die if they received the therapy than those who did not.[40]

Apparently, the benefits of this treatment were unimportant to the Mayo Clinic. Here's an excerpt from the Mayo Clinic memo to Joyner:

> Your use of idiomatic language has been problematic and reflects poorly on Mayo Clinic's brand and reputation....[In addition] your June 2022 comments in a NY Times article were problematic in the media and the LGBTQI+ community at Mayo Clinic....Over the years you have failed to consistently work within Mayo Clinic guidelines related to media interactions and failed to communicate in accordance with prescribed messaging. Currently concerns remain with disrespectful communications with colleagues who describe your tone as unpleasant and having a "bullying" quality to it.... Mayo Clinic prides itself on our values and it is important for you to align your behaviors with those values...You must immediately eliminate any new incidents of behaviors which display a lack of mutual respect and unprofessionalism....Failure to fully comply with the expectations...will result in termination of employment.[41]

It's worth noting that the Mayo Clinic did not exempt itself from the very behavior it accused Joyner of engaging in: "bullying." Nevertheless, the clinic wanted to make sure it was sensitive to the demands of the LGBTQI+ community, which undoubtedly did not want it publicized that a testosterone-infused, natal male body participating in women's sports is unfair. (See Appendix B for details on transgenders in sports.) Equally troubling was the clinic's apparent aversion to eliciting the ire of the NIH, which—given the world "health" in its name—should have been eager to utilize every promising therapy available to treat serious conditions. Three times in 2022, Joyner and dozens of other doctors from Harvard, Stanford, Columbia, and other medical centers sent NIH scientists research materials, urging them to expand their guidelines to include convalescent plasma therapy. The NIH did not respond.[42] As unpleasant as some might perceive Joyner to be, his aggravation was understandable when he talked to the CNN reporter about the NIH's evident desire to selectively promote some medical protocols while ignoring others. One must ask why the Mayo Clinic—presumably in the business of saving lives—did not exhibit more interest in a life-saving therapy, and instead chose to focus on the "idiomatic language" used by one of its doctors.

Sometimes, people who criticize the trans agenda are more than merely reprimanded. Utah state senator Mike Kennedy, who is an attorney and physician and works as a family doctor, sponsored legislation that bans the administration of puberty blockers and surgeries to minors who have not been diagnosed with gender dysphoria. The bill was reasonable and laudable. It did not attempt to regulate the choices of adults, and it addressed *only* those minor children who were *not* found to be gender dysphoric. Who could argue against not treating someone for a particular condition because they didn't have an illness that required the treatment? Yet in January 2023, shortly after the bill became law, Kennedy's home was defaced. The words "These trannies bash back" and "fash" (a loosely spelled abbreviation of "fascist") were written in red spray paint on his garage door. Kennedy shared photos of the damage on Facebook and wrote, "To those who seek to use violence, vandalism, and intimidation to deter me from standing up for what is right, let me be clear: you will not succeed…. I will not be deterred by your cowardly actions. The recent vandalism to my family's home was not just an attack on me, but on the very principles our state stands for. We will not let fear and violence control our destiny."[43]

Some states in the U.S. have passed laws, or are trying to pass laws, that give the state the right to remove children from their homes if the government determines that parents are not "gender-affirming" their children. According to one bill, even using the "wrong" pronoun when referring to a child would constitute child abuse. In California, such a bill—Assembly Bill 957—was being heavily promoted with only one senator, Scott Wilk, objecting to it. "In the past," the senator told his constituents, "when we've had these discussions and I've seen parental rights atrophied, I've encouraged people to keep fighting. I've changed my mind on that. If you love your children, you need to flee California."[44]

Trans intimidation has spread to every venue. Those who speak up against the indoctrination of young people on social media have had their accounts closed without explanation. Some people are finding their bank accounts terminated as well. Mainstream media is generally trans-friendly because it's owned by people who either actively embrace the trans agenda or are being coerced not to criticize it. People who object to the participation of transgenders—and biological males who self-identify as female—in women's sports are also being publicly denounced. The hostility, cruelty, and outright violence from the radical trans fringe, simply because others disagree with them, is almost inconceivable. But we must believe it—no matter how painful it might be to think that such a thing could happen—so we can better protect ourselves and our children.

The denial of biological sex is creating emotionally stunted and intellectually maimed human beings. One way we can help restore sanity is to help young people grow up to become self-aware, confident, compassionate, and discerning. These qualities are the antidote to victimhood, the topic of the next section.

The Cult(ure) of Victimhood

An entire generation of vulnerable young people is being conditioned—*groomed*—to become potential consumers of transgendering. The educational system is one of the primary trans marketing vehicles. Colleges and universities, which should be preparing students to become adults, are instead encouraging young people to regress and remain helpless like children. In the discussion of sex role stereotypes in Chapter 2, we learned that most of the adjectives attributed to males (perhaps unconsciously), such as "independent," are also used to describe adults—while most of the adjectives attributed to females (perhaps unconsciously), such as "dependent," are also used to describe children. However, perhaps for the first time in history, sinister elements in our culture are trying to turn males as well as females into dependent children. Another name for this deliberately fostered helplessness is *coddling*.

College students who are coddled today are encouraged to "express their feelings." But the self-expression is not of a mature, self-aware adult who is responding; it's the temper tantrum of a child who is reacting. Reactions and responses are often regarded as the same, but they are quite different. A *reaction* is instantaneous, usually triggered by an association with an unresolved issue from the past. You might say or do something "without thinking," writes a psychologist. "It's driven by the beliefs, biases, and prejudices of the unconscious mind." A *response*, however, "usually comes more slowly. It's based on information from both the conscious mind and unconscious mind....it takes into consideration the well-being of not only you but those around you. It weighs the long term effects and stays in line with your core values."[45] These distinctions are not surprising, given that reactions and responses are generated in different parts of the brain.

Reactions come from the oldest and most primitive part of the brain that's situated directly above the brain stem. The reptilian brain is concerned with basic functions that keep us alive, including threat avoidance. When the reptilian brain sounds the alarm survival mechanisms activate, including the fight-or-flight outpouring of stress hormones. The threat and danger may be real or only imagined, but what's important is the perception of threat. Responses, although they are based on our immediate senses including the reptilian brain, are further mediated by the cerebral cortex, which is in charge of higher-level thinking and processing. Someone who responds might initially have a reaction, but possesses enough self-control to pause and wait—whether it's two seconds, two minutes or two days—to think about what has occurred and decide the best way to handle the situation. Over time, a child who develops maturity learns how to be responsive instead of merely reactive. Unfortunately, children and teenagers today are being encouraged to remain in their reptilian brain and react instead of respond—which means they will never achieve emotional maturity.

Social media has played a huge role in infantilizing teenagers. Pressing a button—"like" or "don't like," "thumbs up" or "thumbs down," "make a friend" or "reject a friend"—provides an immediate result, sending a surge of the pleasurable neurotransmitter dopamine into the brain. This spike in dopamine is a way of experiencing immediate gratification without the need for patience or long-term planning. That's why dopamine is the biochemical of addiction: Who wouldn't want to constantly experience little bursts of pleasure? The problem is, the more dopamine we get the more we want, at the expense of waiting for more significant or fulfilling rewards. In addition, the electronic screens of computers and especially smart phones—which are now being given to even very young children, some barely two years old—emit harmful radiation (electrosmog).[46]

A large number of studies are finding psychological difficulties resulting from the use of social media, whether it's Facebook, TikTok, Twitter (now X), or some other platform. The longer you stay on it, the less self-esteem you have. In one meta-analytic study, the authors reviewed all prior research that had examined social media use by males and females of all ages. People with lower self-esteem tend to cultivate more online relationships. They fear face-to-face social meetings, which they find awkward because there's more danger of disapproval. Online relationships feel much safer to them.[47] But the more they rely on being online for their social interactions, the less they're able to relate in the real world. Another, even larger study published in February 2023—"A Meta-Analysis of the Effects of Social Media Exposure to Upward Comparison Targets on Self-Evaluations and Emotions"—examined a huge sample of 7,679 participants who had been subjects in a total of 48 studies. The authors reached a parallel conclusion, that social media has a negative effect not only on self-esteem and mental health but also on body image. This pertained to both males and females of all ages.[48] By its very nature—snapshots of one single, picture-perfect moment—social media encourages people to compare themselves unfavorably to others, thereby cultivating jealousy. Someone else has the perfect date, the perfect meal or the perfect vacation, because that's all the public sees. "People don't tend to post about their bad days or upload unflattering photos of themselves. These platforms do not offer much insight into real life, and the perfect lives that we see are nothing but carefully constructed illusions," said Carly McComb, lead author of the study. "It is very important that users are aware of the unrealistic nature of social media…carefully curated, manipulated and idealized self-presentation."[49]

Another level of insight came from an article published in 2021. The goal was to determine how much (if at all) social media and smart phones had contributed to the attitudes, behaviors, and interpersonal interactions of thousands of university students. The results of the study were sobering. After adjusting for the sex of the subjects and the countries in which they lived, the researchers found significant decreases in well-being and self-control. The more often people used social media, the less they acted like adults. Compared to students 15 years ago, the students in this study experienced substantial decline in their relationship skills. They were also less tolerant of others whose views disagreed with theirs. This intolerance was so extreme that the students prevented public figures from speaking on campus and bullied them online if they disagreed with their views. Expressiveness, awareness, discernment, and empathy decreased by 11 percent.[50]

With vastly decreased emotional maturity—the extent of which has not been seen in any generation thus far—the findings of Jean Twenge, a psychology professor at San Diego State University, are not surprising. Twenge compared the behavior, attitudes, skills, and interests of three generations of children (Boomers, Gen Xers and Millennials), factoring in the relatively new and increased exposure to smart phones. She found that 18-year-olds today are comparable in emotional maturity to the previous generation's 15-year-olds, and those 15-year-olds act like the previous generation of 13-year-olds. Childhood ends later, in high school.[51] It's a sobering thought that today's 18-year-olds are behaving like their grandparents did when they were 13 years of age. Lacking confidence in themselves, their relating skills are poor. Seeing insults where there are none, they're unable to tolerate differences in others, taking offense if someone else merely offers an opposing opinion. They are quick to demonize people who have different points of view. These young people have become so mired in exaggerated emotional reactions—such as feeling "unsafe" merely because someone disagrees with them—that they are incapable of behaving responsibly, rationally, coherently, or compassionately. In order to feel "safe," they're demanding that college administrators and professors scrupulously avoid any words, subjects, and ideas that might cause offense or discomfort. To their detriment, these angry, hurt, confused young people are being reassured by many school administrators that their hostility and intolerance toward others is not only justified, but admirable. This coddling allows self-righteous anger to simmer and eventually become rage, the source of many of the demonstrations now occurring on campuses. These students may proclaim the need for tolerance, but they fail to see the hypocrisy of their attitudes and actions when they become violent and destroy the property of others in an effort to prevent speakers from appearing on campus.

College administrators are capitulating to students when they try to avoid *microaggressions*. The co-authors of an article appearing in *The Atlantic*, "The Coddling of the American Mind," write that this term designates "small actions or word choices that seem on their face to have no malicious intent but that are thought of as a kind of violence nonetheless. For example, by some campus guidelines, it is a microaggression to ask an Asian American or Latino American 'Where were you born?,' because this implies that he or she is not a real American."[52] *Trigger warnings*, or just plain *triggers*, are "alerts that professors are expected to issue if something in a course might cause a strong emotional response. For example, some students have called for warnings that Chinua Achebe's *Things Fall Apart* describes racial violence and that F. Scott Fitzgerald's *The Great Gatsby* portrays misogyny and physical abuse, so that students who have been previously victimized by racism or domestic violence can choose to avoid these works, which they believe might 'trigger' a recurrence of past trauma."[53]

Following are several examples of what's passing for progress on campuses.

- Students at Emory University demanded counseling because someone wrote the name of an unpopular politician in chalk on the metal railing of an outdoor staircase and at several other places on campus. The title of a *Washington Post* article says it all: "Someone wrote 'Trump 2016' on Emory's campus in chalk. Some students said they no longer feel safe."[54] Here's a sample of more headlines: "Emory University President Vows to Hunt Down Student Whose 'Trump 2016' Message Wrecked Safe Space." "Word 'Trump' Written in Chalk Terrifies, Harms Emory Students." "Emory University Students Think Donald Trump Is Out to Kill Them."[55] Putting aside the issue of mild defacement (chalk washes off), the lack of "safety" that some students expressed seems excessive for a chalk scrawl consisting solely of a last name and a year. The university administration apologized to the students and immediately had the graffiti removed, but the editor-in-chief of the *Emory Wheel* asked the students to stop and think before becoming hysterical. "Suppose we had a different administration. Suppose it was ruled that protests, such as the one on Tuesday, made Trump supporters feel threatened on campus. Freedom of speech works both ways, and its hindrance affects both sides. It is not the role of an institution that is devoted to the critical education of its students to tell those students which opinions they are allowed to have."[56]

- In the UK, LeedsTrinity professors and lecturers were sent a memo forbidding them from using capital letters when giving students assignments because using uppercase letters might "scare them into failure….Despite our best attempts to explain assessment tasks, any lack of clarity can generate anxiety and even discourage students from attempting the assessment at all." One lecturer responded to the memo by stating, "We are not doing our students any favours with this kind of nonsense."[57]

- The recreation and athletics department of Carleton University in Ottawa, Canada, had trainers remove the scale from its gym because the presence of the scale could be "triggering" for people who were overweight or had eating disorders. Students who did want the scale in the gym objected because they weren't given a choice.[58]

- During the 2014–2015 school year, nine of the ten University of California campuses held faculty training sessions intended to give educators tips on how to avoid offending students. Educators were told *not* to say "There is only one race, the human race," and "I believe the most qualified person should get the job" because these phrases were considered examples of subconscious racism. Other forbidden phrases included "Where are you from?" and "Where were you born?" The deans and department chairs were also told to avoid using application forms and other types of documents that, when asking for the person's sex, contained check boxes for only "male" and "female."[59]

- In her essay, "The Trouble with Teaching Rape Law," Jeannie Suk Gersen wrote that in the current climate, students were more "anxious…about approaching the law of sexual violence...than they have ever been in my eight years as a law professor." Student organizations for women were warning female students that they might be "triggered" by the word "violate" or by any discussion of rape law. It was even claimed that such triggering was equivalent to sexual assault itself. Some students tried to pressure their professors not to teach the subject so they and their classmates could be protected "from potential distress." This assumption of protection is ironic, because the classes were meant to teach attorneys not only how to better defend clients who were raped, but also how to help people communicate consent in order to prevent rape from occurring. Gersen analogized future attorneys who avoid learning rape law to "a medical student who is training to be a surgeon but who fears that he'll become distressed if he sees or handles blood."[60]

♦ In a nod to transgender ideology, students in schools all over the world are now being permitted to self-identify as animals. This might be seen as a macabre parody if it weren't true. "An extraordinary report from a Sussex [UK] school," wrote reporters at *The Telegraph*, "has shed light on the growing trend of pupils insisting on being addressed as animals." Some students "were reprimanded... for refusing to accept a classmate's decision to self-identify as a cat. [They] were told they would be reported to a senior leader after their teacher said they had 'really upset' the fellow pupil by telling them: 'You're a girl [not a cat].'...One pupil at a state secondary school in Wales told *The Telegraph* of a fellow pupil who 'feels very discriminated against if you do not refer to them as 'catself.' When they answer questions, they meow rather than answer a question in English. And the teachers are not allowed to get annoyed about this because it's seen as discriminating [against the child].'"[61]

♦ In an outright nod to political correctness—only this time, the issue was race, and the event took place in 2013—a band scheduled to play at a party at Hampshire College was canceled because students thought that the musicians were "too white." A statement posted on the college's website read in part, "Some members of our student community questioned the selection of [the] band, asking whether it was a predominantly white Afrobeat band and expressing concerns about cultural appropriation and the need to respect marginalized cultures." It's illegal to discriminate because of race. So the college officially responded that its intention for a "safe and healthy" event was no longer possible due to the "intensity and tone" of comments made on the event's Facebook page (which was immediately removed)—and therefore, the performance was canceled. The disappointed musicians were told that they would still get paid, but the keyboard player responded, "Our band is not for profit. It's a labor of love....It just felt like a dirty bribe, you know, 'Shoo, shoo, take this money and go away.'"[62]

♦ The University of Northern Colorado investigated two professors because after they asked their classes to consider diverse viewpoints on controversial political and social issues, students complained online about an "offensive classroom environment." One of the professors had asked his students to read the aforementioned article, "The Coddling of the American Mind." The article addressed the dangers of avoiding issues that students might disagree with because it "deprived them of the opportunity to examine their beliefs."[63]

Let's take a deeper look at the article that created the "offensive classroom environment." The authors wrote, in response to comments that "these developments are a resurgence of political correctness":

> There are important differences between what's happening now and what happened in the 1980s and '90s. That movement sought to restrict speech (specifically hate speech aimed at marginalized groups), but it also challenged the literary, philosophical, and historical canon, seeking to widen it by including more diverse perspectives. The current movement is largely about emotional well-being. More than the last, it presumes an extraordinary fragility of the collegiate psyche, and therefore elevates the goal of protecting students from psychological harm....[In addition] this movement seeks to punish anyone who interferes with that aim, even accidentally....It is creating a culture in which everyone must think twice before speaking up, lest they face charges of insensitivity, aggression, or worse....[Emotionality] dominates many campus debates and discussions. A claim that someone's words are "offensive" is not just an expression of one's own subjective feeling of offendedness. It is, rather, a public charge that the speaker has done something objectively wrong. It is a demand that the speaker apologize or be punished by some authority for committing an offense.[64]

Students who demand a "safe space" are equating emotional discomfort with physical danger. But the two are not equivalent. During an interview at the University of Chicago Institute of Politics, media personality and CNN contributor Van Jones explained the difference between them. On the one hand, there's the justified need to be protected from physical assault or an immediate threat of assault, and of course sexual abuse. However, Jones explained, the second type of safety that students say they require—the need to be safe ideologically and emotionally, and to feel good all the time—is unrealistic because it can never be guaranteed. Moreover, it's "obnoxious and dangerous" because it fails to teach life skills. This mindset also teaches students to become little dictators. It promotes the attitude, Jones continued, "if someone else says something that I don't like, that is a problem for everyone else, including the administration." Directly addressing the students, he explained that a campus is a place "where people say stuff you don't like. [But] these people can't fire you, they can't arrest you, they can't beat you up, they can just say stuff you don't like—and you get to say stuff back! [Yet] this you cannot bear! This is ridiculous." Jones, who is black, added, "My parents marched [during the Civil Rights movement in the U.S. in the 1950s and 1960s]. They dealt with fire hoses. They dealt with dogs. They dealt with beatings. You can't deal with a mean tweet?"[65]

An undergraduate liberal arts student wrote to her fellow millennials:

> I am not going to attack people over social media or on campus trying to tell them that they're wrong. This is a huge problem with our millennial generation, and it's leading us to our own demise.... To those who state their thoughts as facts, rather than opinions, stop trying to push your views on others...[and disregarding] them as your equal if they don't agree with you....[S]top being so damn *narcissistic*....We want to be able [to] prove the baby-boomers generation wrong when they tell us that we're not going to be successful adults governing the world. Truthfully, unless we can learn to agree to disagree, they all might be right.[66]

Passing laws to prevent someone from being offended is a violation of the First Amendment of the Constitution of the United States, which protects freedom of speech. Rather than limit people's exposure to what they fear, why not teach them how to be strong and deal with ideas that are different from their own? A healthy society welcomes debate and does not punish those with differing viewpoints. Mike Adams, the late criminology professor at the University of North Carolina at Wilmington, wrote:

> I need to address an issue that is causing problems here at UNCW and in higher education all across the country. I am talking about the growing minority of students who believe they have a right to be free from being offended. If we don't reverse this dangerous trend in our society there will soon be a majority of young people who will need to walk around in plastic bubble suits to protect them in the event that they come into contact with a dissenting viewpoint. That mentality is unworthy of an American....It is the price you pay for living in a free society.[67]

Despite what students who demand "safety" might believe, pandering to their presumed fragility is not helping them. Trained to see everyone else as potential aggressors, they're becoming helpless and ill-equipped to deal with the outside world. Living in an environment that focuses on finding and eradicating the enemy creates constant anxiety.[68] But students are not the only ones who are anxious. Teachers are no longer allowed to help pupils develop critical thinking skills by exposing them to a multitude of situations and ideas. Instead, they are being censured for doing their jobs properly. And it's taking a toll on them. One professor wrote, "I am frightened sometimes by the thought that a student would complain...[about my] not being sensitive enough toward his feelings, of some simple act of indelicacy that's considered tantamount to physical assault."[69]

I mentioned earlier that an entire generation is being groomed to accept and desire transgenderism. This would not be possible unless they were being encouraged to be *victims*—casualties of the misdeeds of others. Wanting others to feel guilty for oppressing them, victims feel justified doing everything possible to manipulate. To receive special treatment they threaten, lie, con, exaggerate, deny, and ignore. Never satisfied, they create drama where none inherently exists. By whining, crying, banging their fists on the table, yelling, screaming and shouting, victims try to coerce others to capitulate and give them what they want.

What separates victims from non-victims is the belief that they have no control over their actions—and therefore they don't assume responsiblity for how those actions affect others. People immersed in their victimhood are prone to self-pity, self-absorption, and a sense of entitlement. They insist that because the entire world is against them, they are justified in constantly feeling resentful.[70]

A *Scientific American* article explains that "the tendency for interpersonal victimhood consists of four main dimensions," and provides a checklist of thoughts and beliefs of a victim—even if there was never an experience of genuine trauma.

- It is important to me that people who hurt me acknowledge that an injustice has been done to me (*constantly seeking recognition for one's victimhood*).
- I think I am much more conscientious and moral in my relations with other people compared to their treatment of me (*moral elitism*).
- When people who are close to me feel hurt by my actions, it is very important for me to clarify that justice is on my side (*lack of empathy for the pain and suffering of others*).
- It is very hard for me to stop thinking about the injustice others have done to me (*frequently ruminating about past victimization*).[71]

"Victimhood culture rewards us when we are aggrieved, helpless, and weak," writes psychotherapist Lisa Marchiano. "It therefore encourages us to experience ourselves as being at the mercy of external forces beyond our control." Most importantly, this mindset also encourages assigning "diagnoses to ordinary distress, which encourages children to perceive themselves as ill"—perhaps even an "illness" called gender dysphoria. "A diagnosis carries with it a sense of absolution. It isn't our fault that we have anxiety or depression….However, when our diagnosis becomes an important part of who we are, we are encouraged to abdicate responsibility for our plight. We are adrift on life's turbulent currents, without blame, but also without agency." This sense of helplessness in turn can lead to increased anxiety—which makes victims want to feel more powerful, so they try even harder to manipulate others. "Being a victim raises one's standing and confers virtue," Marchiano adds, "in part because it mobilizes protection and support from powerful third parties."[72]

One vicious circle that isn't talked about much is that in order for there to be a victim, there must be a victimizer. After awhile, it can become difficult to tell them apart. At some point in the victim/victimizer dance, the two change places. Victims turn into victimizers, and vice-versa. Schools and universities have the power and authority to say *no*—but considering how much effort they make to please the students and soothe their "sensitivities," you wonder who's acting like an adult. The students aren't, and the school administrators aren't either. School personnel are chronological adults; but because undergraduates aren't adults yet—remember, the brain doesn't stop growing until we're about 25 years old—to some extent, we might give students some leeway for their lack of maturity. So in a very real sense the students *are* being victimized, although not in the way they might think. Educational institutions are actively preventing them from growing up. The students' misplaced righteous anger, poor relating skills, inability to discern what's actually going on, and their disconnection from reality—*and thus from their own bodies*—are all being awakened, cultivated, and rewarded. This ensures that students will gravitate toward whatever promises to take them outside of themselves and give them maximum relief. Oblivion and escape are possible, they are being taught, by becoming another person entirely. Thus today's climate makes them ripe for indoctrination by the trans agenda.

Legal Battles

The state is trying to take over the job of raising children. Parents have lost custody for refusing to allow their child to take cross-sex hormones or undergo sex "reassignment" surgery. Even if parents merely ask for a second opinion about whether their child actually has gender dysphoria, they risk having the child removed from the home.

Take the 2018 case of a 17-year-old girl living in Ohio (unnamed because she was a minor). She was removed from her home because her parents did not believe that it would be in her best interest to take cross-sex hormones.

> The State of Ohio listened to the complaints of transgender advocacy groups who argued to the court that if the young woman did not receive the treatment she would kill herself. With co-occurring symptoms of depression and anxiety—which the transgender advocacy groups noted as the reason to mandate her transition—the parents felt their daughter was in no position to determine her best interests. The court, on the other hand, decided that because she suffered from diagnosed mental health issues, the minor had to receive sex reassignment.

The father—who had told the judge that sexual surgery "goes against his core values"—was accused of being sadistic to his daughter. The transgender advocates who were in court "alleged that the father said the daughter may go to hell and subjected her to six hours of Bible study [for an undisclosed number of days], which the Hamilton County Job and Family Services decreed was tantamount to abuse."[73] Whether or not the girl was being abused, and in the manner claimed, she clearly had problems. An alternative to cross-sex hormones and surgery could easily have been found—such as placing her in a supportive live-in environment and providing her with mandatory psychotherapy. Unfortunately, decisions similar to that judge's are becoming more common.

Of course, not all parents advocate for their children's best interests. Some try to convince them that they are the "wrong" sex and coerce them into receiving surgery. One example is the case of a divorced mother in Texas, medical doctor Anne Georgulas. After being awarded sole custodianship of her fraternal twin boys, she dressed one of them, 7-year-old James, in dresses and called him by a girl's name—even though he had clearly stated on camera that it was his mother who told him that he's really a girl.[74] Whenever James saw his father, Jeffrey Younger, he chose to wear pants and never expressed a desire to wear dresses. In the divorce proceedings, Georgulas had charged the father with child abuse because Younger refused to "affirm" their son as transgender. "Imagine," Younger told a reporter, "that your ex-wife has dressed him as a drag queen to talk to you. He has false eyelashes and makeup. His hair has got glitter in it. He's wearing a dress. Now imagine how you would feel seeing what I believe is actual sexual abuse—I believe this is not just emotional abuse but is the very, most fundamental form of sexual abuse, tampering with the sexual identity of a vulnerable boy. Every. Single. Day."[75]

Georgulas—who had begun to make payments to a clinic that would start James on hormones and later surgery—sought restraining orders against Younger and a termination of his parental rights. In October 2019, a judge ruled for shared custody and said that both parents must make all medical decisions together. But in 2021, the court reversed the ruling and Georgulas was given full custody. She was permitted to be solely responsible for the children's medical, psychiatric and psychological care, but was not allowed to consent to puberty blockers, hormones or sexual surgeries for James "without the consent of the parents or court order."[76]

By this time, James had started identifying as a girl—because, stated his father, school personnel were "actively teaching" him to be female. Jeffrey would bring James to school in pants and a shirt but the school would give the boy a dress to wear. "They use a girl's name," Younger said. "They even make James use the girl's bathroom."[77] Later that same year, after yet another judge granted Georgulas full custody of both boys, she relocated them to California. Younger believes she intends to take advantage of California's new "trans refuge" law, which essentially allows parents who would not have been allowed to "reassign" their children in another state to enter California and do it there. His petition to prevent his ex-wife from moving to California with the two boys was denied by the Texas Supreme Court.

The latest revelation to this sad tale is the reported collusion between Georgulas and one of the three gender therapists to whom she brought James for evaluation. The therapist "recomended that he begin transitioning by wearing dresses and going by [the name of] Luna after his mom said the child requested a 'girl's toy' and wanted to be one of the female characters from the Disney film *Frozen*."[78] To drug a child and chop off his genitals simply because he wants a toy considered unsuitable—based on antiquated sexual stereotypes—and plays at make-believe, defies reason.

College students were not sympathetic to Younger's plight. When he tried to speak at the University of North Texas in March 2022, protestors pounded on tables and screamed profanities. He was eventually forced to leave. The event organizer hid in a janitor's closet in another building before being escorted out by an armed police officer. She told a reporter afterward, "I've received a lot of threats. I've never been scared until last night in that janitor's closet....I didn't know if I would make it out of there."[79] The reporter commented, "With every pound of their fists, these students demonstrate that their views are so fragile, so precious, they cannot even bear the sound of an opposing idea without breaking down into a toddler-esque tantrum....[L]ittle could justify an eruption like this, a cacophony of chaos designed to shut down Younger's speech while claiming he's a fascist."[80]

In Chapter 6, I discussed some lawsuits that were initiated by detransitioners. The right to privacy in bathrooms is also prompting lawsuits, this time by non-trans people. One of the most complex and lengthy cases involves a bathroom in Stone Bridge High School located in Loudoun County, Virginia. The school had a policy of allowing biological males who "self-identified" as transgender or female into the girls' bathrooms. On May 28, 2021, a ninth-grade girl told school administrators that she was raped in the bathroom by a boy in a skirt. Her father, Scott Smith, was called to the school, who told him that the incident would be handled "internally." When he demanded that they immediately report the assault to police—because this was a crime, not a mere disciplinary problem—the school administrators "called the police on him for getting angry and causing a scene."[81]

One month later, a County School Board meeting was held. At the meeting a trans activist confronted Smith and accused his daughter of lying. In the middle of their argument, a police officer grabbed Smith, who was "hit in the face, handcuffed, and dragged across the floor, with his pants pulled down." The prosecutor for Loudoun County held Smith on charges for "disorderly conduct and resisting arrest." Meanwhile Scott Ziegler, superintendent of the Loudoun County Public Schools (LCPS), told the audience at the meeting that "we don't have any record of assaults occurring in our restrooms"[82]—when it was later revealed that in fact, he had sent a confidential email to the Loudoun County School Board members the day of the Smith girl's assault, saying simply that the school would investigate the matter.

Because the entire school district was allowing males into the girls' bathrooms, the incidence of reported sexual assaults skyrocketed. A news outlet reported that "a boy was charged with two counts of forcible sodomy," and "the same student has now committed another sexual assault after being transferred to another school within the same school district." This is believed to have been the same boy whom Smith's daughter accused of sexual assault. Nevertheless, the prosecutor said there was "no reason for the boy to remain in juvenile detention facilities."[83]

Over a year later, a Special Grand Jury that had been convened to investigate the LCPS indicted superintendent Ziegler for lying when he claimed that the school system had no record of the bathroom assaults. The jury also discovered that during the actual rape a staff member had walked in, and through the gap under a stall door, saw a girl lying on the floor with a boy on top of her. But she did nothing, testifying that this was a common occurrence. The boy accused of rape said that school officials "usually don't do anything" about such events.[84]

The Loudoun County school district then proceeded to spend 10.9 million dollars for bathroom renovation in two schools to make them coed. They obtained the money from what would have been spent on special education programs. This pilot program was intended to provide a template for bathrooms in all Loudoun County schools. The stalls were covered floor-to-ceiling, completely blocking anyone from seeing inside them. While a board member boasted that the new stalls would provide "complete privacy," Virginians for Common Sense tweeted that these same cubicles would allow assault, drug use, and other misconduct in complete privacy as there was "no escape route." The cubicles would also force "slower detection/response to unconscious patrons." In addition, lack of air flow made them less sanitary. A board member who resigned just after the rape wrote:

> The first time a child dies in one of those floor to ceiling rooms, the community will revolt. No one actually uses the bathrooms for their purpose in high schools unless they absolutely have to. Principals are already dealing with kids who use the bathrooms to get high, vape, skip, have sex or just meet up. Floor to ceiling "private rooms" are simply going to add to the ease of doing these things without getting caught. Some things that sound good in a think tank are just a bad idea when implemented in real life.[85]

Even after receiving a subpoena from the attorney general's office, the Loudoun County Public Schools refused to release the internal report it had commissioned on how the rape was handled. The Virginia Project tweeted that "the purpose of this bathroom design change is perfectly clear: to lessen LCPS' liability for future rapes in the bathrooms. Not to prevent any rapes; this design clearly increases the risk. This is purely a defensive legal maneuver to protect [the administration]."[86]

Here's an excerpt from the Special Grand Jury report:

> We believe that throughout this ordeal LCPS administrators were looking out for their own interests instead of the best interests of LCPS. This invariably led to a stunning lack of openness, transparency, and accountability both to the public and the special grand jury....LCPS administrators...including the superintendent... failed at every juncture....
>
> According to the LCPS website, the stated mission of the safety and security division is "to provide a safe and secure educational environment for all students, staff, and external stakeholders." [Note that stakeholder "security" can only be financial, which is very different from the physical safety of students.]...Yet on the afternoon of May 28, 2021, the director of safety and security was mainly concerned with the fact that a disruptive parent was in the

front office of SBHS [Stone Bridge High School]—not that a student had been sexually assaulted or that the assailant was at-large in the school....[The director of safety and security] never even asked what caused the parent's disruptive behavior, nor did he make any inquiries about the sexual assault victim or the alleged perpetrator.[87]

So where is everyone now? The assailant was transferred from Stone Bridge High School to Broad Run High School, "notwithstanding the fact that the student was awaiting trial on two counts of forcible sodomy, was ordered to wear an ankle monitor, had been assigned a pre-trial release officer and had a twelve-page disciplinary file."[88] Ziegler, despite the objections of parents, refused to resign from his $295,000-a-year job—until he was finally fired by the school board after the Special Grand Jury report was released. Charges against Zeigler for lying to the school board were dropped.[89] Not surprisingly, the Smith family filed a 30 million dollar federal lawsuit against the Loudoun County Public Schools. In November 2023, male and female students at one of the Loudoun County schools walked out in protest of the bathroom policy. But the bathrooms are still coed. That's not likely to change, because in March 2020 the governor of Virginia had signed a bill requiring school boards "to adopt policies in line with a model policy from the State Department of Education establishing transgender students' rights."[90]

Perhaps 14-year-old Katie Young said it best at one of the LCPS board meetings: "The fact that I have to be here defending my rights to not have your radical agenda shoved down my throat in school is not only concerning, it's upsetting. My peers and I are not tools to further your political agenda."[91]

As terrible as these events in Loudoun County were—especially for the children who were sexually assaulted—if this were restricted to just a handful of schools, the problem might feel manageable. But this is happening all over the United States. It's no wonder that the home schooling movement is rapidly growing. Children, especially girls, no longer feel safe in the public schools.

Self-identified FtM individuals are also making trouble, though so far I have not heard any reports of FtM transgenders sexually assaulting others. In December 2021, a jury in Missouri ordered a school to pay four million dollars to a self-identified transgender student because it had denied her access to the boy's bathroom and locker room. The girl had legally changed her name on her birth certificate, which now read "male." In the state of Missouri, such changes are sufficient to legally recognize the person as the opposite sex. Even though the school had provided her with her own bathroom, the court said this wasn't sufficient.

What else can be done to help children resist the trans agenda? Or reverse at least some of the damage that has been done in the name of "gender liberation"? That will be the topic of the next and final chapter, which focuses on healing.

PART IV

HEALING

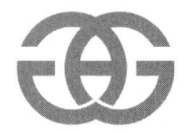

9

MAKING PEACE WITH YOUR BIRTH BODY

Emotional Awareness

The Body-Mind Connection

Every single day the human body performs miracles. The heart beats without our needing to consciously make it happen. Minute particles of ionic (electrically charged) minerals constantly permeate each cell membrane to facilitate hundreds of biochemical reactions. A thought occurs in milliseconds. It travels across a nerve cell in the form of electrical impulses, which propel neurotransmitters across a tiny gap to the next neuron, where another electrical impulse sparks another round of neurotransmitters, and so on.

Our emotions travel in a similar way. Electrical charge and minute amounts of neurotransmitters circulate throughout the bloodstream at lightning speed. "E-motion" is *energy in motion*. There's the *content*, which we experience as joy, anger, sadness, or something else. Then there's the *expression*, which is content made manifest through some act—facial articulation, vocal utterances, and/or obvious body movements. Vocalizations make an emotion easy to spot. We might cry when we're sad, scream with fear, yell in anger, or laugh if something is funny.

What we subjectively experience as an emotion cannot be separated from what's happening in the body. Take love, for example. We feel the charge build up in the heart, and it expands the chest cavity in a pleasurable way. When enough energy accumulates, we feel a need to discharge that energy through an act. Often, it's affectionate touch. The built-up energy flows out from the chest through the shoulders, arms and hands via muscular pressure, which we call a hug. The hug might be accompanied by a vocal utterance such as "I love you," or perhaps an enthusiastic "Uh!" Should we choose not to hug, we might experience love as a warm glow, a fuzzy softness, or tingles that designate excitement. But there's never a lack of movement. Energy is always flowing through the body.

Sadness feels much heavier than love. When we feel sad, our head and shoulders are bowed. Our attention is turned inward; we cannot look at others the way we do when we're happy. Sadness can be expressed by repeated, voiced, rhythmical contractions of the diaphragm and ocular emission—in other words, sobbing and crying (the act) to discharge the energy. Anger, an especially forceful emotion, feels very different, sometimes explosive. If we allow it to engulf us, we might shout or raise a fist to strike (the act). If anger is expressed in a more controlled way, the voice will have an intensity and focus to it and perhaps be louder, although not at the level of shouting. And our gaze may be direct and steady, eyes flashing with a force that can be palpably felt.

When asked what they are feeling, many people say instead what they are *thinking*. A young boy is yelled at for misbehaving. When asked how that makes him feel, he mumbles, "I'm sorry, I won't do that anymore," instead of "I feel ashamed because you yelled at me." A woman is about to divorce her husband. When asked how she feels about him, she tightens her jaw, saying, "It's all for the best," rather than "I feel angry and betrayed." The soon-to-be ex-husband is asked how he feels about divorcing. He remarks with a shrug, "I've had worse days," instead of "I feel hurt, because I tried my best to make this marriage work." Many people don't want to talk about their emotional lives with anyone—not even a psychotherapist—because they're afraid of being negatively judged. They're also fearful of ruining a persona that has been so carefully crafted that after a while, they've forgotten it exists and they now believe that the persona is who they actually are. Plus, they can no longer identify their feelings because they've spent so much time and effort trying to avoid and bury them.

A 2013 Gallup poll showed that only 54 percent of the U.S. population—just a little over half—exhibited emotional self-awareness. Scores for Canada and the UK approximately matched that of the U.S. Scores for awareness in ten countries in Eastern Europe and Asia ranged from 36 to 38 percent, while many African countries scored in the low to high 40s. Western Europe and Scandinavia scored a bit better, in the high 40s, while other countries were right on the 50 percent mark. Interestingly, Singapore—which scored the lowest at only 36 percent—was reported as "the only country in the world to fully incorporate emotional intelligence skill development into its public schools."[1] The survey methodology could have been better. Instead of introducing people to different scenarios in a laboratory setting where their emotional responses could be observed, and then compared to what they *said* they had felt, the survey merely asked participants whether they had experienced five positive and five negative emotions on the previous day. The article citing the survey did not explain what these emotions were or how they were selected for determining emotional self-awareness.

Another factor not considered is that some people naturally possess—or have deliberately cultivated—more genuinely sunny outlooks than others. Rather than hiding from their emotions, they have simply chosen to focus on feelings that are positive and uplifting; and by mindfully changing their focus, they've been able to genuinely transform what they are feeling. Such individuals may not have recalled feeling so-called negative emotions because they truly did not have them.[2] Despite the methodological concerns, that the survey was conducted at all indicates that in general, people's emotional awareness—also known as *emotional intelligence* or *emotional literacy*—is hugely lacking. Some psychotherapists and life coaches even give their clients handouts to help them learn about "feeling" versus "thinking" words. Just a few "feeling" words are *love, angry, excited, happy, sad, grief-stricken, remorseful, afraid,* and *joyful.* Some "thinking" words are *prefer, perceive, think, believe, regard,* and *consider.*

The English language is full of expressions indicating the body's involvement in emotional expression. "I can't stomach this," "I feel sick to my stomach," and "I have butterflies in my stomach" indicate disgust, dislike, horror, or nervousness. All of those phrases are literal translations of our emotions because the digestive tract is intertwined in an intricate feedback loop with the nervous system. The nervous system has a huge reach. It's comprised of the brain, the spinal cord, and all of the nerves that connect the spinal cord to the muscles, organs, glands, and the skin. Even the immune cells are part of this complex. Together, they are called the *gut-brain axis.*

The digestive tract is especially sensitive to emotional states because the large and small intestines, as well as the lining of the esophagus and stomach, contain receptor sites for the same neurochemicals as the brain. The intestines also produce these neurochemicals, including 95 percent of the body's supply of serotonin (which people normally think of as a "brain" chemical).[3] That is why the intestines are often called the *second brain.* It's also why people who are experiencing stress-related emotions such as upset, anxiety, fear, or anger are advised to wait until they calm down before eating. Even extremely high levels of emotions that are considered positive—such as love, joy, and eager anticipation—can upset the body's balance, especially in the digestive tract.[4]

Another common body-related expression is "He has a chip on his shoulder." Still reacting to hurts that occurred in the past, he cannot respond accurately or appropriately to events in the present. Physical manifestations—the "chip"—are a tight upper body and shoulders either slightly or considerably hunched forward. "Keep a stiff upper lip" is another expression. It advises that to keep yourself from crying or expressing anger, bite your lip or don't move it. (While it's actually the lower lip and not the upper one that's chiefly involved in emotional release, this is close enough.) To "get something off your chest" means freeing yourself of worry, fear or hurt by confiding in someone about it. Not surprisingly, this "something on your chest" equals a tense rib cage and diaphragm—which is also linked to a "heavy heart." People typically feel lighter, and can breathe more freely, once they have shared their pain. A chilling (negative) experience manifests in a chilled heart and possibly cold hands, which are extensions of the heart. Conversely, a "heartwarming experience" brings warmth to the area.

What all these expressions have in common are references to physiological and biochemical changes in the body that simultaneously occur with emotional states. "A person cannot be divided into a mind and a body," writes medical doctor and bioenergetic therapist Alexander Lowen.

> An individual's personality is expressed through his body as much as through his mind....Despite this truth, all studies of personality have concentrated on the mind to the relative neglect of the body. The body of a person tells us much about his personality. How one holds himself, the look in his eyes, the tone of his voice, the set of his jaw, the position of his shoulders, the ease of his movements, and the spontaneity of his gestures tell us not only who he is but also whether he is enjoying life or is miserable and ill at ease. We may close our eyes to these expressions of another's personality, just as the person himself may close his mind to the awareness of his body, but those who do so delude themselves with an image that has no relation to the reality of existence.[5]

How do we dodge our emotions? During full respiration, rhythmical waves continually travel back and forth between the chest and the abdomen, with subtle pulsations reaching the base of the spine on the exhale. But to suppress dread, fear, or another uncomfortable emotion, people hold their breath. The lips stiffen or turn inward, the jaw clenches, the throat tightens, and movement in the abdominal muscles and diaphragm is restricted.[6] This tension confines respiration to the chest area. Shallow breathing prevents us from experiencing strong emotions—or experiencing them deeply—because it inhibits the fuelling or "charging" of the feeling. This includes the natural inclination to vocalize that feeling. Psychologist Sean Haldane, author of *Emotional First Aid*, writes that in order to hold the breath we must "suspend the main pulsation of the organism."

> The word *anxiety*, from the Latin word for "narrow," expresses this experience of tightness of the muscles of jaw, throat, chest, and abdomen. Anxiety in its most intense form is fear—a total contraction of the organism. But normally anxiety is a partial contraction against an impending movement of emotion.
>
> When the expansive emotions of joy or rage are blocked, either chronically or in a temporary emergency, the breathing tends to block in a deflated position, with the body area contracted. A depressed person, whose organism resists either joy or rage, tends to be stuck in an attitude of deflation. The body is slumped, hunched, folded forward. The attitude seems to say "I've given up."
>
> When the contractive emotions of grief or fear are blocked, the breathing tends to be held in an inflated position, the chest puffed out. The attitude may seem defiant: "I won't give in."[7]

In someone who breathes freely, the shoulders remain still while the abdomen expands and contracts with the inflation and deflation of the diaphragm. The inhale-exhale cycle is one continual motion, with natural pauses after the exhale.[8] "The depth of breathing," advises Lowen, "is a reflection of the emotional health of a person. The healthy person breathes with his whole body or more specifically, his breathing movements extend deep down into his body. In a man it could be said, broadly speaking, that he 'breathes into his balls'"[9]—or in a woman, into her perineum, the spot between the opening of the vagina and the anus. It's no accident that all ancient healing traditions teach the importance of focusing one's awareness on the breath. Breathing less, but more slowly and deeply, fosters longevity.

Lack of eye contact also corresponds to the avoidance of feelings. We know instinctively that someone who casts their eyes downward is trying to disconnect. Sometimes, though, even if a person appears to gaze in the direction of someone else, the eyes can be fixed and unfocused. This indicates that the disconnection is being denied at the level of the brain. Some people's eyes rapidly flicker from side to side, which is not normal and also serves to shut off sustained contact. However, as Haldane points out, "Cutting contact does not always work. The brain may produce its own inner phantoms. Nothing is more dangerous, for example, than blind rage."[10] With blind rage, the eyes look wild and flash tangibly unpleasant energy. The person seems present but not present at the same time, which can be very frightening. It seems that today, increasing numbers of people are exhibiting glazed-over looks accompanied by blind rage. One might even think that they're acting as though they were possessed. Certainly the person is not acting as though he or she were *self*-possessed. *Self-possession* might be described as possessing, managing, or being in command of our emotions and hence responses, rather than allowing our emotions to overwhelm us and rule our actions. Put another way, to be self-possessed is to respond rather than react. Reacting versus responding was discussed in detail in the previous chapter. Haldane notes that because the eyes reflect what's happening in the brain—and in fact can be regarded as the brain's outer layer—it's important to be able to correctly interpret eye contact.

Large and small motor muscle groups can also be involved when we thwart emotional expressiveness. Psychotherapist-physical therapist Elizabeth Noble writes that when someone's "inner desire to interact with his or her surroundings" is "inhibited by shame, guilt, panic, or defeat...personal resources are not translated into movement." This takes a toll on the body. A muscle may suffer from poor tone, representing "a lost impulse, a giving up before a movement was even begun." Or the muscle may become tense because "the movement was initiated but then suddenly suppressed....Certain muscles become active at specific phases of development, [so] therefore variations in muscle tone provide a map of a person's preverbal being."[11] When muscles contract due to fear or some other emotion, electrical discharge from the nervous system is also curtailed.

When we prevent an emotion from being expressed, we use our voluntary nervous system. But the *autonomic*, or involuntary (automatic) nervous system, is also intimately involved in emotional response. The autonomic nervous system regulates processes over which we have no conscious control, such as digestion and heartbeat. This system contains two divisions. The one that's engaged depends on whether our emotions are pleasurable (positive) or unpleasurable (negative).

The *parasympathetic* nervous system is the relaxation portion. When we're at peace and happy, our digestion is efficient and our breathing is deep and unhurried. Blood vessels widen and the heartbeat is steady, strong and slow. The pupils of our eyes narrow, which promotes clear vision. The *sympathetic* nervous system, which corresponds to unpleasant emotions such as fear and anger, regulates our fight-or-flight response. Our breathing becomes more rapid to increase oxygen consumption in case we need to fight or flee. At the core of the body, blood vessels constrict (which raises blood pressure) to allow blood to flow to large muscle groups involved in running. The pupils dilate, allowing more light to enter the eye. This is the origin of the expression "blinded by fear." The salivary glands slow or entirely stop saliva production, making the mouth literally dry with fright.

Each branch of the autonomic nervous system is associated with distinct biochemicals. With positive emotions such as pleasure and relaxation—which we feel, for example, after a satisfying intimate encounter—the body produces chemicals called endorphins. *Endorphin* means "endogenous morphine," similar in chemical structure to the painkiller drug morphine, except that endorphins are naturally produced by the body itself. During non-crisis situations, GABA is plentiful. *GABA*, short for *gamma-aminobutyric acid*, is a natural tranquilizer that makes us feel peaceful and easygoing. But during a crisis situation, levels of calming GABA and pleasurable oxytocin are reduced, while levels of adrenaline and cortisol, secreted by the adrenal glands, rise. Adrenaline keeps us alert and focused to help us deal with danger, while large amounts of cortisol increase the heart and breathing rates and tense the muscles—again, to help us literally fight or flee. With stress, levels of glutamate—responsible for feelings of dissociation, numbness, addiction, panic and anxiety—also rise, heightening our vigilance and startle responses. There are also higher levels of lactate in the blood, which in excessive amounts can cause anxiety all on their own.

What happens when a frightening, dangerous, or potentially threatening situation passes? The body stops secreting adrenaline. Cortisol levels, which took a longer time to build in the body, take a longer time to return to normal; so after the danger is over, the cortisol volume still rises a bit more and remains at that level for a while before plummeting. The relaxation neurotransmitters again flow and calm the brain. A concentrated supply of blood to the limbs is no longer required for running away from danger, so blood flows back to the core, including the digestive organs which will process any food that's present. Oxygen consumption decreases because we no longer need extra large amounts for combat or running. The pupils in the eyes narrow, and because less light enters the eyes we aren't blinded. Images are more focused and we see more clearly. This translates to being able to more accurately evaluate our situation now that we're calm. All of these changes indicate the body's shift back to the parasympathetic nervous system mode, or relaxation function.

Problems arise if the danger continues. Whether the danger is actually present or if we merely fear it, the body reacts the same (a compelling testimony to the power of thought). But being in constant crisis is a contradiction in terms—as well as an unsustainable condition—because by definition, *crisis* is a sudden, short-term danger. We were never meant to remain in chronic survival mode for a long time without rest and relaxation periods. If the real or perceived crisis continues for too long, the body begins to malfunction. At first the damage is minimal. The adrenals—receiving messages to remain alert to a danger that never leaves—still release cortisol. We need cortisol in small amounts to help the system run smoothly, but during continual crisis cortisol secretion doesn't stop. Eventually, excessive amounts cause inflammation, cognitive impairment, sleep disruption, and other problems. If the danger isn't mitigated, the adrenals finally become fatigued and cannot secrete enough hormones. Finally the depleted glands lose their ability to function altogether and hormone levels are chronically low or even nonexistent. The corollary to physiological exhaustion from constantly being vigilant is emotional drain. This alarm state also depletes the neurotransmitters that help us feel relaxed, creative and optimistic. Over time, the original fear or terror are usually replaced by an underlying unease and low-level anxiety.

This excessive outpouring of fear- and anxiety-ridden biochemicals literally poisons us. Adrenal stress has risen to epidemic proportions in many parts of the world including the United States. People drag themselves around in a state of chronic anxiety, sleep deprivation, emotional overwhelm, and mental fatigue. In this state, one cannot safely operate motor vehicles, make wise decisions, or connect meaningfully with loved ones. Trying to function on such exhausted reserves, it's easy to develop addictions to anything that can act as a stimulant: caffeinated cola and coffee, sugar, recreational and prescription drugs, even dangerous physical activities and violent video games. The craving for stimulation is an attempt to prod the tired adrenals to secrete more vital hormones—a response to a legitimate biological need. Over time, there might be a need to increase the amount and intensity of stimulants in order to produce any adrenal hormones at all. .

There is one more factor that contributes to systemic malfunction in a major way: hippocampal degeneration. The *hippocampus* is a small but complex seahorse-shaped structure in the center of the skull that plays a vital role in contextual and episodic learning. It also helps us form and retrieve memories. When the hippocampus is functioning properly, it's constantly creating new nerve cells that wire themselves in new ways to other nerve cells. The creation of new neurons—which keeps us mentally fit and alert—is possible only when we experience positive and interesting mental and physical stimulation (exercise). In fact, the creation of new neurons and circuits helps prevent Alzheimer's and other degenerative brain conditions. As you might expect, some parasympathetic nervous system-related neurotransmitters that help maintain growth and smooth function in the hippocampus are GABA (proven for its calming effects) and oxytocin (known as the bonding hormone). Together they promote relaxation, well-being, kindness, and sociability. However, sympathetic nervous system-related stress hormones, including cortisol and adrenaline, have the opposite effects. They actively *prevent* neurons from being replenished and connecting with other neurons. Simply put, constant stress impairs memory. This makes it difficult to access and learn from past experiences, which in turn negatively impacts our ability to comprehend, think clearly and creatively, and discern. Moreover, being in this perpetual state causes parts of the brain—the hippocampus, and in some cases also the frontal lobe—to actually *shrink*. And the essence of who we are shrinks as well! Given enough time, the effects are permanent. In *The Indoctrinated Brain*, physician and molecular geneticist Michael Nehls describes the effects of continual, severe anxiety and stress on hippocampal function.

> [During chronic stress] the hippocampal gatweay to our personal memories that define who we are is also shrinking....[E]ustress, or short-term stress in response to challenging situations, has a beneficial effect on hippocampal function by increasing neurogenesis [nerve regeneration]. Chronic and intense stress (distress) has the opposite effect. By reducing synaptic plasticity—the ability of hippocampal neurons to form new connections with each other—intense stress impairs the memory function of the hippocampus. In addition, stress is downright neurotoxic due to the chronically increased release of stress hormones, leading over time to a reduction in hippocampal volume typical of posttraumatic stress syndrome or even posttraumatic stress disorder (PTSD).... [I]n addition to the subcortical hippocampus, the frontal area of the neocortex itself is also affected by chronic stress and has been shown to lose volume as a result. *Thus, not only does the "frontal brain battery" lose capacity, but so does the frontal brain itself—our executive center.* [emphasis added][12]

This state of being is abnormal and not a natural result of aging, despite what the medical establishment would have you believe.[13] Nehls quotes psychiatrist Lise Van Susteren from an article in the *British Medical Journal*: "Chronic stress can permanently affect brain development as well as brain functioning....[D]uring early development [stress] may have damaging life-long consequences, including maladaptive behaviors, memory problems, problems with attention, diminished inhibition, difficulty regulating emotions, impaired decision making, impaired problem solving, behavioral problems, *and priming for future stress events*." [emphasis added][14] Van Susteren was chronicling effects on children who were constantly worried about climate change, but many types of negative stressors can debilitate children: for example, worry about a disease that can suddenly kill loved ones, fear of becoming homeless (due to the financial instability induced by a pandemic), or concerns that one's body is the "wrong" type or defective, which may be catalyzed by fear of impending changes during puberty.

To summarize, constant stress produces a cascade of physical, emotional, and mental symptoms that, if not addressed, become permanent and irreversible. As we have seen, every part of the body is affected by emotions—the nervous system, muscles, glands, organs, lymph, even the brain and skeletal tissue. On a short-term basis, we might experience "only" exhaustion, or aches and pains. But over a longer period, we can also develop the risk of serious disease. Physician Mona Lisa Schulz points out that when cortisol levels remain high, arteries may become stiff and hardened (a condition called arteriosclerosis). Chronically elevated cortisol levels have even been linked to cancer. Schulz also describes the role of stress in immune disorders. Because cells involved in immune function respond to the same chemicals that control emotions in the brain, the suppression of emotions is synonymous with suppression of the immune response.

> The immune system...requires adequate levels of cortisol to function properly....[W]e need a certain amount of stress or stimulation in our lives to function efficiently and to feel alive. Otherwise we go to sleep....Excessive cortisol, however, can rev up the immune system dangerously....You're constantly living on the edge of the cliff of fear and ignoring your body's language of fear—trembling knees, racing heart, and sweaty palms....So your body begins to interpret the whole world...as something to be feared. It secretes more cortisol and begins to make immune cells and molecules against all the dangers out there, real and imagined, reacting as though the outer world were a giant Petri dish of bacteria. You wind up making immune cells against everything....[Ultimately, the excess levels of] antibodies turn against the body itself. The result is autoimmune disease, such as rheumatoid arthritis, lupus, or vasculitis.[15]

In addition to physical manifestations are the horrific mental and emotional repercussions. In fact, Nehls describes how the isolation that governmental and medical authorities worldwide starting implementing in 2020 contributed to—and in many instances, directly caused—the marked rise in depression and anxiety disorders, as well as suicides. Clearly, being in touch with our emotional center—not to mention maintaining our ability to think for ourselves—is essential to a favorable quality of life, if not our very survival.

Although not expressing an emotion begins as a choice, if the issue is not addressed and resolved, the holding back becomes habitual—because contraction cannot be maintained indefinitely through deliberate focus. Over time, what began as conscious behavior, a choice (suppression) becomes unconscious and automatic (repression).[16] Take the example of a little boy who feels lonely, misunderstood and sad. He's constantly told that little men don't cry. He wants to be a good boy and receive positive attention from his parents. So the muscular contractions to prevent himself from crying become automatic, beneath the level of his conscious awareness. Ingrained to embody this stereotypical masculine role, he grows into an adult who does not easily express sadness and many of the other "softer" emotions. He very likely also loses some of his ability to be empathetic—

and perhaps the capacity to receive love. If there's enough stored-up anger in him, it turns into rage. He might become violent toward others. His stereotypical counterpart, the little girl who's constantly threatened with the withdrawal of love if she's not "nice," has a different set of issues. She learns to suppress her own needs and feelings so much that when she's confronted by someone with a self-serving agenda—let's say a sexual predator—who wants to exploit her in some way, she's frozen and has a difficult time defending herself.

Most people find it a relief *not* to be aware of what's being stifled because it's much too painful to keep feeling what cannot be resolved. If they don't have the support to become emotionally aware, they find it easier to be oblivious than mindful. To numb themselves, they might take recreational drugs, drink, or overeat. Or they might try to distract themselves by watching TV, immersing themselves in video games, using social media, or shopping. Even generally positive activities such as exercise and hobbies can be used as distractions. Unfortunately, distractions only create more unconsciousness, and the cycle continues. In *The Body Keeps the Score*, psychiatrist and trauma expert Bessel van der Kolk advises that "The price for ignoring or distorting the body's messages is being unable to detect what is truly dangerous or harmful for you and, just as bad, what is safe or nourishing. Self-regulation depends on having a friendly relationship with your body. Without it you have to rely on external regulation—from medication, drugs like alcohol, constant reassurance, or compulsive compliance with the wishes of others."[17]

Becoming more conscious means confronting painful emotions, overwhelming sensations, and negative beliefs. But self-awareness doesn't mean expressing every single emotion. It's not always appropriate to scream or yell, and it's definitely not appropriate to resolve disagreements by using physical force. We first need to know what we are feeling, and then respond as opposed to react (discussed in detail in Chapter 8). Sometimes it's best not to respond at all, especially if others are being hostile or unreasonable. People who are emotionally literate—that is, who can identify, trust, and appropriately express and communicate their feelings—are far less susceptible to being influenced by people with shady agendas. Emotionally aware people are secure in what they are feeling and are equipped to deal with whatever issues may arise. They have the choice to act on their emotions or not act on them. They also have the ability to release or transmute their emotions in appropriate and productive ways.[18]

Clinical psychologist Travis Bradberry gives an excellent profile of people who possess emotional intelligence (sometimes known as *EQ*, or *emotional quotient*). They are curious about others, have a rich emotional vocabulary, and are aware of their strengths and weaknesses. Because they know who they are, they can accept criticism and don't get offended. But they also have good boundaries and don't allow others to denigrate them. They can "neutralize toxic people" by identifying their own emotions and staying rational, thus averting more chaos in an already stressful situation. "They also," writes Bradberry, "consider the difficult person's standpoint and are able to find solutions and common ground."

Emotionally aware people can let go of mistakes and learn from them because they're aware that holding onto stress keeps the body in fight-or-flight mode. Good judges of character, they understand the motivations of others and read what lies beneath the surface. Significantly, emotionally intelligent people don't aim for "perfection" because they recognize it as an elusive and unrealistic aspiration. "When perfection is your goal," Bradberry points out, "you're always left with a nagging sense of failure that makes you want to give up or reduce your effort. You end up spending your time lamenting what you failed to accomplish and what you should have done differently instead of moving forward, excited about what you've achieved and what you will accomplish in the future." Belief in oneself also means the refusal to limit joy. "No matter what other people are thinking or doing, your self-worth comes from within." Not surprisingly, Bradberry states that emotionally savvy people practice self-care by getting enough sleep, refusing to engage in negative self-talk, regularly disconnecting from smart phones and other electronics, and limiting their intake of caffeine.[19] To this list, I would add avoiding addictions to recreational or prescription drugs, food, alcohol, and compulsive sexual activities.

We function effectively only when our energy flows unimpeded, not when it's stuck. A century ago medical doctor and natural scientist Wilhelm Reich, considered the originator of all mind-body therapies, wrote extensively about how emotional states and physical tension are inextricably linked. Reich referred to stuck energy as *armor*. It forms when we tense up against what we are feeling. In contrast, unarmored people exhibit an efficiency and grace not only in their movements but also mentally—as exhibited by their ability to think "outside the box." People who are unarmored are willing to engage with their emotions but not be ruled by them. In touch with who they truly are, they relate authentically to themselves and others while exercising discernment and refusing to believe everything they are told. People with a strong sense of self-worth will not be at the mercy of fads, trends, agendas, and dictates from authorities who do not care about humanity.

If you are parenting young children or teenagers, helping them get in touch with—and trusting—their bodies will allow them to become emotionally aware. Trusting our bodies helps us experience pleasure at being in the world and ensures the development of a solid foundation, the topic of the next section.

A Strong Foundation in Genuine Pleasure

Many people have mixed reactions to the word "pleasure." They regard pleasure as the indulgence of our most sordid and base instincts, doing whatever we want regardless of the consequences or who is hurt by our actions. Sexual excesses and recreational drug use come to mind as examples. "We fear," writes Alexander Lowen, "that pleasure can lead a person into dangerous paths, make him forget his duties and obligations, and even corrupt his spirit if it is not controlled. To some people it has a lascivious connotation. Pleasure, especially carnal pleasure, has always been considered the main temptation of the devil....[Some doctrines regard] most pleasures as sinful."[20] Yet all the disapproval imposed by morality teachings cannot change the fact that pleasure is an innate human need. The guilt and shame surrounding pleasure are not natural. They are emotional gatekeepers that human beings are taught.

Pleasure is always rooted in the body, mediated via the five senses. It's characterized by a sense of fulfillment and connection. We feel pleasure when we view a colorful flower or a breathtaking seacoast. We can feel pleasure at completing a task such as hitting a home run, figuring out a difficult math equation, cleaning the house, or listening to a complex sonata on the piano (or learning to play it or even create one). And we feel pleasure when making love with a cherished partner. Pleasure can be rooted in a short-term event or in the accomplishment of long-term goals, such as preparing for a coveted career.

Reich pointed out that when we feel pleasure, our energy moves from the center of the body outward, indicating a desire to reach out to the world. Conversely, a lack of pleasure causes us to retract our energy from the periphery of the body inward, indicating a desire to withdraw. "These two basic directions of biophysical…current correspond to the two basic affects of the psychic apparatus, pleasure and anxiety."[21] In other words, genuine pleasure is the equivalent of expanding our energy (which feels good), and anxiety and depression correlate to contracting our energy (which feels bad). Significantly, anxiety can often be sexual or nonsexual positive excitement held back, which means the energy of the feeling is turned inward. Once pleasure is not suppressed, the anxiety can dissipate. When we are balanced, we're drawn to people who feel good inside their own skins and we're deterred by those who don't feel comfortable with themselves. Even sensing the contraction in someone else's energy—whether or not we're conscious that we sense it—doesn't feel good.

One of the chief ways to exert control over other human beings is to disconnect them from their anchor and their ability to feel pleasure—the body. Living is not a pleasurable experience for those who have not learned emotional intelligence, who are under constant stress, and who lack the tools to eliminate or transmute that stress. Physical dissociation always corresponds to mental and emotional dissociation. The more cut off from themselves people are, the easier it is for external agendas to be inserted into their psyches.

The populations most susceptible to being controlled are those who have been severed from the most basic connection to their bodies. This includes children and young adults who have been made to feel confused about whether they are boys or girls. Adolescents are particularly vulnerable. Many parents don't talk to them frankly and in-depth about sex and maturation. Ill-prepared for puberty, these young people are frightened by new and intense physical and emotional changes. And they can be overwhelmed by sexual sensations that society frequently tells them they're not supposed to have (or enjoy). As for older high school and college students, many of them are struggling with depression and anxiety. Plus, they're actively discouraged from cultivating emotional resilience and critical thinking skills. All of these populations, who for different reasons are not integrated with their physical selves, can be seduced by the trans agenda. Without a foundation in purpose or *genuine* pleasure—which amount to the same thing—it's easy to feel that our bodies are defective. From there, it's a logical step to fear or imagine that we were born into the wrong body. Hating the body that has not given us— and which we believe will never give us—genuine pleasure can only lead to its inevitable mutilation, under the guise of correcting its inherent flaws.

It's no accident that transgendering seems to be occurring with the most frequency among those who lack a spiritual focus. I am referring to a meaningful sense of belonging, regardless of whether one follows an organized religion. In many cultures, the body was (and is) considered a sacred temple. Primitive cultures regarded all of nature, including ourselves, as animated with a living force that some called God, Source, the Creator, or other names. This energy—which permeates all matter, from the distant stars to our bodies—has allowed humans to feel connected to everything around them: animals, plants, minerals, the very air we breathe. Having this sense of belonging provides a strong spiritual foundation. In fact, someone who meets the world in an engaged, curious, compassionate and expansive manner is sometimes said to "have soul," or to be "soulful."

Modern civilization—which considers itself rational and scientific, and thus superior to so-called primitive cultures—largely lacks soul. We may be able to see cells under a microscope and even split atoms. But for this heavily mechanistic orientation we have paid a steep price: feelings of being disconnected and alienated, from ourselves as well as others. The need to acquire material possessions has replaced oneness with the cosmos, just as the search for status (rank in the eyes of others) has become a substitute for one's inner knowing, self-confidence, and rootedness on this planet. Such a materialistic approach—which by definition shuts down our connection to the Earth and to our bodies—deprives us of the ability to feel genuine pleasure. In the U.S. and other highly industrialized parts of the world, emphasizing the supposed superiority of the mind over lowly emotions relegates the body to little more than a mobile unit designed to transport the esteemed head. People are taught that their own bodies are not the major—or even a valid—barometer of their experiences. Children are trained and encouraged to mistrust their perceptions, emotions, and even their sensations. The educational system and media push children to become consumers of other people's "facts," fantasies and beliefs, instead of experiencing their own truths.

The trans agenda deliberately tries to discourage everyone from connecting to the truth of their own body. Being "in our heads," we are filled with ideas that are baseless—without a base, or foundation. Dissociated from our bodies, we learn concepts that seem like truths because our physical senses—which include powers of observation—are no longer able to guide us. When thoughts become delusional and spin out of control, it's easier to believe that we are different from what the reality of our body tells us.

When a girl pretends she's a mermaid or a boy imagines he's an astronaut (or *he's* a mermaid and *she's* an astronaut), this is healthy make-believe. The child, who is creatively exploring possibilities, always returns to his or her foundation and grounding in reality. But *I am different from what my body actually is* indicates a break from reality. Such children resolutely ignore the truth of their own body due to some form of trauma. But even if no obvious trauma exists, if the child lacks a supportive foundation, being in the world feels too painful—and it's natural to want to escape reality. Buoyed by social media and repetition, the trans agenda is easily assimilated by the child's neuroplastic brain. Sometimes it's the parent who convinces the child that he or she should actually be the other sex, or actually *is* the other sex, because that's what the parent wants—again, another fantasy.

Deep breathing is the first way to get back into the body and reclaim one's sense of self. People who have panic attacks are advised to take full, slow breaths. Some people are afraid to do this, however, because this type of breathing can elicit emotions and sensations—including sexual charge. Lowen points out:

> Breathing cannot be dissociated from sexuality. Indirectly it provides the energy for the sexual discharge. The heat of passion is one aspect of the metabolic fires, of which oxygen is an important element. Since the metabolic processes provide the energy for all living functions, the strength of the sexual drive is ultimately determined by these processes. The depth of respiration directly determines the quality of the sexual discharge. Unitary or total breathing, a respiration that involves the whole body, leads to an orgasm that includes the whole body. It is common knowledge that breathing is stimulated and its depth is increased by sexual excitation. It is not generally recognized, however, that shallow or inadequate breathing reduces the level of sexual excitation. Restricted breathing prevents the spread of the excitation and keeps the sexual feeling localized in the genital area. Conversely, sexual inhibition, the fear of allowing sexual feelings to flood the pelvis and the body, is one of the causes of shallow and limited breathing.
>
> The respiratory wave normally flows from the mouth to the genitals. In the upper end of the body it is connected to the erotic pleasure of sucking and nursing. In the lower end of the body it is tied to the sexual movements and sexual pleasure. Breathing is the basic pulsation (expansion and contraction) of the whole body; it is therefore the foundation for the experience of pleasure and pain. Deep breathing is a sign that the organism experienced full erotic gratification in the oral stage and is capable of full sexual satisfaction in the genital stage.
>
> Deep breathing charges the body and literally makes it come alive. And one of the self-evident truths about an alive body is that it looks alive: The eyes sparkle, the muscle tone is good, the skin has a bright color, and the body is warm. All this happens when a person breathes deeply.[22]

Getting out of the head and back into the body is a major line of defense against indoctrination of any type, no matter what the source. There's a saying that the body has a mind of its own. When we deny its messages, it's easy to make up things that aren't true. These untruths ultimately hurt us more than if we had faced what our body was trying to tell us in the first place. If children are being taught that everything is relative—*including their bodies*—and that there's no such thing as absolute truth, then there's literally nothing that they can rely on or trust, because they have no foundation. If you believe that your body has betrayed you, if you have no sense of biological "rightness," if you believe that you are a mistake of nature and have to "transition" into something else—how can you trust yourself? Your mind then becomes open to whatever message is hammered into it, as long as it's loud and is repeated enough times.

In Chapter 5, I mentioned a video in which Jazz was crying and saying to his mother, "All I want is to be happy and feel like me, and I don't feel like me, ever."[23] This lack of feeling "like me, ever" is understandable. Jazz's neurological, biochemical and energetic pathways—which ordinarily would deepen, expand, and evolve during an entire lifetime—were more than merely altered. The body's innate genetic tendency towards growth and change (puberty) was suddenly halted, the energy irreversibly suffocated.[24] Jazz's very genes were unable to express themselves naturally and organically because of outside interference. "No child is born in the wrong body, their bodies are just fine," observes psychiatrist Miriam Grossman. "It's their emotional life that needs attention and healing."[25]

In Chapter 6, unhappy detransitioners described childhood suffering that made transgendering so appealing. Below is an account of a traumatized young woman who was influenced by the trans agenda in a different way.

Confronting Trauma

A friend's 23-year-old daughter, whom I'll call Tracy, pulled her father aside during the last face-to-face talk they would have for many years. "Dad," she said earnestly, without smiling, "I'm non-binary." Her father, whom I'll call Robert, recalled being stunned by the conversation. "I didn't say much, except 'okay.' Inwardly I was thinking, *So what?* At some point in the conversation I told her I'd love her no matter what. I don't know if that's what she needed to hear from me, but the topic didn't come up after that."

Tracy's father Robert had traveled all over the world for his career, after which he was employed for several years as a police officer. "I've been in some really unusual and dangerous situations," Robert told me, "and I thought nothing could surprise me anymore. But Tracy's declaration truly startled me. I don't know why she thought it was such a big deal, but it seemed to be really bothering her." I wish that Robert had thought to ask his daughter what being non-binary meant to her and why she felt it was so important. But knowing some of this young woman's history, I could venture a guess.

Tracy's parents had acrimoniously divorced when the girl was very young. Custody was awarded to Tracy's mother, who tried to control every aspect of her daughter's life. Plus, she often denounced Robert in front of Tracy. So the girl hardly ever saw her father, who lived far away. When Tracy was in her teens, she was staying with Robert for a rare extended visit when she was assaulted. For months, she had been stalked by a slightly older man who wouldn't take no for an answer; and finally, he attacked her with repeated kicks to her abdomen. Tracy was so physically and emotionally traumatized that for a year afterward, whenever she had her monthly period, she suffered intense cramps and an abnormal amount of bleeding. A few times, she bled so heavily that she ended up in the emergency room. Even though the man had caused serious internal damage, Tracy would not press charges. "She shut down sexually after that," Robert recounted. "She wouldn't even leave the house. I tried to get her into therapy, but she refused. Tracy is asexual at this point, but I don't think that's her real nature. She never dealt with the trauma, and instead escaped into a world where she didn't have to deal with males. It's very sad. But because she doesn't live near me anymore and won't even pick up the phone when I call, there's nothing I can do."

Had Tracy remained with her father after the assault, she might have had a chance to heal. Instead, insisting that she had family obligations, she headed back to her mother's unstable and unloving home, where she received no support for what she'd been through. It was years after the attack, during a very brief visit with her father, that Tracy told him about being non-binary.

In modern trans-suffused lingo, *non-binary* means that an individual does not identify with the "gender" that was "assigned" at birth. This is further broken down into various sub-categories. Some people say they don't identify exclusively as a male or female, while others state that they experience themselves as both male and female. Still others say they don't identify as either male or female. If "non-binary" were simply a fancy way of saying "I don't subscribe to sex roles," that would be fine. But because trans activists have insidiously conflated biology (sex) with cultural roles (gender), it's a small step from shunning sex roles to believing that with a simple declaration, one's unwanted natal biology can be changed or erased. If this sounds confusing, it is. It's impossible to make sense of a concept that's fundamentally flawed and intrinsically *doesn't* make sense.

In some ways, Tracy's upbringing was free of stereotypes. Her father, despite having always worked in traditionally masculine occupations, had been a loving, attentive, and devoted father when Tracy was small. Before Robert and his wife divorced, he had taught his young daughter how to use power tools for woodworking and set design. They went camping in the woods, where he taught her survival skills. And he encouraged her considerable artistic talent. "I never told her that she couldn't do something because she was a girl," Robert recalled. "I encouraged her to go beyond what she thought her limits were. If she made mistakes I told her it was okay, because we can't learn to do better unless we fail." Although Robert never insisted that his daughter assume a stereotypically feminine role, her mother did. So it's no surprise that eventually Tracy felt a need to identify as non-binary, instead of simply allowing herself to be who she was without the need for labels. After she was assaulted, identifying as non-binary in her system of logic gave her the excuse to renounce intimacy and sexual pleasure.

Some young people renounce their biology if they feel threatened by the sexual maturation process. But for Tracy and others like her who have experienced outright trauma, emotionally dissociating from their body makes them feel safer. Being stalked and attacked catalyzed Tracy's desire to escape her body, perceived as the source of her pain rather than the repository of it. I hope that one day, Tracy will find the courage and support to confront her fears and suffering so she can move on and enjoy a more fulfilling life. Because it's in her nature—and because her father had exposed her to a variety of engrossing activities during an earlier, happier time—Tracy is indeed "fluid" in her interests. But she's still very much a woman, rather than the neutered, one-dimensional person she tries so hard to convince herself she is.

Bessel van der Kolk points out the differences between someone who's in touch with their body and someone who has unresolved trauma.[23]

> Our gut feelings signal what is safe, life sustaining, or threatening, even if we cannot quite explain why we feel a particular way. Our sensory interiority continuously sends us subtle message about the needs of our organism. Gut feelings also help us to evaluate what is going on around us. They warn us that the guy who is approaching feels creepy, but they also convey that a room with western exposure surrounded by daylilies makes us feel serene. If you have a comfortable connection with your inner sensations—if you can trust them to give you accurate information—you will feel in charge of your body, your feelings, and your self.
>
> However, traumatized people chronically feel unsafe inside their bodies: The past is alive in the form of gnawing interior discomfort. Their bodies are constantly bombarded by visceral warning signs, and, in an attempt to control these processes, they often become expert at ignoring their gut feelings and in numbing awareness of what is played out inside. They learn to hide from their selves.
>
> The more people try to push away and ignore internal warning signs, the more likely they [the warning signs] are to take over and leave them bewildered, confused, and ashamed. People who cannot comfortably notice what is going on inside become vulnerable to respond to any sensory shift either by shutting down or by going into a panic—they develop a fear of fear itself.[26]

"Shutting down" after a trauma involves every means possible to prevent movement in the body, whether that's deep breathing, sensations, energy flow, or motor activity. The less movement there is, the less accessible emotions are. "In such cases," writes Haldane, being frozen "is functional; it is of help to the organism *not* to react....The problem here is not that the person has become frozen...but that as the frozen state thaws out, all the emotions of terror that have been suspended during the crisis flood to the surface."[27] The person may appear to be nonreactive, but that doesn't mean everything is fine. She or he needs time to process the event, and dealing with the threat can occur only in a supportive atmosphere. The pain, which doesn't leave, is stuck until it can be released. "The challenge here," advises Haldane to the layperson,

> is to try to jolt the person out of their frozen state without giving them a shock....Opt for standard methods of treatment such as providing warmth and rest....[A]fter a severe emergency...that has shocked the person without injuring them, try to make sure that there is the possibility of contact and comfort at hand for the person for some days ahead. The trouble is that the longer the person stays out of contact and copes mechanically with the aftermath of the crisis, the more intense the eventual thawing out may be (more like an overwhelming spring flood [than a dip in a calm pond]).[28]

Tracy has remained frozen. Until she confronts her trauma from having been terrorized and assaulted—along with the earlier strife between her parents when she was growing up—she will continue to avoid intimate contact with another adult. Meanwhile, by refusing to confront her conflicting emotions, Tracy is vulnerable to noxious external influences. There are many people like Tracy. But by getting the support they need to admit and release their pain, access their ability to feel pleasure, and confidently express their emotions in appropriate ways—that is, rediscover their foundation in the physical self—they will be able to become complete human beings. This includes resisting the assurance of salvation, or escape from the body, that gender "reassignment" falsely promises.

How to Help Children (and Adults) Considering Transition

If you are a parent seeking counseling for your distressed son or daughter, keep in mind that psychiatrists are trained as medical doctors. Therefore, as with almost all medical doctors, their "therapy" of choice will be drugs. And for trans-oriented physicians, their "therapy" of choice will be cross-sex hormones. There's always an M.D. after the psychiatrist's name. On the other hand, psychologists, psychotherapists, social workers, marriage and family counselors, and non-medical mental health professionals have different degrees. If a counselor or psychotherapist is also an M.D., those initials will likely be emphasized because physicians earn more money (and have more prestige) than non-medical counselors. So regardless of other credentials that someone might have, an M.D. degree usually indicates that drugs will be considered first. Of course, not all psychiatrists are proponents of cross-sex hormones and surgery. Dr. Miriam Grossman is one example of an ethical and skilled psychiatrist. In *Lost in Trans Nation: A Child Psychiatrist's Guide Out of the Madness*, she explains how she works with young would-be transitioners to get to the root of their problems so they can embrace true change and self-acceptance. She also offers excellent advice to parents on how to remain calm when speaking to their trans-identified offspring. If you're seeking genuine help, find someone like Dr. Grossman. How?

Learn about the professional's approach and treatment philosophy before you bring your child to their office. Mental health workers associated with gender "reassignment" clinics, medical centers or hospitals that perform transition surgery have only one agenda in mind—so if you want your child to remain intact, avoid them. Even if a clinic is not licensed to dispense hormones or physically equipped to perform surgeries, it may adhere to the ideology that transitioning is always the answer to psychological problems and refer the client to a place that *is* equipped for hormones and surgery. Ask the counselor if he or she is affiliated with "reassignment" institutions or pharmaceutical companies. Even if a facility isn't affiliated, it might fire a staff member who simply *questions* the need for gender "reassignment." So you may need to look for a therapist in private practice.

As of this writing, almost two dozen states in the U.S. have laws forbidding surgery and cross-sex hormones for children under 18. If you live in a state that's heavily pro-transgender, seek mental health assistance in another state—via online sessions, if you have to.

A good therapist will know when to send the client for a complete medical workup. If there's a serious or ongoing medical condition, it might be due to sexual abuse, an undiagnosed health problem, or a genetic variance. For example, a girl with high levels of adrenal hormones who presents in a more masculine manner might have a life-threatening type of CAH. Only an experienced doctor can treat such a condition. Also, due to the higher rates of suicidal ideation, actual suicide attempts, post-traumatic stress disorder, and other mental health issues in people presenting as gender dysphoric as compared to the general population, the therapist should investigate trauma before even discussing gender "reassignment."

Dr. Grossman describes her therapeutic approach:

> We'll talk about gender, of course, but instead of automatic affirmation, we will look deeper. We will try to determine what living as the opposite sex accomplishes. How will it make life better or easier? Is the new identity about becoming someone new, or fleeing who they are?
>
> I look at my patient's family. Is there conflict in her home, an ill parent or sibling? I determine if she has a psychiatric condition such as anxiety, depression, OCD [obsessive-compulsive disorder], ADD [attention deficit disorder], psychosis, or if she's on the autism spectrum or has some other form of neurodiversity.
>
> Is there a history of adoption, trauma, or abuse? Social awkwardness or bullying? Attraction to the same sex? Is the trans identity a way of exploring themselves separate from their family, a normal task of adolescence, taken to an extreme?[29]

Some techniques are specifically designed to help people cope with trauma. They include EMDR (Eye Movement Desensitization and Reprocessing), EFT (Emotional Freedom Technique), and similar mind-body modalities that eliminate pervasive, distressful, and repetitive "stuck" reactions to traumatic events. While EMDR requires a trained therapist, EFT can be self-administered. The manual is free from Gary Craig at www.emofree.com. Be aware, however, that although EFT can always be helpful, for serious problems I recommend consulting a skilled professional as well.

The following questions are designed to help people clarify the differences between biological sex (which is fixed) and gender role stereotypes (which are based on fluctuating cultural beliefs)—and the impact that such stereotypes may have had on their lives. The questions are not intended to take the place of psychotherapy, but they can be used as an adjunct. Appropriate for both children and adults who are thinking about transitioning, they are a starting point, designed to get to the roots of how, when and why biological sex became conflated with gender. If deeper issues hiding behind the self-diagnosis of "gender dysphoria" arise, please see a qualified psychotherapist.

****

1a. *To Boys:* What does it mean to you to "feel like a girl"? What do you think a girl feels like? What do you believe you can do as a girl that would be impossible for you to do as a boy? What in your life do you think that being a girl would fix? [Additional questions for older children and adults:] Define "feminine." Do you feel "feminine"? What does it mean to you to be "feminine"? How do you feel about being "feminine"?

1b. *To Girls:* What does it mean to you to "feel like a boy"? What do you think a boy feels like? What do you believe you can do as a boy that would be impossible for you to do as a girl? What in your life do you think that being a boy would fix? [Additional questions for older children and adults:] Define "masculine." Do you feel "masculine"? What does it mean to you to be "masculine"? How do you feel about being "masculine"?

2. What kind of toys did you play with growing up? If it was "opposite sex" toys, why do you think this makes you the opposite sex?

3. Did you ever dress up in "opposite sex" clothing? If yes, why do you think this makes you the opposite sex?

4a. *To Boys* [Tread carefully]: How do you feel about your upcoming changes from being a boy to becoming a man? Might this have anything to do with your wanting to be the opposite sex?

4a. *To Girls* [Tread carefully]: How do you feel about your upcoming changes from being a girl to becoming a woman? Might this have anything to do with your wanting to be the opposite sex?

Someone with counseling experience may also ask:

5. Have you ever been bullied or picked on? By whom? Under what circumstances? For how long? Did anyone ever intervene? What are your feelings about this? Might that experience have anything to do with your wanting to be the opposite sex?

6. Did you ever experience rape, sexual assault, or inappropriate touching? When? By whom? Under what circumstances? Have you ever told anyone? If yes, what happened when you told?

    Investigate this thoroughly. If necessary, enlist the assistance of a professional who specializes in post-traumatic stress disorder (PTSD).

7. Have you had any romantic or sexual relationships? When, and for how long? If you haven't had any romantic or sexual relationships, why do you think you haven't?

8. Do you think you might be gay / homosexual / lesbian / bisexual? If so, why? How do you feel about your sexual orientation?

******

If you're the parent of a child who's drawn to transgendering, now is the time to discard any attachment to sex role stereotypes that you might have. Your child's life may literally depend on it. Does your boy like fashion and sewing? Encourage his talents; he might grow up to be the next Calvin Klein. Does your girl like fast cars and tinkering with engines? Get her into a vocational school for auto repair. She'll end up thanking you when she gets a well-paying job in the real world instead of being unprepared with a college education that nowadays isn't worth much (and which might have a toxic environment). Is your son self-conscious about his appearance? Reassure him that more or less facial and body hair than other boys, a smaller or larger penis, less developed muscles, or any other variation does not make him any less of a man. Is your daughter sensitive about *her* appearance? Reassure her that smaller than usual or large breasts are perfectly fine. Also tell her that there's no such thing as the "typical" vagina or labia, and that women's genitals are all unique and different. Let her know that what's important isn't how she looks, but that she's healthy and happy. Emphasize that the most important thing is for her to feel connected to her body and feel good in it, rather than trying to measure up to some unrealistic beauty standard.

Does your child express needs timidly? Encourage him or her to speak out by asking questions. And listen to their answers without judgment. Reassure the child that he or she is fine—and that compassion, integrity, healthy relationships, and the development of their talents and skills are what count. If your child has an issue with excessive anger, do what a handful of schools are doing today: Teach the child breathing exercises and meditation. Children appreciate this "time out" that allows them to calm down, collect their thoughts, and manage their emotions.

If your child is gay, let him or her know that as long as he or she is comfortable in the world, happy, and ethical when dealing with others, a loving, kind, caring relationship is more important than the genitals of the partner. You don't want to give your child an excuse to think that they have to change their body in order to become acceptable. If you have issues with your child being gay (or being gay yourself), please seek help from a qualified professional. Bottom line, the sex of the romantic partner is unimportant compared to the insanity of body mutilation.

Social psychologists are aware that support outside the home environment is important too. Your child's peers, the kindness and closeness of your community, and the media to which your child is exposed—films, printed materials, social platforms—also need to reflect the goal of self-acceptance. Try to expose your child to activities with other like-minded children and their families. The more positive role modeling your sons and daughters consistently receive from many sources, the more they'll be comfortable with and accept themselves. In addition to guiding what they watch and read, you will also need to heavily restrict their social media access, or—better yet—not allow them to use it at all. Parents are increasingly reporting that severing contact with social media, which includes trans support groups, is critical to restoring sanity in their children's lives.

Beyond Stereotypes

What Equality Really Means

Today a war is being waged between science and fantasy, common sense and dogma, health and delusion—keeping one's body intact versus chemically and surgically transforming it to such an extent that it become unrecognizable. More people than ever are fighting back against the trans agenda. They come from all points on the political spectrum, and have varied ethnic, religious, and financial backgrounds. That is a good thing. But there's still a problem. Even among those who agree that the trans movement is dangerous and harmful, and especially exploitative of vulnerable children, some people are still adhering to traditional gender stereotypes. Unversed in the scientific literature and without any knowledge of the neuroplastic brain, they make irrational claims about what's "proper" or "natural" for males and females. Here's an example of what I'm talking about, from a newspaper article written by a stay-at-home mom.

A woman named Shelby Lancaster who (reasonably enough) didn't want to leave her 3-month-old in daycare because he was colicky, quit her job to stay home full-time. Once home, Shelby discovered the joys of canning and other traditional homesteading skills that have almost become a lost art. She writes about her decision to stay home for her son, daughter, and impending third child.

> Because of the feminist agenda...we've been told we need to be like men, get out there in the job market in order to be valuable to society, but I think we've lost what valuable really means...

> For millennials especially, there's this view of the 1950s homemaker....posh and pretty and quiet, and dinner is supposed to be on the table at 6 p.m. sharp. Well, that's not exactly what a homemaker is....Women have been made to seem unvalued, like something that's no longer special...Skills that were once obtained by women and passed down through the years have been completely demolished. For instance, herbalism, midwifery...Plus, we don't have aunts and sisters and grandmothers rallying around us and guiding us through motherhood and womanhood....
>
> If a woman wants to be a CEO and climb the corporate ladder, then sure, homemaking might not be the best thing. It could restrict your growth. If you're looking at it [staying home with the children] from a materialistic viewpoint, it might not fulfill you. But if you're wanting to look at life a little bit different than just money or what society deems as valuable, it can be wonderful.[30]

Lancaster is indeed correct that having a community—whether it's one's family of origin, partner, or group founded on a common goal—is vital to leading a rich and fulfilling life. Studies have shown that people live longer when they have a strong social network of real people, not online contacts.[31] And it's true that skills required for homesteading—which relate to self-sufficiency and living in greater harmony with the natural world—can bring enormous satisfaction because they are related to real and basic needs. Ultimately, humanity will be better off spending a lot less time on cell phones and computers, which although convenient, can disconnect people from themselves and from each other.

Without discounting Lancaster's obviously positive experiences, like many people not only does she harbor misconceptions about feminism, but she also believes in gender stereotyping. In American society, men's work outside the home has always been valued more than homemaking skills for two reasons: it's men and not women who are doing the work, and they're receiving a paycheck. Industrialized societies tend to value money more than skills. Housework, along with the women who provide it, is often taken for granted and dismissed as insignificant because women are involved and they're not being paid with dollars. But it isn't the fault of women—or feminism—that the larger culture has consistently undervalued unpaid work performed by women in the home. Even today, housework is still not considered a real job, despite the fact that a stay-at-home mom provides the services of cook, cleaner, launderer, chauffer, and nurse for children who require care when ill.[32] So if a woman needs to feel appreciated by being paid for her work, and the only way to earn an actual wage is by securing outside employment, who can blame her?

Furthermore, Lancaster's equating women working outside the home to "being like men" reveals a strong sexist bias that women's work *should* center in the home, just as men's work *should* be outside the home. Feminism has always been about options. Women don't want to feel limited in their choice of work or profession. And some don't even want to be mothers—after all, just because a woman possesses the apparatus to give birth doesn't mean that she should. Also, some fathers are happy staying home with their children, doing tasks that Lancaster and many others still believe should be performed by women. Finally, the author doesn't consider that being employed at a job outside the home can feel just as demoralizing and unfulfilling to men as staying home with the children might feel to women. Having meaningful work, whatever its source, is important to both sexes. Work dissatisfaction in any sphere is an indictment of the lack of humanity in our social institutions and corporations, not of feminism.

Of course, choice doesn't mean that we're all equipped to perform the same jobs. Reviewing the definition of *feminism* illustrates this point. *Merriam-Webster* defines it as "the theory of the political, economic, and social equality of the sexes."[33] But the *Cambridge Dictionary* definition is more complicated and open to debate: "The belief that women should be allowed the same rights, power, and opportunities as men and be treated in the same way, or the set of activities intended to achieve this state."[34]

What makes the second definition tricky is the suggestion that women and men should be treated "in the same way." Women are not merely smaller men. And men are not simply larger women. Given the very real biological and physiological differences between the sexes, it would be terrible indeed if men and women were treated as though they're exactly alike. Imagine a woman who has just given birth. Should she be expected to return to her outside job the following day, and treated as though she'd merely suffered a cold that had run its course? Should her unique reproductive role—not to mention the infant's needs—be ignored so that she's not given time off to breast feed (not "chest feed") and bond with the baby? In the U.S. and most other technologically developed countries, an infant's critical needs are generally eclipsed by marketplace demands because not surprisingly, relationships with very young children are still regarded as feminine and are thus devalued. Plus, the importance of fatherhood is rarely considered at all. Contrast this attitude with the social practices in Sweden, Denmark, and Norway. After a child is born, both parents share a paid parental leave to assume child rearing tasks and bond with the infant. Studies have shown that fathers' involvement with their infants can have a permanent positive impact later on the children's self-esteem, emotional security, peer relationships, and even cognitive abilities and IQ.[35] Close intimate contact with both parents is critical for a newborn. Once we eliminate the sex typing of different kinds of work, we can strive toward values that are not masculine or feminine, marketplace-heavy or home-oriented, but human.

Here's another example of how men and women should be treated differently— not because they don't deserve equal opportunities, but because certain jobs are more suited to specific body types. Imagine a petite woman who's five-foot-two and possesses the physical strength typical of females her size, not the one in twenty women who's as strong as the average man. She submits an application to be a firefighter. A typical firefighter who battles blazes in buildings wears basic protective gear (helmet, boots, thick coat, pants, gloves, and an oxygen tank) and carries heavy equipment (an ax, radio, flashlight, and sometimes a thermal imaging camera). The weight of protective gear is about 45 pounds. The weight of the additional heavy equipment can range from 66 to 77 pounds.[36] Although she's unable to wear and carry all that gear, she indignantly sues the fire department for discriminating against her because she's a woman. But sexist prejudice is not the issue here. Shouldn't she be held to the same standards that are required of men for this type of highly specialized work? If your house were on fire, would you want assistance from a firefighter who cannot do the job properly because some gear, deemed too heavy, was left behind?

Firefighting certainly requires physical strength, which is far more typical of males than females almost all of the time. But assigning the labels "masculine" or "feminine" to such labor invites us to categorize work according to sex—which I've been arguing against doing throughout this entire book. So we are presented with a more complex challenge: to accommodate probabilities (that men are more suited than women to be firefighters) without assuming that those probabilities are permanently and innately fixed for every single situation—and, most importantly, *without giving those probabilities gendered labels*. Such an outlook requires mental flexibility that can handle not only black and white, but also many shades of gray. It's to our advantage to be adaptable—because, to use the firefighting example, the moment we sex-type heavy lifting, we start reinforcing other sex role stereotypes as well. And what happens? We're back to limiting people all over again. The areas that actually *require* an acknowledgement of masculinity and femininity are directly related to reproductive functions, secondary sex characteristics, and body structure and metabolism.

Some people mistakenly think that purposely not genderizing a career field is the same as capitulating to quotas, otherwise known as *affirmative action*. But quotas, rather than genuinely "affirming" people, give certain individuals and groups preferential treatment that's unfair to everyone else. (There's that word *affirm* again, being twisted for a political purpose.) Should a woman be given a particular job simply because there aren't "enough" females in that field? It's like saying that more people of color, or transgenders, or blind people should be hired—not because they are better at or more suited to a job, but because they are underrepresented in that profession. It's one thing for historically and circumstantially disenfranchised people—who have been prohibited access to education and training—to request assistance that had been prejudicially denied to them, after which they would apply for a job like everyone else. But it's not reasonable for someone to demand special favors because of sex, skin color, ethnicity, religion, or any other feature that's being exploited to claim victimhood. Equal opportunity does not mean—or guarantee—equal outcome. And sacrificing quality is never a wise practice.

Feminism does not mean that women want to be men or want to do everything that men do. Nor does it mean that women *should* do everything that men do simply to even up the numbers. This important distinction is missed by those who unjustly feel entitled, and who (mis)use feminism to embrace their victimhood and demand favored treatment. Entitlement is not feminism! Yet some people conflate the two, which gives feminism a negative reputation.

"Is A World Beyond Stereotypes Possible?" is the title of an article that appeared online several years ago. The authors got straight to the point:

> We grew up with the perception that somehow pink is every girl's favourite colour...and that a woman on the front cover of a magazine represents every female in society....We can't ignore the stereotypical images depicted through the TV screen....clichéd gender roles. The main character, Regina [in *Mean Girls*], is a self-centred and superficial high school girl who only owns pink cardigans and miniskirts. She has zero intellectual abilities and is only concerned about her physical appearance. Then we have the stereotypical male image of a high school football player who happens to be one of the most popular guys in school.
>
> This is only one among thousands of examples of stereotypical images found in our society. What is clear is stereotypes destroy individuality. And often, it can be difficult to express our true self when the sources that we look to everyday are feeding us with the complete opposite image.....
>
> We are all raised with filters that determine the content and severity of biases, preconceptions, and prejudices. *Scientists are unlikely to agree how much of "gender" roles are learned and how much is based in biology. In the end, it doesn't matter as long as we give people equal opportunities to learn, grow and advance according to merit and aptitude.* [emphasis added][37]

A Stereotype-Free World

To many people, gender roles feel so natural that it's difficult to imagine a world without them. Moreover, the extremes of masculine-appearing males and feminine-appearing females are so tightly bound to cultural roles that often, there doesn't seem any other way to be.

Fortunately, not everyone is tethered to appearances. During a Young America's Foundation speaking engagement on June 15, 2022, American lawyer and columnist Ben Shapiro was challenged by a student in the audience who claimed that "gender"—by which he meant one's biological sex—is subjective. "For all of human history there was an objective standard between male and female," Shapiro responded. "In 99.8 percent of cases you absolutely can gender [determine the sex of] somebody based on looking at them...if you can see their genitals....The problem I have with the transgender argument...[is] that no objective standard exists by which I can determine sex...'I can determine my own gender [sex] based on no biology, and in fact in abeyance of biology. I can have every single biological characteristic of a male and if I say I am female, then I am female.' This is anti-scientific nonsense."

Shapiro, who is an Orthodox Jew, displayed a great deal of tolerance. "If you want to say that there's a genetic male with feminine characteristics...That's cool, who cares? But that doesn't make you a woman....Or a woman with...masculine characteristics is a man. That's nonsense too....It actually ends up [misclassifying] a lot of people who are just butch women or effeminate men."[38]

This is the heart of the issue: accepting men and women as they are, even if they don't fit a typical version of what we think "masculinity" or "femininity" should be. It's no accident that after women made inroads in the professions and began to succeed in their own sports, more men became involved with childrearing, rape of both sexes started to be dealt with more openly and fairly, and same-sex-attracted people became more visible and socially accepted—war was declared on humanity by trans activists. Rather than encouraging people to express themselves according to their inclinations and preferences, trans activists seek to restrict them. Rather than respecting people's bodily autonomy, trans activists violate it. Rather than truly affirming people's rights, the trans agenda negates them. Promoting itself as the liberation of human beings, the trans agenda has flourished. This is thankfully starting to change, but much more needs to be done to stop the destruction of humanity.

The question is simple but the issue is profound. Can we accommodate people's individuality *without the need for labels*? Can we refrain from coercing others to act a certain way in an effort to help us feel more comfortable? And can we avoid trying to induce people, including their genitals, to *look* a certain way—again, because we'd feel more comfortable if they were different? *No one is born into the wrong body. We are born into the wrong mindset.* Our slavish adherence to stereotypes is what needs to change, not our sexual organs.

Extricating ourselves from sex role stereotypes also means resisting the tendency to judge the sex of someone's romantic partner. Why should it matter to us if a woman loves another woman, or if a man loves another man? It looks strange only to those who are unaccustomed to it. One way that trans proponents manipulate parents is to ask, "Would you rather have a trans child or a dead child?" But as I discussed in Chapter 4, studies have shown that suicidal ideation and actual suicides in transgenders are not caused by cultural prejudice or rejection, but by serious emotional problems they had before they transitioned. A more valid question to ask parents is, *Would you rather have an unusual or gay child, or an irreversibly mutilated one?*

Clearly, adherence to gender roles is not working. We need to rethink our slavish acceptance of these stereotypes, no matter how innocuous we believe them to be. All stereotypes, no matter whom they target, limit who we are and who we can become. The trend toward transgenderism—no matter how preposterous and harmful it is—is presenting us with a hidden gift: a vital wakeup call to confront our narrow-minded view of gender. Confronting our hidden biases will allow us as a species to become sane and whole—not to mention remain physically intact.

Jennifer Bilek comments:

> The acceptance of the diversity of bodies appears to be the core issue, not gender dysphoria; that and unmooring people from their biology via language distortions, to normalize altering human biology. Institutionalizing transgender ideology does just this. This ideology is being promoted as a civil rights issue by wealthy, white men with enormous influence who stand to personally benefit from their political activities.
>
> It behooves us all to look at what the real investment is in prioritizing a lifetime of anti-body medical treatments for a miniscule part of the population, building an infrastructure for them, and institutionalizing the way we perceive ourselves as human beings, before being human becomes a quaint concept of the past.[39]

As limiting as sex role stereotypes are, though, breaking free of them can be a slow process. And there are some aspects of living that freedom from these roles may never erase. For instance, someone perceived as female from birth has a different experience from someone perceived as male from birth. As a woman, I am unable to embody the experience of being male, just as a man cannot know what it means to be a woman—regardless of how long he might take cross-sex hormones or how many surgeries he might undergo. As long as each sex is perceived differently and is treated substantially differently by others, it's important for them to have their own space. Division of space by sex is not that different from other groups—pilots, birdwatchers, teachers, or alcoholics—that assemble based on their commonality of experience.

As for people who identify as "non-binary," we need to read between the lines to understand what they are trying to tell us. Might they be saying that they don't want to be encumbered by the sex role stereotypes they see our culture trying to enforce on them? In some ways, their message is similar to that of feminists in the 1970s and 1980s, albeit in different language. If we can get past the language, the issue is really about choice in self-expression and pursuit of interests. It's possible to have a non-binary mind in a binary body.

Some members of the trans community are perfectly comfortable taking cross-sex hormones and receiving top surgery while leaving their genitals intact. They claim that it's unnecessary to subscribe to a "binary system" of "gender." But whether they are referring to biological sex or gender roles—or a convoluted, imprecise and illogical merging of the two—the question I ask is the same: If a binary system is unnecessary, why bother to change the body at all? Furthermore, isn't self-acceptance better than being drugged and sliced?

If people had permission to be themselves without worrying about what type of body is expressing which aptitude or behavior, the transgender movement would fall apart tomorrow. But if enough young people decide to make their bodies "non-binary" to match their "non-binary" minds, the ability of humanity to reproduce itself will be in danger. We are sterilizing ourselves out of existence.

All human beings have talents and skills they need to be utilizing in order to fulfill themselves. Everyone experiences the same emotions, including the need to feel valued and loved. And everyone needs to have their bodily autonomy respected. Males and females and yes, intersexuals are more alike than they are different. But as long as gender stereotypes exist—as long as we continue to believe that all men are naturally a certain way and *should* be that way, and all women are naturally a certain way and *should* be that way—we will fail to stop the onslaught of the trans agenda. And the ones who will be harmed the most will be vulnerable children.

You can call this emancipation from sex role stereotypes feminism, being humane, an implementation of the Golden Rule, scientifically sound, or plain common sense. It doesn't matter what you call it as long as human beings are free to discover who they really are. Imposing gender roles on people is not only limiting, but cruel. Yet stereotypical masculine and feminine roles are exactly what today's trans activists are embracing, celebrating, and promoting. And not only do they want everyone else to pigeonhole themselves into those very same stereotypes, they want people to mutilate themselves in order to do it.

Do we really want to fall into the gender trap? Or will we hold on to our humanity?

It's time to decide.

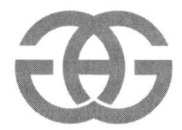

Appendix A

Highlights of the Gender Wars

First Wave Feminism

Every aspect of life—work, home, relationships—touches men and women very differently. Today in the Western world, women can own land, apply for a loan and receive a line of credit, work outside the home, and run for political office. They can also obtain a divorce, receive sole custody of their children along with alimony, and initiate lawsuits. But until relatively recently, women were treated as second-class citizens. There were few social or legal protections for females because they were considered property—first of their fathers, and later of their husbands. It may seem unbelievable to us now, living in the 21st century, but not too long ago women were forbidden to own land, either through purchase or inheritance. They were not allowed to engage in trade outside the home (except in special circumstances, decided by male officials). And they were definitely not welcome in the public sphere, which included politics. Moreover, the children to whom they gave birth and raised were considered property of the father. Schooling for boys lasted much longer than schooling for girls. The more rigorous and extensive boys' education was designed for activity and commerce outside the home, while girls were educated primarily to learn how to run a household and please others, especially their future husbands.

Because women were men's property, their bodies were not their own. In 19th century United States, many states defined "rape" as the "carnal knowledge of a woman when achieved by force *by a man other than her husband.*" [emphasis added][1] Thus if a husband wanted "carnal knowledge" of his wife, even if she did not want to be carnally known it was his right to demand it. A raped woman elicited concern for the honor of the man who owned her, not the honor or feelings of the woman who had been sexually violated. "A Feminist History of Rape" advises that "The origins of the word rape are found in the ancient Greek—to steal. The etymology of the word alone underscores the cultural assumptions...[that] until very recent history, the rape of women has been constructed as a property crime whose redress was directed to the husband or father of the victim."[2] A woman was not regarded as deserving restitution or healing, so in most cases the man who raped her was not punished. Stanford University history professor Estelle B. Freedman writes that because only men could be judges and attorneys, and juries were comprised solely of men, it was often assumed that "once a woman had consented to sex, any subsequent sexual activity was consensual. Usually an unwanted sexual encounter could be classified as rape only if the woman was white and chaste, the perpetrator was black, and the act was violent."[3] But because the act had to be seen as overtly violent in the men's eyes, this made rape even more difficult to prove.

In most parts of the world, centuries passed before women were regarded seriously enough to be given legal protection. For example, in England it took until 1994 for the law to finally acknowledge that it was possible for a husband to rape his wife. Even so, after the laws were changed, in many cases social attitudes lagged behind legal gains. Today, many women as well as men still believe that if a woman was raped, she must have done something to provoke it. "She was wearing revealing clothing." "She was walking in a sexy way." "She was smiling at me." "She looked as though she wanted it," and so on. In other words, the woman is responsible for being attacked, and the perpetrator, no matter how brutal, is not accountable for his actions.

Laws concerning rape were not the only ones that women lobbied to change. They wanted to play an active role in the creation of all laws so that their lives would be better. Women began to organize. The official women's rights/suffrage movement in the United States is often credited to have been launched with a presentation by Elizabeth Cady Stanton and Susan B. Anthony at a Seneca Falls, New York convention in 1848. The reality, though, is much more convoluted and in some ways ignoble. Anthony hadn't even attended the convention, but it was a good marketing tool and soon myth was accepted as fact. In truth, there were hundreds of white and black women, and a few men such as the freed slave Frederick Douglass, who worked to obtain voting rights for all women. The names of most of the very active black women have been forgotten by all except those exceptionally well versed in women's or black history.[4]

There have always been overlapping interests and disagreements among people who campaign for societal reforms. The early supporters of women's voting rights were divided. Some wanted to campaign for white women first and bring in black women later, while others wanted to include all women from the beginning of their suffrage campaign. Also, some public figures were more acceptable than others.

Anthony and Stanton almost got kicked out of the suffragist movement because of their association with Victoria Woodhull (1838–1927). Demonstrations for the right to vote seemed tame compared to Woodhull's deeds. The first woman to own a brokerage firm on Wall Street with her sister Tennie, Woodhull proved to be a savvy stockbroker and made a fortune. She was the first woman to start a weekly newspaper and run for the U.S. presidency (in 1872). She caused a scandal by divorcing her abusive first husband—declaring that despite the laws of that time, women had the right to deny their husbands sexual access and should be able to divorce as easily as men did. She publicly advocated free love, maintaining that women were sexual beings and deserved pleasure equal to that of men—and that they could, and should, marry for love. Woodhull also stated that men and women should be held to the same moral standards. She was so far ahead of her time, unafraid to challenge unfair cultural and legal dictates, that it's easy to see why Anthony and Stanton wanted nothing to do with her.

To get women the vote, organized meetings, protests, and letter-writing campaigns were initiated all across the United States. This process was gradual, occurred in many stages, and took decades. "By the time Stanton and Anthony died in 1902, and 1906, respectively," writes one journalist, "the movement over the next decade took on more urgency. Women were becoming a social force, riding bicycles, wearing pantaloons and challenging society's normative views of how they should act."[5] It wasn't until August 26, 1920, that the 19th Amendment of the United States Constitution was finally passed, which gave everyone the right to vote. However, loopholes in that Amendment still prevented many people from voting, mainly blacks. It wasn't until the Voting Rights Act was passed in 1965 that most people were free to cast a ballot.

One major disagreement besides including black and white women together in the campaign for suffrage was the necessity for temperance laws. Some women fought to pass laws limiting or entirely eliminating the sale and consumption of alcoholic beverages, while others felt that promoting those laws weakened any support for women getting the vote. It's true that the temperance movement was infused with unwanted moral overtones; religious leaders often preached about the immorality of drink. But the reason many women wanted temperance laws passed was that husbands would come home drunk, having spent the money for food, and sometimes rent, on alcohol. The men would also beat up their wives and children without fear of legal reprisal, having little to lose in terms of their social standing in the community. So even though many men were against the unpopular temperance laws, women wanted them for their own protection.

Another disagreement among the early feminists involved the moral character of women. One faction believed that women were morally superior to men because they were more stable emotionally and had the ability to endure more suffering—an idealized notion that was also associated with sexual purity and, of course, celibacy until marriage. This paradigm was used as a rationale for conferring more legal rights to women. Then there was the opposite faction, which insisted that nurture and not nature had molded women into this unrealistic archetype. But that was why, this second faction argued, women deserved to be given equal social and legal rights. These arguments were versions of older debates. Historically, women had either been lauded for their inherent compassion and saint-like ability to suffer, or denounced as incapable of being virtuous due to their inherent moral deficiencies. To use an old expression, females were either Madonnas or whores, mothers or monsters. There was no middle ground. Women continued to be deified or denigrated, but they were rarely human.

Second Wave Feminism

World War II gave thousands of women in the United States the opportunity to become part of the workforce. This included women who were racial or religious minorities, married, and mothers. While the men were out fighting overseas, women became liberated from the private (feminine) sphere of the home to the public (masculine) sphere of the workplace. It turned out that women could excel at the heavy-labor jobs in industry. Aside from liking the added income, social prestige and greater freedom to travel, they gained satisfaction from their work because they were making tangible contributions. The ubiquitous "Rosie the Riveter" poster was featured everywhere, showing a physically strong women in a red head scarf—an inducement for women to take jobs in factories that manufactured warplanes and weapons. But after the war, the advances women had gained were withdrawn. The men returned, forcing the women to relinquish their paying jobs and return to their homes. The employers rationalized that because men had families to support, they needed the work more than women did. Until 1964 in the U.S., it was legal for employers to fire a woman or refuse to employ her if she was married. It was assumed that because the husband was the breadwinner, the wife's job was to be responsible for the running of the household—and thus her working outside the home was not only superfluous, but an invasion of the male realm. In the U.S., married women weren't even allowed to apply for credit cards in their own name until legislation was enacted in 1974.[6]

Back in the home, women followed their social mandate to produce babies— hence the term "baby boomers" for children born between 1944 and 1964. An upsurge in advertisements for labor-saving appliances featured women pushing vacuum cleaners, opening ovens, and wiping sparkling windows with spray bottles in their hands. The women in the ads were always smiling, suggesting that they were where they were supposed to be and doing exactly what made them happy.

In 1950, in the 16- to 64-year-old age group, a little over 30 percent of women and just over 80 percent of men earned money in the workforce—contrasted with 2015, with closer to 70 percent for women and the high 70s for men.[7] In the 1950s, so-called women's work was comprised mostly of nursing, secretarial duties, and teaching. Women were limited to those occupations due to the stereotyped belief that their minds were unsuited for the sciences, but they naturally excelled in the role of caregiver, . It was also believed that women were unequipped to handle the stress and responsibility of being business leaders. Opportunities in high-echelon, high-paying professions such as law, politics, engineering, electronics, heavy industry, mechanics, construction, and the medical field including surgery—which required higher education, special training or skilled labor—were almost nonexistent for females. It was no secret that a woman earned half the salary that a man earned. Today, the situation is considerably less disparate,[8] but even in 2022, women earned an average of 82 percent of a man's salary for doing the same job.[9]

Betty Friedan is credited with having sparked the second wave of the feminist movement, which began in the mid-60s and continued well into the 1980s. In 1963, Friedan's book *The Feminine Mystique* hit the best-seller list with her in-depth discussion of "the problem that has no name." The problem was housewife malaise. Friedan described how women were becoming increasingly dissatisfied with their roles. Women were not only expected to be housewives and homemakers, child bearers and child rearers, but doing these jobs was supposed to bring them more satisfaction and enjoyment than anything else. However, cleaning dirty dishes with the newest products and dusting the latest in matching furniture did not offer the ultimate in fulfillment. Many women felt insular and isolated, stuck with boring domestic chores. Also, spending so much time around babies afforded them little intellectual stimulation. Lacking purpose, with limited opportunities for engaging interactions outside the home and unable to contribute to the marketplace in ways that utilized their intellect and talents, more and more women were feeling trapped.

Alcoholism and other addictions among women became rampant. Psychiatrists started seeing many more female clients who were diagnosed with depressive disorders. Electroconvulsive Therapy or ECT, also known as electroshock—and misleadingly labeled "therapy"—was popular in the 1950s. Although it fell out of favor in the 1960s and 1970s, it was resurrected in the 1980s. No matter what decade we review, though, for the most part the figures remain consistent. Over 60 percent—and sometimes closer to 70 percent—of subjects receiving this protocol were female.[10] In fact, stated one psychologist, "Women are subjected to electroshock 2 to 3 times as often as men."[11] This figure is not surprising, considering that women's lack of status in the world—a lack that directly impacts a person's feelings of self-worth—directly contributed to their feeling more depressed than men. A smaller percentage of candidates for ECT, but still a significant population, was gay men, and to a lesser extent lesbians. The politics of electroshock, as well as the horrific damage it causes, is discussed in great detail in Chapter 8.

The unpaid labor of housework was usually taken for granted. By extension, so were the women who provided it. Housework was not considered a "real" job, despite the fact that women performed the services of cook, cleaner, launderer, chauffer, and nurse (children tend to get a lot of scrapes and bruises, and require constant care when they're ill). When a woman's services were assigned the monetary value of equivalent jobs outside of the home, her worth as a housekeeper/

mother in 1965 was estimated to be worth about 22,000 dollars a year.[12] This is comparable to just under 211,000 dollars in 2024. Yet because she was not bringing home actual money, her job didn't count—at least not in the eyes of the larger culture, not in the eyes of her husband, and by extension, not in her own eyes either.

Women were in a no-win situation. They felt they needed to measure up to men; otherwise, they wouldn't be taken seriously. But the "measuring up" was according to stereotypically male standards. These standards were partly based on men's physically stronger bodies, and partly based on values of the commercial workplace—considered more important than the stereotypically feminine values of home and family. Although women did enter the business world, even if they managed to secure a position they were paid half of what their male counterparts earned. And they had to work twice as hard to prove themselves. This sent a clear message, reinforced daily, that they would never be esteemed as much as men.

One area of life that underwent huge changes was sexual relationships. Heterosexual intimacy had been defined primarily according to what pleased men. Penis-in-vagina sex—usually with the man on top in the so-called missionary position—was the ultimate goal and main event. If women were lucky, there was enough stroking and fondling before intercourse to arouse them. However, even if a woman was aroused, sexual intercourse alone was often insufficient to bring her to orgasm. Many women—whose parents had been raised under repressive Victorian morality—were still ignorant about the structure and function of the clitoris. Their male partners, who didn't spend much time (if any) stimulating that most vital organ, were likewise ignorant. Once the man ejaculated and his penis became soft, not only was sexual intercourse over but so was the entire experience. This left women sexually and emotionally frustrated. Feminist educators began teaching women about their anatomy. Classes sprang up during which women examined the genitals of other women and viewed their own genitals using plastic speculums and mirrors. A burgeoning sex toy industry evolved that allowed consumers to purchase vibrators through the mail.

Professionally, women were still discouraged from entering male-dominated occupations. Men typically became doctors while women trained as nurses, unless they were especially persistent. Medical doctors, mostly men, had status but the women who were nurses were typically undervalued and underpaid. Feminists called this *male privilege*, and because black people were more likely than whites to be economically disadvantaged, the phrase was refined to *white male privilege*. A less incendiary name for this—and one that's certainly more encompassing, minus the references to sex and race—is simply *entitlement*.

If grown women and men had a difficult time casting off stereotypes, children were helpless to do so. Already in school, children were being conditioned for their future roles. Boys took classes in woodworking (building bookcases) while girls had to take home economics courses (cooking and housekeeping). Feminists from all over the world, including the U.S., France, the UK and Canada, continued to bring women's rights to a mainstream audience with their unique perspectives on matters that affected not only women and men, but also children. They kept saying that if children grew up unrestricted by antiquated ideas of sex-based limitations, they'd have much more self-confidence and be kinder adults.

As feminists asked others to be tolerant and inclusive, they strove to do that themselves. Activists were divided about including homosexuals and lesbians in the women's liberation agenda. Some argued that the freedom to be sexually active without shame or fear of reprisal automatically incorporated the freedom to love whomever one chose—and thus the movement should include women who loved other women, and by extension men who loved other men. Other feminists didn't want to include gay people in the struggle. While they weren't against same-sex intimacy, they felt that the different (though related) concerns of gays diluted the goals of women, and might alienate members of the public who were sympathetic to women's needs but not ready to accept homosexuality. Also, some gay men—whose world was insular and did not regularly include women in social interactions—did not care about women's rights, and in fact were outright misogynistic. Being part of a sexual minority did not make them allies of women, either gay or straight. Ironically, some gay men called themselves and other men "girls" or "ladies" as part of an exhibitionistic tendency to act like stereotyped females. Some of the portrayals consisted of the most unflattering, unrealistic, and exaggerated feminine caricatures, which understandably offended many women. But despite these fundamental differences, after many heated debates gays and lesbians were ultimately embraced under the umbrella of feminism. So were bisexuals, but not before sparking an entirely different debate among lesbian feminists, who regarded bisexual women as avoiding their truer lesbian natures and betraying their sisters by playing both sides of the fence.

Thanks to a steady diet of publications and speeches by feminist authors and leaders, women of all ages were repeatedly told that if being a housewife and mother wasn't fulfilling—despite what psychologists and the media told them they should feel—it was okay to explore other ways of being in the world. Women were also assured that it was okay if they enjoyed being mothers and centering their lives around the home; but bottom line, they deserved to have a choice.

Second wave feminism was largely about equal opportunity and options, but society didn't always want to cooperate. The myth persisted that females should embrace and enjoy their presumably feminine role. Thus, married women who worked outside the home felt pressured (as did their husbands) to maintain conventional roles. Ironically, the small percentage of women who were earning more than their husbands sought to downplay the perception of being undesirably masculine by doing even *more* than their share of the housework. The more those women earned, and the greater the gap was between their salaries and the salaries of their husbands, the more housework those women did. The researcher who studied this concluded that such an arrangement was very advantageous to the husbands—but for the wives, not so much.[13]

While women have made visible progress in the last century, they are still heavily burdened with sex role stereotypes that are slow to change. Limitations preventing not only women, but also men, from reaching their full potential were discussed in depth in Chapter 2.

Despite the lingering effects of sex role expectations and unequal pay for women in the marketplace, the second wave feminist movement did help many women become more independent and strong, with greater self-esteem and a sense of purpose. It also helped many men become happier, freer to more fully express their many sides and not just the more socially acceptable macho roles.

Third Wave Feminism

Phony Feminists

Groups pushing for reform have always been infiltrated by people with hostile agendas. In the last decade, some very vocal women—whom I call counterfeit or phony feminists—have insinuated themselves into our culture. Their unreasonable demands, sense of entitlement, and attacks are so reminiscent of the complaints and tactics of trans activists that these complementary agendas appear to be backed by the same sources—if not financially, then certainly ideologically. Counterfeit feminists are trying to destroy not only the personal and professional advances that women have made, but also any good will between the sexes. These phonies have become so hateful that many men, understandably angry, have classified all women perceived to reside under the feminist umbrella as "femi-nazis." There's no way to determine the actual numbers of these hijackers because their high media visibility may make them seem more numerous than they actually are.

In this section on the current state of the feminist movement, I will describe some serious problems that both men and women are facing. But first, I want to discuss some issues that are causing enormous conflict. I see them, rather than being endemic to feminism, as part of a much larger agenda to create discord, divide humanity, and prevent real solutions from being implemented.

Toxic Masculinity

A great deal of publicity has been given recently to a phrase attributed to third wave feminists: *toxic masculinity*. For the record, *toxic femininity* is just as real, and as damaging, as toxic masculinity—although in different ways. I will discuss toxic femininity in the section immediately following this one.

"Toxic masculinity" does *not* mean, as one *New York Times* reporter explains, "that all men are inherently toxic."

> For decades, we used terms like "macho," "red-blooded" or "machismo" to describe the kind of hulking masculinity that men were, on some level, expected to aspire to....So what does "toxic masculinity," or "traditional masculinity ideology," mean? Researchers have defined it, in part, as a set of behaviors and beliefs that include the following:

- Suppressing emotions or masking distress
- Maintaining an appearance of hardness
- Violence as an indicator of power (think: "tough-guy" behavior)

In other words: Toxic masculinity is what can come of teaching boys that they can't express emotion openly; that they have to be "tough all the time"; that anything other than that makes them "feminine" or weak....It's these cultural lessons, according to the A.P.A. [American Psychological Association], that have been linked to "aggression and violence," leaving boys and men at "disproportionate risk for school discipline, academic challenges and health disparities," including cardiovascular problems and substance abuse. "Men are overrepresented in prisons, are more likely than women to commit violent crimes and are at greatest risk of being a victim of violent crime," the A.P.A. wrote.[14]

Henry A. Montero, a counselor who is committed to helping men explore and express their emotions, writes that even young boys "who express feelings are compared to girls in a negative context. Common responses to young males who become emotional include *Boys don't cry! Man up! Don't be such a baby! Be a man—get over it!*...In the American culture, and others, many men have difficulty expressing emotion...Toxic masculinity refers to actions that discourage displays of emotion—other than anger—in men while also encouraging behavior that will deem the male 'dominant' in a given situation."[15]

Sociologist Michael Flood, who writes about gender-related issues including fathering and sexuality, discusses the need to "diminish the policing of gender and gender boundaries....Narrow and stereotypical norms of masculinity constrain men's physical and emotional health, their relations with women, their parenting of children, and their relations with other men." However, Flood acknowledges, the phrase "toxic masculinity" has its drawbacks as it may elicit defensiveness in some men who feel attacked simply for being men. It's important to remember that individual men are not being accused of a personal failing. Rather, the phrase indicates violent attitudes and behaviors that are culturally entrenched both in individuals and institutions. This a social problem—that is, the institutionalization of violence and entitlement.[16]

In a few remaining areas of the Middle East, whose cultures are thoroughly saturated with violence and entitlement, women are legally property. If a woman wears her garment incorrectly, if she walks outside unaccompanied by a male relative, if she works outside the home, or if she engages in a relationship with a man of her own choosing, she's accused of dishonoring her family and is likely to be put to death. This is gendered masculinity *carried to its ultimate extreme.* Fortunately, Westernized societies do not condone this type of behavior and most people would be appalled by it. However, sometimes the atrocities approach it to some degree. Jaclyn Friedman describes a series of rapes that occurred in 2013 in Steubenville, Ohio. These rapes indicated how what some call "manly" can be heavily distorted. The rapes were instigated by two young football players (ultimately convicted) who "carried the unconscious body of a local girl from party to party, violating her in ways you'd probably prefer not to think about."

> This rape is like most in that it was enabled by a...masculinity that defines itself not only in opposition to female-ness, but as inherently superior, drawing its strength from dominance over women's "weakness," and creating men who are happy to deliberately undermine women's power; it is only in opposition to female vulnerability that it can be strong. Or, as former NFL quarterback and newly-minted feminist Don McPherson recently put it, "We don't raise boys to be men. We raise them not to be women, or gay men."...
>
> Toxic masculinity has its fingerprints all over the Steubenville case. The violence done to the victim was born out of the boys' belief that a) sexually dominating a helpless girl's body made them powerful and cool, and b) there would be no consequences for them because of their status as star athletes (if you want to see stomach-churning first-hand evidence of this, check out this video of one of their friends gleefully talking about how "raped" and "dead" the victim was). The defense is basing their entire case on it, arguing that this near- (and sometimes totally) unconscious girl's body was the boys' to use because "she didn't affirmatively say no." The football community's response—by which I mean not just the coaches, school, and players, but the entire community of fans— [treated]...the athletes and the game as more important than some silly girl's right to both bodily autonomy and justice. Steubenville residents have been quick to rally around the team, suggesting that the victim "put herself in a position to be violated" and refusing to talk to police investigating the assault. The two players who cooperated with police were suspended from the football team, while the players accused of the rape have been allowed to play.[17]

Had these football players not been conditioned to prove their manhood (read: self-worth) by hurting others, the rapes would not have occurred. Flood discusses the need to "to redefine what it means to be a man, encouraging visions of a healthy, positive masculinity....There is value...in getting men to care less about whether they are perceived as masculine or not, to feel less anxiety about 'proving' themselves as 'real men.'"[18] Former National Football League player and self-identified feminist advocate Wade Davis delivers a similar message. He began a public speaking career on issues relating to sexism, homophobia and racism (Wade is black) after coming out as gay in 2012. "Patriarchy has benefited us like crazy," he told a reporter, "but it's killing us at the same time....If we truly believe in a fair and just world, we all have to give up something....Men will lose something, yes, but what we will gain, what everyone will gain, is so, *so* much more than we can even imagine."[19]

Unfortunately, accusing men of behaving in a "toxic masculine" manner has become a weapon of choice that some women unfairly use when they want to manipulate men into doing their bidding. Phony feminists are doing their best to convince people to target males simply because they exist, thus decreasing the incentive for men and women to work together for everyone's betterment.

Syb, a young man in his 20s—who was given puberty blockers, hormones and surgery before detransitioning—explained on Substack that he became a vulnerable target for transgendering because he had learned to hate his very maleness.

> I had no friends in high school and spent a lot of time online, and I was exposed to the burgeoning social justice/woke movement before it entered the mainstream. When I connected to the internet, I was inundated with messages about the violence of maleness. This wasn't just "toxic masculinity"—I saw feminists saying all masculinity was toxic, that all men were rapists, all men were oppressors, all men should be killed. As a white man, I was directly responsible for all of the oppression experienced by women and people of color. I was fourteen years old and had never been in a fight in my life or said a racist or misogynistic word to anyone, but I believed that the circumstances of my birth made me a monster. I wasn't mentally mature enough to think critically about these ideas, or to take them as anything but literal fact. (Literal thinking is common among autistic people, and I would be diagnosed with autism a few years later.) I believed, all the way down to my core, that all men were evil and all women were unimpeachably virtuous. This was black-and-white thinking; it's one of the reasons why so many autistic people are transitioning. I believed that my very existence was sinful.[20]

It's tragic and cruel—though unfortunately not surprising—that such a message would be given to a young person. As we have seen, masculinity that is distorted ranges from hating oneself for the real or imagined potential of being violent to actually perpetrating violence against others and being reluctant to relinquish that raw power. Both sides are extremes, and each requires very different kinds of treatment. Males like Syb need reassurance, encouragement, and loving support to appreciate the good in themselves. Males like the football player-rapists are unable to respond to gentleness because they are arrogent and entitled. Invested in their glorified status, they will keep perpetuating the ultimate masculine stereotype unless they are forcibly restrained. Women can stand up to such men if they are sure of their physical safety; but ultimately, power-hungry men will be stripped of their "right" to abuse only if decent men join the fight to stop them.

Males are not the only ones who are invested in their gender roles, however. *Toxic femininity* is not in the common vernacular because phony feminists are interested only in denigrating males. But there cannot be toxic masculinity without its counterpart, toxic femininity. That is the topic of the next section.

Toxic Femininity

Just as some men have taken their stereotyped roles to an extreme (being hyper-masculine), some women have taken *their* stereotyped roles to an extreme (being hyper-feminine). In a gendered society, toxic masculinity cannot exist without toxic femininity. Each negatively offsets, contrasts, and opposes the other.[21] However, the negative traits of each are very different.

The first rule that most girls learn is to be "nice" (as discussed in Chapter 2). Nice means smiling, even if they don't feel like it, to make others feel better. Nice is keeping quiet about what they need, especially if saying something might hurt someone else's feelings (others always come first, they are taught). A nurturer isn't selfish, and women are nurturers. And if a woman is *really* nice, she won't express anger if she doesn't get what she needs because it's not feminine. Besides, being angry doesn't look "nice." Common phrases that girls hear are "Don't rock the boat." "It's not as bad as you're making it out to be." And of course there's the classic guilt trip, "How could you do that to your mother/father?" To keep quiet, girls are either rewarded with praise, intimidated by the withdrawal of love, or threatened outright with punishment. This strong childhood conditioning ultimately backfires in the worst way possible. Girls grow up believing that if they cannot get their needs met by being direct, they'll have to manipulate. The coping skills they develop, sometimes referred to as "feminine wiles", are tricks to get others to do what they want—either without appearing pushy, or without appearing as though they are asking for anything at all. This manipulation is a major feature of toxic femininity.

Another classic manifestation of toxic femininity is martyrdom. While martyrdom is usually recognized in a political or religious context—someone sacrificing their life for a cause—when it pertains to day-to-day relationships, the psychological term is "having a martyr complex." In this paradigm, martyrs believe that because they're supposed to be "nice," the only way they can be accepted and loved—and get their own needs met, albeit surreptitiously—is to selflessly take care of others. The catch is, no one can continually give and deny their own needs without eventually feeling resentful. Martyrs typically blame others for the sacrifices they make. And they never let others forget it. Imagine the following scene between a woman and someone else. In this example it's a male romantic partner, but it could involve a female romantic partner, friend, or family member. Hurt or angry about something he did or didn't do, instead of being direct she's silent—shoulders dropped, eyes cast down. He asks her what's wrong but is told, "Nothing. I'm fine," when she clearly isn't fine. Or she says "It doesn't matter," when he can tell that it really does matter. She might also say, "After all I've done for you, you don't care," and then list her grievances. Whether the behavior is overt complaining or sulking, he rightly experiences it as manipulation. Crying—a more acceptable expression for females than anger—might be perceived as manipulation too. The common denominator of all of these scenarios is that they feature woman as victim.

Victimhood can be regarded as the logical outcome of gendered femininity *carried to its ultimate extreme.* When it's fueled by anger, victimhood can manifest as an aggressive sense of entitlement. (Victimhood was addressed in detail in Chapter 8.) Toxic-feminine entitlement is what we see in highly materialistic women who are often referred to as "gold diggers." Sometimes they are seen as stereotyped spoiled princesses who make unreasonable demands and expect their husbands, wives, or male or female lovers to cater to them. A partner who is kind-hearted may try hard to please such a woman, but end up only feeling frustrated, hurt, and angry. Sadly, this caricature of a woman is not only supported in our culture, it's encouraged. Her victimhood—a combination of entitlement and childishness, because she cannot make her own way in the world as a mature adult—ends up victimizing those who feel guilty and responsible if she doesn't get what she says she needs. In this dynamic, the woman-as-victim ends up victimizing her partner. The lines between victim and victimizer eventually become so heavily blurred that the roles are reversed.

Another way in which toxic-feminine women may manipulate is by using sexual charisma—the most potent, and only, power they feel they have left. Because women as a group still have less influence in the world than men, if a woman can use her sexiness to entice, taunt, persuade or influence susceptible men or women, she will do it. In return for her allure or explicit sexual services, a woman assumes the right to acquire material goods. Stereotyped masculine-identified males (and an occasional butch lesbian) are especially susceptible to willingly provide these for her. A man may give her trinkets and she gives him sex—often without feeling gratified herself—but neither one is capable of a mutually satisfying, loving relationship because for the extreme stereotypical female and the extreme stereotypical male, this is the only way they know how to connect. A man who wants an honest and authentic relationship with a woman—no game playing, not saying "yes" when you really mean "no" (or vice-versa)—is going to be disappointed if the only type of woman he meets is a woman immersed in toxic femininity. A superficial pickup at a bar comes to mind.

It's not only culturally permissible for a woman to exploit or flaunt her sex appeal, it's often expected—so expected in fact, that even underage girls are sexualized. Hence, some beauty pageants feature girls as young as five years old in makeup and ballgowns, apparently designed to elicit inappropriate sexual desire in others.[22] A former child contestant, who as an adult judged a juvenile pageant, wrote that "one of the contestants…was a lovely girl, but her wardrobe was horrific….She looked like a prostitute."[23] Suffusing the sexiness of toxic femininity is a woman's learned helplessness. Some men find this appealing and even sexually arousing. In others, this distorted character trait elicits their desire to dominate, even rape. And in others, it taps into their preferred role as protector.

Occasionally, girls have parents who actually do prefer girls over boys. Such girls are raised to feel as though others should meet their needs simply because they demand it. This is another form of entitlement, though more direct.

Toxic femininity, which originates in learned passivity, relies on subterfuge and manipulation. Toxic masculinity, which originates in learned aggressiveness, is fueled by the quest for power. As long as men and women are trapped in a polarized, gendered world, they'll continue to be toxic.

Male Bashing

As a group, men in the U.S. deal with higher rates of school dropout, homelessness, suicide, deaths in the workplace and from war and crime, and a reduced life expectancy. Men are often incarcerated longer than women for the same crimes. Also, when parents divorce, today's courts tend to give custody of a child to the mother, even if she's the less fit parent of the two.

Despite the fact that in today's world many men are having a hard time, some women use the phrase "toxic masculinity" to criticize *all* males—irrespective of their capacity to love, their good intentions, or how they're behaving—for being the enemy. *Bashing, no matter who is doing it, is an act of hostility and aggression.* Women who bash men simply for being male—yet object when men do the same to women—apparently don't recognize the double standard. Trained to perceive themselves as victims, such women feel justified in blaming everyone else. Men suffer as a result, because they are villified no matter what they do.

It's difficult to determine what percentage of the general public has come to associate male-bashing women with third wave feminists. However, to see the growing number of articles and commentary on social media and in podcasts and videos, the number seems to be growing. But feminism is not about male-bashing or female-bashing; it's about equal opportunity for both sexes to learn, grow, and develop according to their interests and capabilities. The feminist movement has become infiltrated by a nasty agenda that wants to turn everyone into victims—and thus turn people against each other. Being aware of this ploy can help stop it.

The Aborting of Girls

Independent of the unusual difficulties that modern males are starting to face, females are still devalued. The premium placed on male lives began causing a huge population problem worldwide in the 1970s as sex-selective abortions eliminated hundreds of thousands of female fetuses. Normally, the number of females and males are roughly the same, each comprising about half the population. But in some countries, so many females have been aborted that populations are becoming unbalanced with many more males than females. In many parts of the world only males are desired, including in India, China, Vietnam, Thailand, South Korea, Taiwan, and some countries in the Balkan peninsula of Europe. People in poorer countries who practice female infanticide do so because men are seen as having greater earning power. Also, only men and not women are allowed to perform religious ceremonies. Sometimes the costs of being a bride are a factor. In India, when girls get married their parents are expected to offer the groom and his family a dowry of large sums of money and valuable possessions. Aborting a female fetus solves the problem if the parents aren't well off financially. China's "one child per family" policy makes it an easy decision for many parents to decide to abort female fetuses, especially because (as in other countries) elderly parents live with their sons rather than daughters, who live with the husband's family when they marry. Clearly, having a daughter is a huge liability—so much so, that even some live female infants are killed after they're born.[24] As a general rule, males are given better medical care and are more well-nourished than females. Males also receive education while females aren't educated at all.

In a 1975 study of 99 pregnant mothers who were informed of the sex of their children (53 percent were boys and 46 percent were girls), one mother aborted her boy but 29 aborted their girls.[25] According to another set of data, parents whose nationalities are Chinese, Korean, or Indian "are selectively aborting female fetuses—right here on U.S. soil."[26] More recently in the UK, with greater numbers of immigrants arriving there, an analysis of the 2011 National Census found "widespread discrepancies" in the sex ratio of children being born, indicating that "girls are being aborted....[The] illegal practice of sex-selection abortion is so prevalent that up to 5,000 females have disappeared from the latest national census." One general practitioner said "she is a strong supporter of women's right to choose but that this practice reinforces a very misogynistic view that girls are less valuable than boys."[27] The skewed ratio of males to females has become such a huge problem that *Plos One* published an article in August 2020, "Probabilistic projection of the sex ratio at birth and missing female births by State and Union Territory in India." The sex birth ratio of India, unbalanced since the 1970s, is projected to result in 6.8 million fewer female births by the year 2030 due to the availability of sex-selective abortions. "Our study," the researchers wrote, "highlights the need to strengthen policies that advocate for gender equity and the introduction of support measures to counteract existing gender biases."[28] In 2019, a research analyst at the Population Research Institute wrote, "In India alone, I have found that approximately 15.8 million girls have been eliminated through sex-selective abortion and other forms of prenatal daughter elimination since 1990."[29] This number is equivalent to about the combined populations of Portugal and Finland.

In an attempt to help change the cultural attitudes toward girls, some government officials are visiting the homes of families who have just had baby girls to congratulate them. In Sikar, a particularly sexist province in India, the girl's name is engraved on a nameplate and hung outside the house to show that she is worth as much as a boy. However, beliefs that girls are of no value are slow to change. Since the legalization of abortion (for any reason) in 1971, and the popularity of tests to determine the sex of the fetus, there have been 63 million fewer women born in India. Not surprisingly, India and China perform more than 90% of the world's sex-selective abortions.[30] In the parts of the world where females are so blatantly devalued, how can girls and women be expected to develop self-esteem, autonomy, and skills?

Anyone who believes that females have achieved equal status worldwide with males has only to look at who is being aborted. Humanity has become polarized by gender roles. Chillingly, though, men are beginning to catch up to women in what had previously been seen as a women's issue: rape. See below.

Rape

Of all the forms of bodily harm that one human being can inflict upon another, the invasion of another person via the genitals is the most traumatic. Having one's boundaries invaded in that way—which includes being forced to touch someone else in that most private of areas—cannot be compared to, for instance, being punched in the stomach, as painful as the latter might be. Many people think of rape as forced sex, but "forced" and "sex" is a contradiction in terms. Rape is never about sex. It's about exerting power, domination, and control over another in the most extreme way possible. When one person dominates another physically, it's known as violence. But when someone dominates another and the violence involves the sexual organs, it's rape. Rape is a whole other level of aggression, personal in a way that a punch could never be.

Sexual communion is a physical expression of love and affection—or at the very least a mutual sharing of potentially intense pleasure—that involves the genitals, breasts, and other areas of the body. These are known as *erogenous zones* because they contain the greatest number of nerve endings that are especially sensitive to being touched. Therefore, they are a focus of pleasurable sexual arousal. During sexual excitement between two people who care about each other and are involved in mutual satisfaction, the body releases powerful hormones including *oxytocin*. Known as the "love hormone" or "bonding hormone," oxytocin inspires warm feelings for another person. When private sexual parts, normally connected to an intimate act of sharing pleasure, are associated with a violent and hate-filled act like rape, this creates cognitive and biological dissonance. Furthermore, being raped is physically painful. The delicate nerve endings in the genitals and anus (where men are often raped) are exquisitely sensitive. For all these reasons, rape is traumatic and is rightly considered the ultimate violation. Whether the victim is a woman, girl, boy or man, rape is a terrible desecration not only of someone's body but also their mind and spirit.

In 1927 in the United States, "forcible rape" was defined as "the carnal knowledge of a female, forcibly and against her will." Back then, no one even considered that men could be raped. Rape was generally recognized as the penetration of the vagina by a penis or object through the use of outright force, the threat of physical violence, or emotional intimidation (such as a threat to harm the woman's child or other loved one). In 2012, to ensure that rape included men as well as women so it "will be more accurately reported nationwide," the United States Attorney General issued a new definition of rape that encompassed every possible intrusive behavior: "The penetration, no matter how slight, of the vagina or anus with any body part or object, or oral penetration by a sex organ of another person, without the consent of the victim."[31] Legal definitions in each state can vary, however. Some specifically state that it can occur inside or outside of marriage, or that the victim can be either a woman or a man. In most states, the absence of force is not considered relevant if the person lacks the ability to consent—if they are mentally impaired, or unable to refuse due to the effects of drugs or alcohol. Statutory rape refers to sexual intercourse with a minor (the age of whom varies according to locale), or someone whose age makes consent impossible. Further refinements include the age gap between the two parties.

The rape of women is still tolerated today, primarily in places such as Middle Eastern countries whose laws severely restrict women's movements and rights, and give men a privileged status simply for being male. However, in the industrialized and presumably more enlightened West, rape is still a huge problem. One especially troublesome venue is the military. Female military personnel have increasingly reported being raped—or coerced into having sex with, which is basically the same thing—by their superior officers.

Most rape statistics focus on who is raped. The data may vary slightly depending on who's compiling the data, but the information generally remains consistent. The Rape, Abuse & Incest National Network (RAINN) has compiled the following statistics from various databases, including the Department of Justice and the Department of Defense. Every 73 seconds an American is sexually assaulted. Younger people, especially ages 12–34, have the highest risk of being sexually violated, and women and girls experience the highest rate of sexual violence (one out of six). Eighty-two percent of all juvenile rape survivors are female, and 90 percent of adult rape survivors are female. A surprising 4.3 percent of active duty women experienced unwanted sexual contact. Statistics for males say that about 3 percent of American men, or 1 in 33, have experienced an attempted or completed rape in their lifetime.[32] Another data analysis, this one from University of Michigan, shows that by age 44 at least 25 percent of American woman (one in four), and 8 percent of men, are raped.[33]

Rape has customarily been viewed as a woman's issue, especially by feminists. And most of the publicity surrounding the act has involved females as the victims. However, throughout history more males have been raped than is normally publicized. In 2010, *The Primary Care Companion to the Journal of Clinical Psychiatry* published a letter from a doctor about the rape of men. She pointed out that the effects of sexual abuse have been studied much more extensively in women than in men, but from her experience men suffer just as much, albeit in different ways. Like women, men feel humiliated and ashamed, and they tend to blame themselves. But they're even less likely than women to report sexual assaults—probably because in most cases males are raped by other males, particularly in the military and during wartime, where there's no accountability or restitution. One of the doctor's patients admitted to her that he never told his wife of 30 years that he'd been raped because to him, the act brought so much dishonor. This brings me to another, perhaps more important reason a man doesn't report being raped: He perceives it as a loss of his manhood, because being raped is perceived as "feminine."[34] If a male is overpowered by another male, he's not living up to cultural expectations that he demonstrate power. Being less powerful makes him less manly. Therefore, he's judged to be in the same caste as a less powerful woman. Moreover, a man who is raped and believes that only women can be raped, sees himself—or fears that others will see him—not only as less manly, but as similar to *or the equivalent of a woman*. Without trivializing the disgrace and suffering of males who are raped, there's an ugly subtext here worth noting. In a gendered society, part of what gives a man his identity is that he's not a woman. His selfhood and self-worth are based on his not having presumably "lesser" traits ascribed to females. So when a male is raped and he feels shame because this makes him "feminine" or at the same level as a female, that stereotype sends a clear message to women of their own inferiority.

Most women are vaginally raped, although the anus can also be an avenue of violence for a penis or hard object. Most men are anally raped. They can also be forced to have genital contact with other men's or women's genitals as well as inanimate orifices. A male's physiology allows him to achieve enough of an erection that will allow the penis to enter a vagina or other orifice—even if the boy or man doesn't want that type of contact and doesn't derive pleasure from it. Male physiology may also make ejaculation possible, even under stressful or downright unpleasant circumstances. Anal penetration alone can exert enough pressure on the prostate gland to lead to unpleasurable physiological responses of erection and ejaculation.[35] It's understandable that men feel ashamed and bewildered over having had an erection while being coerced into unwanted sexual contact.

During wartime, the rape of men can be a regular occurrence—although reporter Will Storr, who traveled to Uganda to survey the situation first-hand, wrote that "It is usually denied by the perpetrator and his victim." One man who had been raped by his captors three times a day, every day for three years, was in constant pain and continually exuded pus from his penis. He told Storr, "There are certain things you just don't believe can happen to a man...But I know now that sexual violence against men is a huge problem. Everybody has heard the women's stories. But nobody has heard the men's." The rape of men has occurred in many places besides East Africa, among them Kuwait, Russia, Chile, Greece, Coatia, Iran, and the former Yugoslavia. Storr wrote, "Twenty-one percent of Sri Lankan males who were seen at a London torture treatment centre reported sexual abuse while in detention. In El Salvador, 76% of male political prisoners surveyed in the 1980s described at least one incidence of sexual torture. A study of 6,000 concentration-camp inmates in Sarajevo found that 80% of men reported having been raped."[36]

Boys are another group specifically targeted for rape. In the last few decades, a large number of courageous males disclosed that their perpetrators came from an unexpected sector: the Catholic Church. Since at least the 1950s, Catholic priests were molesting young children, many of them alter boys. Based on what we now know about human trafficking and sexual abuse, it's not unreasonable to think that this type of abuse may have been occurring for a century or more. Many of the boys who had been abused came forward only when they were adults. Other men who had been abused as boys died before restitution could be made. The molested boys number in the hundreds of thousands, despite the Church's best efforts to silence them.[37] Clearly, we have work to do to surrounding the abuse of power.

Even if a child (of either sex) is molested without penetration, it's still traumatic. Sexually violated girls and boys are additionally victimized because they're still maturing, and are mentally and physically dependent on adults for love and support. If the parents deny that abuse has taken place, the child is more traumatized. And if the sexual abuser is a close relative, family friend or the child's own parent, the repercussions are devastating.

The stigma of being thought homosexual can be strong for men who are raped, particularly those who aren't comfortable with same-sex attraction. Therefore, many male rape victims don't report abuse. Those that do seek treatment may prefer to talk to a female, rather than a male, therapist. Men's fear of being judged for being homosexual by male counselors may be justified, because mental health professionals are not immune from personal bias and it's possible that they have not overcome their homophobia. Unfortunately, when doing intake evaluations the majority of mental health professionals, particularly if they are male, still fail to ask men about a history of rape or other forms of sexual abuse. Storr pointed out that "silence about male victims reinforces unhealthy expectations about men and their supposed invulnerability."[38]

As more men overcome their shame at what they perceive as a threat to their masculinity and are willing to report being raped, an unexpected picture of potential rapists emerges. Although the majority of sexual assaults on men are committed by other self-defined heterosexual males, women can be perpetrators too. Although historically women and girls have been the targets of rape, and people commonly perceive men as the rapists and women as the victims, more accurate recent reporting as well as convictions show that women can, and do, sexually assault men, other women, and children. Men are now coming forward to relay accounts of getting drunk or force-fed Viagra and other drugs, being tied up, and brutalized by women. While most women are unable to employ physical force to sexually assault a man—unless he is drugged—they can utilize blackmail, threatening to disclose something in the man's life if he doesn't comply.

An article published in 2017, "Sexual victimization perpetrated by women: Federal data reveal surprising prevalence," stated that a much higher number of women than had previously been thought had perpetrated nonconsensual sexual events, and that those on the receiving end were mostly men. "Stereotypes about women...include the notion that women are nurturing, submissive helpmates to men," the authors wrote. "The idea that women can be sexually manipulative, dominant, and even violent runs counter to these stereotypes. Yet studies have documented female-perpetrated acts that span a wide spectrum of sexual abuse, which include even severe harms such as nonconsensual oral sex, vaginal and anal penetration with a finger or object, and intercourse. Despite this reality, the minimizing of female perpetration persists."[39] The authors took great care to reassure their readers that focusing on the abuse of men did not negate the fact that women are abused. Also, they stated, by acknowledging that women can be perpetrators, they were not being misogynistic but were imparting a more in-depth picture that women, far from being passive, can be forceful—although of course this particular manifestation of aggression was hardly condoned.

The study, enthusiastically picked up by the media, had the benefit of giving more men permission to publicly acknowledge their sexual abuse, to notify law enforcement, and to seek psychological help. However, one extremely troubling aspect of the paper was the authors' report of a study that had a very broad definition of rape. "Nonconsensual sex," which included nagging, begging, and other verbal pressure, was regarded as rape.[40] But if having intercourse because someone yielded to verbal pressure is equated with rape resulting from overt force or violence, this automatically increases both the number of male victims and the number of female perpetrators, which is what the study focused on.[41] Of course all acts of violence, sexual or not, are reprehensible, and perpetrators should be punished. But whining and pestering someone for sexual intercourse—when the man might simply walk away, and the woman might walk away too if she's not being physically threatened or overpowered—is a far cry from rape. Men, who as a group have the advantage of greater physical strength than women, need to give themselves permission to remove themselves from an emotionally manipulative situation—in contrast to women as a group, who tend to be more easily coerced due to the very real fear that the man could become physically violent. It's a reasonable question how much this change in definition detracts from the seriousness of actual rape—of both females and males. It should be noted that after reading the paper, I emailed one of the authors and asked him if he, and/or his co-authors, subscribed to the broader definition of rape. He never responded. So it's quite possible that they included the broader definition when citing their statistics—which would then invalidate the entire study.

Another danger of broadening the definition of rape is that rather than empower people, the precise opposite will occur. Being encouraged to verify, "My spouse harassed me for sex and wouldn't leave me alone until I acquiesced—and now I'm a rape victim," discourages the supposed victim from implementing proactive behavior, including walking away. While any form of emotional abuse is cruel and should never be ignored or excused, having someone whine at you for sex can hardly be equated with someone pointing a weapon at you or using physical force. To offer people legal "protection" against being pestered creates a mindset of being a victim. And convincing people that they're powerless lowers their self-esteem and doesn't teach them how to take care of themselves. This broadened definition of rape feels similar, in both intention and agenda, to coddling college students so they perceive themselves as victims (discussed in great detail in Chapter 8). On the other hand, threatening to stop a spouse's allowance unless there's compliance, kicking the refusing party out of the house, or leaving and taking the kids, is an entirely different scenario and needs to be dealt with differently.

The person who has been raped is responsible for promptly reporting it. But she or he sometimes avoids doing so out of shame, fear, or guilt. Thus the reporting might be delayed, which means that any DNA evidence could degrade or wash away. Understandably, a woman who has been brought up to think that her body should be available to anyone who wants it—and then faces the prospect of dealing with law enforcement personnel who believe this as well—might be reluctant to file a report. And a man burdened by his stereotyped role—that men are always able and willing to have sex, and what's wrong with him if he doesn't want it?—might also be reluctant to file a report. Thus both women and men underreport sex crimes, though for different reasons.

Once a report is filed, the person who is raped must be interviewed. Not all interviewers are trained to handle this sensitive crime. If the interviewer is the same sex as the person who perpetrated the rape, this places additional stress on the interviewee. Then there's the exam. A thorough exam must be performed (again, with someone of the appropriate sex), which includes the collection of saliva, semen, vaginal fluids, perhaps blood or hair, and any other materials that could yield DNA. But in some states, people who are raped are required to pay for their own rape kits. This communicates to them that their experience was not important, and they must bear their burden alone.

Police treatment of people who have been raped is not always kind. In 2015, an 18-year-old woman named Marie reported that she was sexually assaulted by a masked man who broke into her Washington state apartment and stood over her bed wielding a knife. She was not only ridiculed by the authorities when she described the masked man, but she was charged with false reporting and branded by the media as the perpetrator of a massive fraud. Because there were slight inconsistencies in her account—which commonly occurs with people who have been traumatized—the detectives handling her case treated her as a suspect. Under pressure, the young woman recanted. She was subsequently prosecuted for false reporting and was ordered to pay $500 in court costs, get mental health counseling, and be on supervised probation for one year. It was only two years later in Colorado, when the police arrested a serial rapist and found a photograph of Marie proving that he had indeed raped her, that she was finally exonerated and her name was cleared. But a great deal of damage had already been done. Marie's story of not being believed is regrettably typical. Although there are many wonderful police officers who are sensitive to the needs of sexually traumatized people, Marie's situation is hardly unique—because, write two reporters in an article "Charged With Lying," "the victims hadn't acted the way the police thought a victim should act. Their affect seemed off, or they declined help from an advocate, or they looked away instead of making eye contact"—all of which are reasonable and normal reactions after having gone through a traumatic event. "As a result, their stories became suspect....The police should be wary of stereotypes; they should not, for example, find an adolescent victim less believable than an adult. Some victims will be hysterical, others stoic; police should not measure credibility by a victim's response."[42]

Most people who are raped don't receive effective help, or enough of it. If proper treatment is not consistently available, the negative effects can be devastating. Effects on physical health range from immune malfunction and increased susceptibility to infections to chronic pelvic pain and constant head and back pain. There's also the possibility of venereal disease, pelvic inflammatory disease, and urinary tract infection directly resulting from the rape. Psychologically, victims may experience chronic anxiety, hypervigilance, excessive anger, and long-term depression. Sleep and eating disorders may erupt, and flashbacks and nightmares are common. Motivation, self-confidence, and one's sense of self-worth decrease. Intimacy in personal relationships is avoided because it's too scary or emotionally painful. In severe cases, a person might become suicidal. Thirty-one percent of rape victims develop PTSD (post-traumatic stress disorder), and 11 percent still have PTSD today—an estimated 1.3 million people.[43, 44]

At what point does a rape subject become a victim? Without the proper treatment, his or her view of the world orients around danger and unkindness because brain circuits and neurochemical output have been permanently altered. Because the person was likely too terrified or intimidated to say "no" during the rape—especially if the perpetrator was physically overpowering, threatened the victim with violence or blackmail, or showed a weapon—supportive counseling is always indicated. The therapist must make it clear that not having said "no" does *not* mean that the victim was complicit, invited it, or wanted it. If PTSD symptoms appear, more than talk psychotherapy may be required. Chapter 9 addressed the biochemistry of PTSD in detail.

In the past several decades, laws have been passed that offer rape survivors more protection and legal recourse. According to some statistics, incidences of rape, sexual assault, and other violence against intimate partners have been declining for decades.[45] But it's difficult to know how to interpret those figures. We don't know if rape survivors always reported the abuse, if accused rapists were prosecuted, or if rapists were convicted and jailed. Also, rape is not always defined consistently. In surveys where men are asked if they ever raped anyone, they tend to respond no—but if asked if they ever coerced someone to have intercourse by physically restraining them, they respond yes. The same holds true for the women who are coerced into yielding to sexual intercourse.[46] Thus the incidence of rape is not only higher than what's being reported, people's awareness of what constitutes rape is much lower than you might think. It's troubling that men would not allow themselves to be held accountable for sexual violence.

This brings me to society's attitude toward females who are raped. One 1998 study found that both men and women believe the following: *A woman claims rape to protect her reputation. Women unconsciously want to be raped, so they put themselves in a dangerous situation (including going out alone at night). If a woman's intoxicated, she's usually willing to have sex. Women who wear revealing clothing or act flirtatiously are inviting rape. Sexually experienced women cannot be damaged if they're raped. One should be skeptical of accusations of rape by women who work in bars, as dance hostesses, and as prostitutes. Women who accept rides from strangers and are then raped, get what they deserve. An able woman can resist being raped if she really tries. Some women need to be raped, it would do them some good. Most women secretly want to be raped, and in most cases if a woman was raped she deserved it.*[47] Have attitudes changed since then? A small sample of 208 participants responded to more recent surveys. Some common ideas about rape were: *She asked for it. He didn't mean it. It wasn't rape. She lied.* More males than females blamed rape victims for both their behavior and character, and believed that women were responsible for being raped. More women than men thought that rape was traumatic.

Persistent gender role stereotyping makes everything worse, the authors continued. Men equate sexual expression with dominance, thus justifying rape and other forms of violence. And women who are trained to be sexually passive—and thus blame themselves for being raped even when it wasn't their fault—may fall into patterns that provide a foundation for rape to occur. In fact, women who are quick to blame themselves may even doubt that a rape has occurred, and they may not even be certain whether or not the man was violent.[48]

Sometimes, however, women *are* at fault—but not in the way one might think. It has become increasingly common for women to make false accusations of rape, usually against high-profile and wealthy men. In some cases, the women were later proven to have lied. One example, which allegedly occurred in 2006 at Duke University, was said to have involved three lacrosse players. The woman who falsely accused them was later convicted of child abuse and criminal damage to property. Another example is a gang rape that had presumably taken place at the University of Virginia. It was reported as factual in the *Rolling Stone* article, "A Rape on Campus," but the following year the magazine was obliged to retract the entire story. We don't know how many false rapes are reported. According to the FBI database, the number of false allegations is 8 percent, but these statistics are from 1996, and the FBI is no longer compiling rape statistics (we need to ask why).[49] A more recent study—supposedly after a detailed investigation—estimates the number of falsely reported rapes to be between two and 10 percent.[50] But even those statistics are unreliable. Either there's insufficient evidence, the accuser is characterized as "uncooperative" (due to trauma or untruth), or those charged with determining fact from fiction are biased.

Regardless of how often rapes are falsely reported, in today's climate accusing someone of rape is a highly effective weapon to extort money or destroy their reputation. A false accusation is not only unjust, it's illegal. The act of falsely accusing someone of committing any crime, including rape, is a misdemeanor that could result in incarceration for at least one year. So why would a woman place herself in such legal jeopardy by knowingly making a false accusation? Is she acting alone out of vindictiveness? Or is she being paid off by someone? Even if the accused is eventually exonerated of the crime, the publicity itself can cause social, professional, and psychological damage. Every time a woman falsely accuses a man of rape, she not only makes it difficult for the man, but she invalidates women for whom sexual violence is a reality. She also makes it more difficult for actual rape victims to receive the empathy and services they urgently need because people no longer take them seriously. The high media profile of false accusations has made it more difficult for even law enforcement personnel to believe women who are raped.

One more thing. Most men regard their genitals as an expression of manhood and their personal worth. Similarly, most women regard their genitals—including their internal reproductive organs, capable of creating new life—as an expression of their womanhood and personal worth. If being genitally violated (raped) can cause massive trauma to a person's psyche, imagine what the actual loss or mutilation of these literal and figurative symbols of personhood does. When people undergo genital surgery for whatever reason, it's a violation. Perhaps this is one reason why the majority of trans adults, even though they identify as the opposite sex, keep their genitals.

The Enemy Within

In the United States, the issue of gender has become so polarized that even some men who are sincerely sympathetic to the problems that women face react negatively to the word "feminism." Conversely, some women who are still grappling with the way they are still viewed and treated by this culture find it difficult to relate to men as human beings.

In 2017 in California, American film director Cassie Jaye—who directed the 2016 documentary "The Red Pill" about the men's rights movement—gave a talk about how, as a feminist, she needed to learn to let go of certain assumptions about men. "Being pro-woman doesn't mean being anti-male," she pointed out. "It's not a contest...When you dehumanize your enemy you feel more justified in attacking them....We need to work together....Equality should not be about punishing the other side, it should be about lifting each other up. We have to stop expecting to be offended and start truly, sincerely, listening."[51]

Sometimes it's difficult to listen to the other side—precisely because we see them as "other." It's time to call a truce. Erroneous beliefs and expectations prevent us from developing compassion. Gender—the word that many still insist on using to indicate biological sex—isn't the problem. Gender *roles* are. The sooner we understand this, the sooner we can heal.

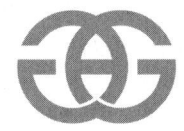

Appendix B

Transgender Athletes in Sports

Biology and Physiology of Male and Female Athletes

Before puberty, when another surge of testosterone will saturate the bodies of boys, children who engage in physical activity in mixed-sex groups have a more level playing field. Even so, in most cases the athletic prowess of the sexes is not equivalent. As a group, boys are more energetic. They tend to play rougher than girls—unless the girls are particularly athletic. The organization Gays Against Groomers created a sticker that reads, "Save The Tomboys." This refers to the better-than-average athletic prowess of some girls who love physical activities and prefer the company of their high-energy male counterparts. As long as the girls can keep up, most boys don't mind playing with them. They regard their female playmates as "one of the guys."

After puberty, the differences in physiology between females and males are much more pronounced. Testosterone not only gives men as much as 40 percent more muscle mass than women, but men's skeletal muscle fibers contract more quickly, and with more force.[1] In upper body strength, men are more than 30 percent stronger than women.[2] The bone mass in men can be up to 50 percent higher than in women.[3] Adjusting for differences in size, men's hearts and lungs are larger than women's, allowing for a higher intake and delivery of oxygen. Translated into jogging performance, a woman will need to work at over 70% of her capacity to keep up with a man who's jogging at about 50% of his. *Sports Medicine* researchers—after examining body fat percentage, hormones, cardiovascular adaptations to aerobic training, high density lipoprotein and cholesterol levels, and even women's menstrual cycles—concluded that males have an advantage over females in sports,[4] which is a very good reason why sports for girls and boys, and women and men, are segregated.

Articles comparing women's and men's athletic performance aren't new. Back in 2010, an article in the *Journal of Sports Science and Medicine* analyzed 82 sports events that had been in existence since the first Olympics games. These events included cycling, swimming, weightlifting, speed skating, and many other types of track and athletic events. After a thorough comparison of male and female performances for identical events, the authors concluded that men were faster than women.[5] Dozens, if not hundreds of such papers, exist. No impartial or reasonable researcher could dispute these findings. The fact that today we seem to require studies to prove what mere observation would have confirmed to our grandparents is another issue.

What about adult men who take estrogen, or take estrogen *and* suppress their testosterone production? Are there differences in exercise and running between them and biological women? A study in the *British Journal of Sports Medicine*, "Effect of gender affirming hormones on athletic performance in transwomen and transmen: implications for sporting organisations and legislators," examined 29 FtM and 46 MtF people who were taking cross-sex hormones while in the United States Air Force. Air Force troops were a good choice for the analysis because of the superior fitness standards required in order to be admitted into service. Pre- and post-hormone fitness test results were compared, along with body composition and athletic performance. The MtF transgenders, before taking estrogen—which means they still had their natal blood hormone levels—did 31 percent more push-ups and 15 percent more sit-ups in one minute than natal women. They also ran a mile and a half 21 percent faster than natal women. After two years of being on estrogen, the number of push-ups and sit-ups were the same as those of natal women. However, the MtF running times were still faster, at 12 percent. Even testosterone suppression could not equalize the running times between the MtF individuals and biological women.[6]

What about differences in strength between MtFs and natal women? Think about the effects of testosterone on a male body *in utero*. Not only are bones denser and stronger, but the unique muscle fibers formed by testosterone, along with their greater mass, confer advantages for swimming, running, hitting, lifting, cycling, and all other types of weight-bearing activities. Inherently wider shoulders, due to a different skeletal structure, add to the strength advantages conferred by the muscles. The authors of the afoementioned article wrote:

> Exposure to testosterone during puberty results in sex differences in height, pelvic architecture and leg bones in the lower limbs that confer an athletic advantage to males after puberty. These anatomical differences do not respond to changes in testosterone exposure among post-pubertal adults. These pretreatment anatomical differences

may explain why transwomen retained an advantage in 1.5 mile run times over CW ["cis" women, or natal women] after beginning oestrogen as an adult, while push-up and sit-up performance, which are less influenced by differences in skeletal architecture, declined to the level of CW after two years on oestrogen....[7]

The authors also pointed out that on average, male-bodied MtFs weigh more than natal females—so any reduction in MtF individuals' strength due to estrogen is still not enough to level the playing field between them and actual women. The researchers admitted that they may have underestimated the strength advantages of MtFs—differences that even years of taking cross-sex hormones could not erase.

Only a tiny number of studies allege no performance differences between MtFs and natal women. Nevertheless, trans activists claim that estrogenized males have less physical strength, period. The mass media disseminates this view.

Simply put, it's a lie that a male-bodied individual who is taking estrogen and/or testosterone blockers for one year has nullified any benefits of testosterone in his natal male body. The title of this journal article concisely summarizes the data: "Muscle strength, size and composition following 12 months of gender-affirming treatment in transgender individuals: retained advantage for the transwomen."[8] In another article, New Zealand physiology professor Alison Kay Heather (who herself is a long-distance runner and has competed in triathlons) conducted an extensive review of every article on the athletic performance of biological men, biological women, and transgender athletes up until 2022. Heather first summarized men's and women's athletic abilities, and then compared the performances of MtFs to those of biological women.

> Without the sex division, females would have little chance of winning because males are faster, stronger, and have greater endurance capacity. Male physiology underpins their better athletic performance including increased muscle mass and strength, stronger bones, different skeletal structure...[and] better adapted cardiorespiratory systems....Testosterone secreted before birth, postnatally, and then after puberty is the major factor that drives these physiological sex differences, and as adults, testosterone levels are ten to fifteen times higher in males than females. The non-overlapping ranges of testosterone between the sexes has led sports regulators, such as the International Olympic Committee, to use 10 nmol/L testosterone [nmol/L is nanomoles per liter, so the measurement is 10 nanomoles of testosterone per liter of blood] as a sole physiological parameter to divide the male and female sporting divisions. *Using [blood] testosterone levels as a basis for separating female and male elite athletes is arguably flawed. Male physiology cannot be reformatted by estrogen therapy in transwoman athletes because testosterone has driven permanent effects through early life exposure.* This descriptive critical review discusses the inherent male physiological advantages that lead to superior athletic performance and then addresses how estrogen

therapy fails to create a female-like physiology in the male. *Ultimately, the former male physiology of transwoman athletes provides them with a physiological advantage over the cis- [biological] female athlete.* [emphasis added][9]

A few MtF athletes have been honest enough to publicly admit that their natal biology allowed them to become champions. Now 55 years old, retired Danish golfer Mianne Bagger supports legal changes that "would have stopped her from competing earlier in her career." The fact that "male-bodied" competitors are allowed to compete, Bagger stated, is a "slap in the face to women." The golfer was in favor of "inclusion" in "everyday society" as well as "equal access to life and services and work." But athletics is different, Bagger declared. "Sport is about physical ability....If you've got one group—males—that are on average stronger, taller, faster, as opposed to women, there has to be a divide."[10]

Another highly accomplished athlete—who transitioned after retiring from sports—has also spoken many times in favor of keeping women's sports for natal women. Bruce Jenner was a world-class athlete and Olympic gold medalist, seeming to embody what one might envision as a model of masculinity. However, Jenner has confessed that as a young boy, he never felt right in a male body and secretly tried on dresses belonging to his mother and sisters. Born in 1949, Jenner finished transitioning very late in life—taking estrogen briefly in the late 1980s, resuming it in 2014, and completing surgery in 2017—and at the age of 65, came out to the world as Caitlyn Jenner.[11] One might think that Jenner's fame, accomplishments, and unbiased MtF trans perspective would be enough for people to seriously consider the issue of unfair competition between biological women and MtFs. But even Jenner has experienced backlash from highly vocal trans activists who make unfounded and implausible accusations of transphobia.

Professional tennis player and biological female Wimbledon champion Martina Navratilova has also objected to MtF trans participation in women's sports. One of her Twitter posts read, "You can't just proclaim yourself a female and be able to compete against women. There must be some standards, and having a penis and competing as a woman would not fit that standard."[12] In 2019, she wrote in England's *Sunday Times*:

> Letting men compete as women simply if they change their name and take hormones is unfair—no matter how those athletes may throw their weight around....A man builds up muscle and bone density, as well as a greater number of oxygen-carrying red blood cells, from childhood....To put the argument at its most basic: a man can decide to be female, take hormones if required by whatever sporting organisation is concerned, win everything in sight and perhaps earn a small fortune, and then reverse his decision....It's insane and it's cheating.[13]

As punishment for speaking up, Navratilova has been denounced and accused of transphobia by trans activists and the mainstream media.[14] To her credit,

Navratilova stated that before publicly commenting, she had researched the issue first until she had enough data to make an informed opinion. One irony—which trans activists conveniently overlooked—is that Navratilova is hardly a stranger to the so-called LGBTQ+ community. She herself is an "out" lesbian, has participated in lesbian rights groups for years, and is friends with not only trans tennis player Renée Richards but also intersex track star Caster Semenya, both of whom are discussed a bit later.

Many other female athletes, both high school and professional, object to men competing in women's sports. But few have come forward because they've been psychologically intimidated and even warned that they'd be blacklisted if they spoke up. Some have been physically threatened. Martina Navratilova is retired, so she does not have to fear financial retaliation. Nevertheless, the negative press against her has been very hostile and disturbing, and would dampen the spirits of anyone.

Male-Born Transgenders (MtFs) Who Compete Against Women
The First MtF Trans Athlete

The earliest known existence of a transgender person in sports was in 1975, when American Richard Raskind underwent sex "reassignment" surgery to become Renée Richards. Regarded as one of the best male college tennis players in the country, Raskind received training as an ophthalmologist while continuing to play competitive tennis, ranking sixth out of the top twenty men over 35 years of age. After surgery, Richards sued the United States Tennis Association to be allowed to compete in women's professional tennis. The USTA, the United States Open Committee (USOC), and some other tennis associations were requiring all female competitors to verify their sex with a Barr body test of their chromosomes. Richards did not want to take the test. In a court document, the Tennis Association emphasized that men—even those who had completed sex "reassignment" surgery—have a competitive advantage due to their initial development and physical training as males.

> We have reason to believe that there are as many as 10,000 transsexuals in the United States...Because of the millions of dollars of prize money available to competitors, because of nationalistic desires to excel in athletics, and because of world-wide experiments, especially in the iron curtain countries, to produce athletic stars by means undreamed of a few years ago, the USTA has been especially sensitive to its obligation to assure fairness of competition among the athletes competing in the U.S. Open, the leading international tennis tournament in the United States. The USTA believes that the Olympic type sex determination procedures are a reasonable way to assure fairness and equality of competition when dealing with numerous competitors from around the world.[15]

Richards finally took the chromosome test. Although results proved inconclusive (the public record does not state why), in August 1977 a judge ruled in Richards's favor, and the tennis player continued to compete and win a large number of women's tournaments. Significantly, many years later Richards conceded—and, one might infer, contritely—that having the foundational physiology of a man had conferred advantages in the sports field. "I know if I'd had surgery at the age of 22, and then at 24 went on the tour, no genetic woman in the world would have been able to come close to me. And so I've reconsidered my opinion....Maybe... not even I should have been allowed to play on the women's tour. Maybe I should have knuckled under and said, 'That's one thing I can't have as my newfound right in being a woman.' I think transsexuals have every right to play, but maybe not at the professional level, because *it's not a level playing field*." [emphasis added][16] Richards is on record as opposing the 2004 ruling of the International Olympic Committee (IOC) that transgender people can compete after they've had surgery and two years of cross-sex hormones. The most recent guidelines of the IOC are much more lax, which I'll be addressing shortly.

Same Privilege, New Package

Until recently, it was instinctively and rationally understood that it's unfair to force women to compete against generally stronger men. Again, only one in 20 women is as strong as the average man. But in today's climate, males who take estrogen are allowed to compete in women's sports. Having retained their heavily muscled physiques, and with their genitalia intact, they appear male in every respect. This means that after growing their hair long and applying a little lipstick to prove their "identification," they get to keep their reproductive organs—and then outperform their competitors, stealing the prize money and trophies from the women and girls who had trained so hard for so long.

Cycling is one of the pro sports that has been very insensitive, if not hostile, to the needs of actual women. In 2022 Rachel McKinnon, a biological male who says he identifies as female, won the women's Masters Track Cycling World Championships sprint title for the second year in a row, setting a new world best time. McKinnon won 35,000 dollars, stealing titles and money from the woman who came in second. This isn't the first time that McKinnon had unethically acquired prize money and awards. In 2019 on a Manchester, England track, he won a second consecutive Sprint gold and a silver in the Time Trial event, and set a world record. In response to these upsets, someone tweeted, "Sorry to all female athletes who spent their lives mastering their games. [The headline should have read,] Transgender Cyclist Who Set Women's World Record Wouldn't Have Qualified For Men's Championship."[17] In defense mode, McKinnon posted on Twitter, "3rd place (Jennifer Wagner) claims it's unfair for me to compete. At Masters Worlds, she beat me in the 500m TT. She beat me in 6 of 7 races at the 2017 Intelligentsia Cup. In 2016 she beat me in all 3 Speed Week crits [sic]. She's won 11 of our 13 races...and it's unfair? Excuse me?"[18] However, one exceptional woman who can out-compete McKinnon does not compensate for all the other pro female cyclists whose livelihoods are threatened. They would have won more money and the next highest medal had McKinnon not raced.

About McKinnon's win, Martina Navratilova—who even made a concession by using the pronoun "she"—wrote, "McKinnon has vigorously defended her right to compete, pointing out that, when tested, her levels of testosterone... were well within the limits set by world cycling's governing body. Nevertheless, at 6 ft tall and weighing more than 14 stone [196 pounds], she appeared to have a substantial advantage in muscle mass over her rivals."[19] Cyclist Victoria Hood, who was not competing at the time due to an injury, told BBC Sport:

> The world record has just been beaten today by somebody born male, who now identifies as female, and the gap between them and the next born female competitor was quite a lot. The world record was two tenths of a second. I know that doesn't sound like a lot but it is. The gap between them and the next female competitor was four tenths, which to put into perspective in a sprint event like this, that would be 15m [meters] of the track, when sprint events are usually won by centimetres. It is a human right to participate in sport. I don't think it's a human right to identify into whichever category you choose.
>
> If people want to push this through some misguided idea that they are being inclusive, it is not inclusive. *It is excluding women and girls from their own category.* It's not fair. The IOC [International Olympic Committee] need[s] to make fair policies that are based on the science that we have, because if they can't then they are not fit for [the] purpose [for which they exist]. They are washing their hands of it and it is becoming more political than it is about science and biology. [emphasis added][20]

In response to the accusations of biological advantage, McKinnon posted on Twitter, "Well, no, I'm still forced to have an unhealthily low endogenous testosterone value...it's virtually undetectable it's so low...way below the average for women."[21] With these statements, McKinnon was unwittingly admitting the truth. Being "forced" to lower his testosterone meant that McKinnon did not want to do it. That the hormone dropped to an "unhealthily low" level meant that McKinnon *knew* his male body was not inherently designed for such a drastic, artificial lessening of a hormone required for him to function optimally. In natal males, the dangerous long-term effects of suppressing the body's natural testosterone production—alongside supplementing with estrogen—includes heart problems and brittle bones that will inevitably break. I wonder if, two or three decades from now, the short-term benefits of winning will be worth the health problems for such men. The many negative effects of taking cross-sex hormones was discussed in detail in Chapter 3.

I have not seen reports that McKinnon parted with his penis and testicles. However, it's reasonable to assume that they are intact, because there was no mention of surgery in McKinnon's biographical data or in any news reports. McKinnon's one concession to the appearance of stereotypical femininity seems to be growing long hair and wearing dainty jewelry and a dress, as seen in a stock publicity photo on Wikipedia.[22] However, another photo of him wearing a gold medal, received at the 2018 UCI World Masters Track Cycling Championships in Los Angeles, reveals a masculine-looking guy with shorter hair, shaped so that it's long only at the back of the neck but still above the shoulders. It could be a haircut that any man would wear. Heavily muscled, McKinnon shows a clearly masculine chest, with no breast implants or feminine breast growth.[22] McKinnon is a man, no matter what rules a sports organization concocts.

"There's a stereotype," McKinnon complained, "that men are always stronger than women, so people think there is an unfair advantage." The reality of biology and physique could hardly be called a "stereotype"! But let's move on. "By preventing trans women from competing or requiring them to take medication, you're denying their human rights."[24] What about the "human rights" of women who are excluded from their own category to make room for a man? And if someone is a "trans woman," as McKinnon claims he is, he would not only by definition be on medication, he'd *want* to be taking cross-sex hormones.

Not all female athletes objected to McKinnon's wins. The second-place winner of the 2018 Los Angeles cycling event, Dutch competitor Carolien Van Herrikhuyzen, posted on Twitter her belief that "No one is a transgender to steal anyone's medal. We had an honest race under UCI rules. If you compete you accept the rules, otherwise, don't compete. I can only imagine what she [sic] had to go through in her life to be where she is now, how hard it is to fit in."[25] What about others who had a hard time "fitting in" when they were growing up? Should they be given special dispensation, too? Perhaps Van Herrikhuyzen is the one in 20 women who is as strong as the average man—but what about the other 19? Another cyclist, Austin Killips—a biological male who says he identifies as female and began racing in 2019—was allowed to participate in women's events, winning three races (one by a full five minutes). In Knoxville, Tennessee, during the June 2023 USA Cycling Pro Road National Championships, an angry crowd objected to Killips's presence. The "Our Bodies, Our Sports: Keep Women's Cycling Female" rally included the Independent Women's Network (IWN), Independent Women's Forum (IWF), and the Inga Thompson Foundation. All protested the rules of Union Cycliste International (UCI) and USA Cycling, which permitted male competitors in the women's division. Three-time Olympic cyclist Inga Thompson stated to the press, "Women's sports were created for women. Women fought for years to have sex separated sports. No amount of testosterone suppression mitigates the advantages of being born male. Sports exist on the premise of fairness. There is no fairness or equal opportunity in sports for women if men with gender dysphoria are allowed to compete against women."[26]

A photo of Killips, standing next to second- and third-place natal female winners of a women's elite cyclocross cycling race, shows forced smiles on the women's faces, with Killips looking triumphant. His skin-tight pants clearly show the bulge of his penis and testicles. Even though Killips had complied with the UCI's current rules—that he suppress his serum testosterone levels to 2.5 nanomoles per liter for a 24-month period before racing[27]—that alone could not mitigate the athletic advantages he enjoyed as a biological male. Typical of those who demand special treatment, Killips was oblivious to the feelings of his female competitors. After a victory at the Tour of Gila in New Mexico, he told *Cycling News*, "It's exciting. I'm over the moon about it. The win was incredible, and we were all so happy."[28] Just who is this "we"? Surely not the women who received second and third places—and the unlucky fourth place winner who would have been third if Killips hadn't taken advantage of the new cycling rules.

Swim meets have also been a battlefield for the integrity of women's sports. In 2021, after taking some cross-sex hormones, natal male William Thomas, a swimmer on the University of Pennsylvania men's swim team, changed his name to Lia—excerpted from his birth name—and joined the women's swim team. In response, sixteen of Thomas's teammates sent a letter to the college directors, asking them not to allow the six-foot-tall Lia to compete because the "biology of sex" created an "unfair advantage."

> We fully support Lia Thomas in her [sic] decision to affirm her gender identity and to transition from a man to a woman....However, we also recognize that when it comes to sports competition, the biology of sex is a separate issue from someone's gender identity. Biologically, Lia holds an unfair advantage over competition in the women's category, as evidenced by her rankings that have bounced from #462 as a male to #1 as a female. If she were to be eligible to compete against us, she could now break Penn, Ivy, and NCAA Women's Swimming records; feats she could never have done as a male athlete.[29]

It's appropriate to question Thomas's motives in joining the women's swim team. During the two full seasons when he had previously competed in the male category (until 2019), he was merely mediocre. But by insisting that he was female, he could now shine. Although he took testosterone-suppressing drugs for one year—the minimal amount of time the National Collegiate Athletic Association (NCAA) required in order for a man to compete against women—he did not undergo any surgical alterations to his genitals. Plus, he retained his male chest.

Cynthia Millen, a USA Swimming official who had overseen swimming meets for over three decades, resigned her post in protest of the decision to let Thomas join the women's swim division. "All these women who worked so hard before Title IX [major equity legislation enacted in 1972] when they didn't have the opportunities that men had, it would be such a shame, such a travesty to throw it away now....The statement for women, then, is you do not matter, what you do is not important, and little girls are going to be thrown under the bus by all of this."[30]

Swimming in the women's division, Thomas set a new Ivy League record with a time of 4:34.06 in the finals at the Zippy Invitational at the University of Akron in Ohio. He also finished more than 38 seconds ahead of the second-place contender in the 1,650-yard freestyle. In January 2022, John Lohn, editor-in-chief of *Swimming World*, wrote a piece called "Without NCAA Action, the Effects of Lia Thomas Case Are Akin to Doping." Lohn's comparison—that allowing a biological man to compete against women is similar to doping, even if the man's body currently contains less testosterone than usual—is astute.[31] *Doping* is the term used for athletes of either sex who take testosterone and other steroid hormones to augment strength and overall athletic performance. In the last several decades, doping was a huge problem because athletes who did it enjoyed a disproportionate number of wins. (Although the use of steroids and other drugs in sports was made illegal, that hasn't stopped—and is not stopping—some athletes from breaking the law.) Lohn pointed out that the enhanced strength of male-bodied swimmers not only enabled them to push off the wall of a swimming pool with greater force, but their strokes were more powerful than those of their natal female competitors. They also had greater endurance. "Thomas enjoys similar advantages," Lohn wrote. While Thomas was not doping in the strict sense of the word—that is, currently ingesting steroids to enhance performance—"the *effects* of being born a biological male, as they relate to the sport of swimming, offer Thomas a clear-cut edge over the biological females."

> The NCAA's one-year suppressant requirement is not nearly stringent enough to create a level playing field between Thomas and the biological females against whom she [sic] is racing….Thomas' male-puberty advantage has not been rolled back or mitigated an adequate amount. The fact is, for nearly 20 years, she built muscle and benefited from the testosterone naturally produced by her body. That strength does not disappear overnight, nor with a year's worth of suppressants….
>
> For Thomas to suggest she does not have a significant advantage, as she did in one interview, is preposterous at best, and denial at worst. It is on the NCAA to adjust its bylaws in the name of fair competition for the thousands of swimmers who compete at the collegiate level. It is also on Thomas to acknowledge her edge. The suppressants she has taken account for an approximate 2% to 3% change…[not enough to even the] time difference between male and female swimming records…[which is] roughly 11%.[32]

Capitalizing on the failure of the NCAA to advocate for female athletes, an unnamed biological man—undoubtedly heartened by Lia Thomas's success—joined the women's swim team at a private liberal arts Roanoke College in Virginia. He had been on the men's team at the college, but like Thomas, after switching to the women's team his record seemed better than it actually was for his natal performance class. The man was permitted to leave practice early, senior captain Bailey Gallagher told a reporter, "because they [the unnamed man—clearly Gallagher didn't want to use the pronoun "she"] said they were overstimulated because they were in heat because of their estrogen levels."[33]

Gallagher quickly organized a public protest. On October 5, 2023, ten of the seventeen swim team members held a press conference in a Roanoke hotel. "I felt unheard and unseen," Gallagher stated. "Our comfort was undervalued and discarded. Numerous times we asked the school for support. Each and every time we were told to deal with it ourselves or told nothing at all....[W]e were informed that even if our entire swim team decided to stand together and not swim, in the name of...fairness...our coach would have a one-athlete swim team."[34] Nevertheless, the young women's unified front made a difference, and the man eventually withdrew from the team.

In 2022, the University of Pennsylvania nominated Lia Thomas for the 2022 Woman of the Year award. He lost to an actual woman, fencer Sylvie Binder.

Men in Women's Spaces

Unfair competition isn't the only problem when a natal male insinuates himself in women's sports. One of Thomas's teammates spoke about how frightened she felt sharing a locker with a biological male. Sometimes Thomas failed to cover himself with a towel, which made his genitals clearly visible. Many of the women started changing in the bathroom stalls, which they never did until Thomas joined the team. "It's definitely awkward because Lia still has male body parts and is still attracted to women," an unnamed teammate told a reporter.

> Multiple swimmers have raised it [to officials at the university], multiple different times. But we were basically told that...there's nothing we can do about it, that we basically have to roll over and accept it, or we cannot use our own locker room....The school was so focused on making sure Lia was okay, and doing everything they possibly could do for her [sic], that they didn't even think about the rest of us....It's really upsetting because Lia doesn't seem to care how it makes anyone else feel. The 35 of us are just supposed to accept being uncomfortable...[for] the feelings of one....It just seems like the women who built this program and the people who were here before Lia don't matter. And it's frustrating because Lia doesn't really seem to be bothered by all the attention, not at all. Actually she seems like she enjoys it. It's affected all of us way more than it's affected her.[35]

Shockingly, the women who complained were told by university personnel, "Don't talk to the media; you will regret it....Lia's swimming is non-negotiable."[36] The university did offer counseling services, but with the stated goal of getting them to accept the situation. Note the incongruity of the female swimmers referring to a clearly biological male with visible genitalia as "she." They were doing their best to comply with the university's—and Thomas's—demands, despite their discomfort and the very real threat to their physical safety. But as journalist

Megyn Kelly has pointed out, once you use language that accepts unreality, this indicates that you're in agreement—which opens the door for even more delusion to become entrenched.[37]

Athlete Riley Gaines is noted for speaking publicly about how it feels to be marginalized as a woman in a woman's sport. The twelve-time All-American swimming star had been a student at the University of Kentucky, so she did not have to share a locker room with Thomas. But she did have to compete against him. In March 2022, the two tied for fifth place in the 200 Freestyle finals at the NCAA Swimming and Diving Championships held in Atlanta. Despite the tie, an official from the NCAA told Gaines that Thomas would be the one to get a picture taken with the fifth-place trophy. Gaines was told to pose for a photo with a sixth-place trophy. She would receive her real one in the mail.

In response to Thomas's claim that his teammates had an "implicit bias against trans people," Gaines said, "we are fighting for our right to privacy, safety, and fairness, as well as the essence of Title IX rights....Lia Thomas attempted to gaslight women for feeling uncomfortable with men taking our spots on the podium, taking our titles, taking our scholarships, and taking away our opportunities. It's selfish, and it's wrong."[38]

Gaines's interview and public speaking schedule included a talk in April 2023 at San Francisco State University. "I was invited," she wrote, "to do exactly what I've been doing the past year: sharing my personal experience competing against a biological male and explaining why it's critical that we protect the female category in sport." Welcoming a civil dialogue and the opportunity "to open eyes and change minds," Gaines was not prepared for what happened after her talk. She was ambushed, physically assaulted, and barricaded inside a room for over three hours by a mob of trans rights protestors. "In those hours," she wrote, "the mob screamed, chanted, and yelled." She heard them yell "You did this to yourself," "You come on this campus and think we're not going to start a riot?"—and, to the uniformed campus police, who were at the scene but did nothing to disperse the crowd—"Let her out so we can handle her, we aren't letting up."[39] Gaines could also hear the crowd demanding money from her in exchange for her being allowed to leave the campus. The incident caused her to miss her scheduled flight. She was able to exit the room only after the San Francisco police became involved, encircling her and pushing through the mob to get her outside. "I was still in desperate fear for my safety," Gaines wrote, "the entire time I was in San Francisco and until I was eventually able to board a plane for the return flight home."[40]

This widely publicized incident had one positive outcome: It garnered massive support for Gaines and her message. It strengthened her resolve even further. And it encouraged more women, including Thomas's teammate Paula Scanlan, to speak out. However, being public about one's opinions is not without risk when physical threats are constant and hostile. "People always wonder why more women aren't speaking up (especially the female athletes who have first hand experience competing against a male)," Gaines wrote.

This is why. They don't want to be faced with an angry mob who wants to silence them, harass them, and hurt them. They don't want to be labeled as transphobic, or a bigot, or hateful, but it doesn't make you any of those things by acknowledging [that] women are biologically different than men and deserve respect, safety, privacy, and equal opportunities....To be targeted for standing for women just shows I must be doing something right.[41]

So far there have been no arrests, even though some of the mob actions were captured on videotape (which includes audio proof of the threats). Gaines, who pointed out that the dean of students was present but did nothing, was reported to be pursuing legal action. In the meantime, her speaking schedule is fuller than ever. In June 2023, she told the Senate Judiciary Committee that some of the biological female swimmers were extremely uncomfortable sharing the same locker room with Thomas—who had been caught on various occasions staring at them and "exposing [his] male genitalia." During a recent tournament, Gaines reported, "There was even a group of girls who undressed in the janitor's closet because they felt more comfortable undressing in that environment than they did undressing next to someone with male gaze. They were doing it because they were violated." Gaines was clear that women's need for their own space is not a personal attack on men. "I don't believe trans athletes should be banned from sports....I just want everyone to compete where it's fair and where it's safe, and I don't understand how that's overly controversial."[42]

In 2022, the Federation Internationale de Natation or Fina—the world's governing body for swimming, water polo, synchronized swimming and open water swimming—finally voted to bar MtF transgenders from elite female competitions if they had already gone through any portion of puberty. The vote, to which 71 percent of the members agreed, was made after a Fina scientific panel reported that MtF transgenders enjoyed a "significant advantage" over biological female swimmers even after reducing their testosterone levels through medication. "We have to protect the rights of our athletes to compete," the Fina president said, "but we also have to protect competitive fairness at our events, especially the women's category." He also mentioned efforts to create an "open" competition that would solve the complaint that the organization was anti-transgender.[43] This is a good start, but it doesn't help Riley Gaines and others who have already been forced to compete against men. Also, there are a great many sports organizations and they all have different rules. Some professional sports associations are beginning to stand up for natal women, but universities and colleges are the worst offenders.

Significantly, many categories of athletics, including weightlifting and wrestling, have strict and reasonable rules about who can compete against whom. Divisions are based on body weight, mass and size, because it's understood that athletes with more body mass, and people who are taller, have an advantage. "Male and female athletes are divided for similar reasons," a reporter for *Gender Identity News for the Mainstream* writes.

No matter what, a man will never be a biological woman....These delusional men have no problem cheating women in sports....[and] are destroying women's rights. What they're saying is that women have no right to enjoy success from competing in sports, period, and should set aside their self worth in order to satisfy these selfish men's desires....[L]etting these men compete as women...excludes women from part of public life...No matter how hard or long women train, they will never be able to compete with these selfish, disrespectful men....[Many males] can cry that they're being discriminated against, based on gender. But who are the real victims here?...Stop robbing women of their chances of being champions.[44]

Injuries

There's another problem when natal males invade women's sports, wrote a sports performance coach in 2019.

> This could be apparent in boxing and combat sports, where the higher levels of strength and power could lead to devastating consequences....If we choose to believe that trans women are biological women (which the evidence would disagree with), then the gap between the current sports categories of men and women will cease to exist....[I]t is clear what that would do to most of the women currently competing in professional sports....[It] would likely result in far fewer women actually being able to compete at the professional level.[45]

As it turns out, the above statement proved prescient. Natal women are now being seriously injured by men who force their way into women-only sports. In 2022 in North Carolina, a female high school athlete was seriously injured after a MtF trans member of the opposing team whacked a volleyball into her face. The ball was thought to have been traveling at an unusually fast speed of 70 miles per hour—so fast, in fact, that after hitting the girl in the face it ricocheted back into the net. According to one report, the girl developed a serious, long-term concussion. Because she had vision problems among other symptoms, doctors advised against her returning to play. After the injury, the Cherokee County Board of Education voted 5–1 to cancel all future volleyball games against the school where the trans athlete was a student, citing a "safety issue." A Cherokee County board member told a reporter, "A coach of 40 years said they'd never seen a hit like this."[46]

Severe injuries to female athletes are now occurring in many sport categories. During a 2022 rugby match at Tiyan High School in Guam, a "biological male identifying and playing as a female" was reported to have injured three biological female players. The head coach for the girls is quoted as saying that the male athlete's "body size, body strength...completely dominate any girl that I have on my team. The aggressive nature that was witnessed clearly showed that it's a definite issue that we have to deal with."⁴⁷ Ironically, the guidelines issued by the World Rugby working group state, "Transgender women may not currently play women's rugby. Why? *Because of the size, force- and power-producing advantages conferred by testosterone during puberty and adolescence, and the resultant player welfare risks this creates.*" [emphasis added] The rugby group clearly says that it is "following research into available scientific literature, detailed and extensive consultation where the working group heard from independent experts in the fields of performance, physiology, medicine, risk, law and socio-ethics, and subsequent research and consultation on matters arising from the meeting."⁴⁸ In other words, everyone carefully considered all the data before making the recommendation, which is commendable. Unfortunately, even though professional female rugby players are protected, girls in high school—who need this protection at least as much—are not, because there's no requirement that non-pro players follow the World Rugby guidelines.

Also in 2022, during a National Hockey League (NHL) tournament, a natal female player was seriously injured when playing against Team Pink (all of the teams were identified with a color). Team Pink, which won the tournament, consisted of the biggest MtF players, one of whom had played college hockey when he "identified" as male. Jonathan Kay, who originally broke the story, wrote:

> Should naturally bigger, stronger, faster biological males who self-identify as girls or women be permitted to compete in leagues and tournaments with (on average) smaller, weaker, slower biological females?..."There [was] just an enormous difference in size between the two teams—height, weight, shoulder width, muscles—the differences were plain to even a child," is how one rink-side observer described the finals to me.⁴⁹

In hindsight, the most interesting and peculiar aspect of this event is what the injured player said about how the accident occurred. The player claimed to have fallen head-first into the boards, which caused a concussion and muscle strains in the back, shoulder, and left side of the neck. However, what Jonathan Kay actually saw on the video he viewed was completely different.

> While the video plainly shows #91 [the participant who was injured] *being struck by a Team Pink player*, the victim reports that, "I was playing the puck, and I took a very odd fall into the boards." There's no mention of any opposition player—though the post also notes, cryptically, that this part of the story is "sensitive." Reading this self-blaming narrative reminded me of those stories about women in troubled relationships who tell friends they got their black eye from walking into a door.
>
> One is left to wonder if the "sensitive" nature of this tale helps explain why details about the tournament went unreported... Ignoring or hiding the importance of biological sex may align with the publicity needs of NHL executives and the ideological demands

of trans activists. But it does a grim disservice to every female hockey fan who skates up to play. [emphasis added][50]

This event might also have been considered "sensitive" because the injured player, who self-identified as a FtM transgender, didn't want to risk calling attention to potential future problems involving trans sports players.

There was one more bit of information Kay reported he'd received from that same rink-side observer, which other news media did not disclose:

> Team Pink players even called a meeting during the second period in order to discuss whether it would be best to end the game prematurely. (Some of their deliberations are audible on the video I viewed.) Two players floated the idea of simply announcing that the tournament was over and that "everyone" had won...."I don't know how the teams were made," that aforementioned rink-side source told me. "But any [fan] could see that this couldn't possibly be fair, and that someone could get hurt—and someone did."[51]

Rights that women had gained are now being revoked with a vengeance, and once again they are second-class citizens and expendable. This is becoming particularly evident in the world of sports.[52]

Female-Born Transgenders (FtMs) Who Compete Against Men

When I began research for this section, I had initially thought that there would not be much incentive for FtM transgenders to compete in men's sports—especially those who transition after puberty—due to the absence of prenatal testosterone. (So far, all of the FtM athletes currently in the news have transitioned after puberty.) But as it turns out, there are a few FtM transgenders who are competing against biological men and winning. Testosterone and other steroid hormones are so powerful that the athletic benefits can be impressive. For FtMs, the effects from the hormones far surpass what a normal female would experience if she were doping, because the amounts of steroids that FtMs take are much higher. But where it's illegal for female athletes to dope, it's legal for a FtM to take exhorbitant amounts as long as she calls herself transgender.

A study I mentioned earlier, "Effect of gender affirming hormones on athletic performance in transwomen and transmen: implications for sporting organisations and legislators," yielded some interesting results. As the authors had done with MtF transgenders, pre- and post-hormone fitness tests and athletic performances with FtM transgenders were compared, as well as body composition. Before taking masculinizing hormones (testosterone and other androgens), the FtM transgenders—still possessing the hormonal makeup of biological women—were 15 percent slower than biological males when they ran 1.5 miles. They also scored 43 percent fewer push-ups than biological males. But after one year of being on the androgens, there was no difference in the length of time it took to run 1.5 miles. In addition, there was no difference in the number of push-ups they could do compared to natal men.[53] The authors pointed out that because FtM transgenders tend to exercise the upper body even more than biological males do (in order to simulate a masculine appearance), the FtM individuals might be more athletic than usual. Nevertheless, only time will tell if the majority of FtM athletes will be able to outperform the majority of the most elite biological male athletes who are at the top of their game.

A few FtMs transgenders are currently participating in men's sports with some success. This includes bodybuilder Shay Price and Taekwondo gold medalist Jordan Jackson. The history of FtM champion wrestler Mack Beggs is worth noting. At the age of 18, the wrestler competed in the Texas girl's Class 6A 110-pound division, where for the second time in two years she won against Chelsea Sanchez. Beggs, a biological female, was in the process of transitioning to male, so was taking what was reported as a "low" dose of testosterone. But any amount would have given her an advantage. Beggs did ask to wrestle in the boys' division, but her high school required athletes to compete according to the sex listed on their birth certificate. So Beggs entered the state tournament against young women. With a 32-0 record, thanks to testosterone, Beggs beat three female wrestlers. Astonishingly, Beggs's mother stated to the press, "He [sic] has so much respect for all the girls he wrestles"—and then added, "People think Mack has been beating up on girls...The girls he wrestles with, they are tough. It has more to do with skill and discipline than strength."[54] A true sign of respect would have been not to compete at all—considering that in effect, Beggs was doping. If she had "identified" as her natal sex, the steroid drugs would have been illegal.

Perhaps the most well known of FtM athletes is Chris Mosier. In January 2020, the 39-year-old became the first openly FtM trans athlete to compete in a 50-kilometer race walk, held in San Diego, California. An All-American duathlete and Hall of Fame triathlete, Mosier had just begun to race walk, winning a national championship. A month later she finished twelfth in a race, thus qualifying for the Olympic Trials. (A knee injury made it necessary to withdraw midway during the race.) Significantly, Mosier lobbied the Olympic Committee to remove the requirement that FtM transgenders have surgery in order to compete. This means that a natal woman who is taking hormones to become stronger and acquire some masculine features—while simultaneously possessing the reproductive organs of a female—can still be considered male. From an athletic performance standpoint, this makes sense: Ovaries don't produce much testosterone, and under normal circumstances the adrenals produce androgens in only limited amounts. So keeping a female reproductive system intact does not particularly confer an advantage in athletics because it's the testosterone injections that make the difference. Another consideration is the difficulty that surgeons still have in constructing a penis-like appendage, let alone a functioning one. To create the artificial organ, tissue must be removed from other parts of the body, usually the thigh or forearm. This is not only excruciatingly painful, but the resulting damage requires months of rest. And the loss of vital tissue could interfere with athletic prowess.

One issue I have not seen addressed publicly is how natal males feel about FtM transgenders competing against them. Perhaps most biological males believe that the possibility of a FtM winning is not that high, so no threat is perceived. But one article I did find, "We need a conversation about transmen in sports," indicated that there are problems—at least from the perspective of the author, who is a FtM soccer player. The player wrote, "When playing soccer with men, I've found them to be ultra competitive and threatened by a trans man's dominance on the field. Most cisgender men I play with can't believe that a trans man would beat them to the goal, or dribble faster, and smarter, and juggle better. They become envious, or angry, or, at its worst, violent."[55] The author did not state the nature of the violence. The lack of publicity about FtMs on male athletic teams makes it difficult to tell if biological males are threatened by capable FtM athletes. One might assume, though, that there are issues. Just as women rightly value their own space of camaraderie—due to shared experiences in a society fraught with sex role expectations specific to them—men would likewise value *their* own space, as they have unique experiences based on what's between *their* legs. It's a reasonable guess that natal male athletes would not want a female-bodied trans athlete invading their space. They would be justified in their resentment.

I am unaware of any intact biological women who are not taking androgen hormones, but are declaring that they "identify as men" in order to compete in high-stakes athletic men's events. The reasons for this are obvious.

Intersex Individuals Who Compete in Sports

As established in Chapter 1, intersexuality is very different from transgenderism. However, the participation of intersex individuals in sports—particularly women's sports—has raised some problematic issues due to the enhanced performance benefits of testosterone. The most widely publicized debate so far has involved Caster Semenya.

Caster Semenya, a South African middle-distance runner, was born in 1991. Listed as female on the birth certificate and raised as a girl due to the presence of an external vagina-like structure, Semenya always identified as female. Dedicated and passionate about excelling, the athlete trained extremely hard, even running barefoot as a teenager on bush tracks in South Africa.[56] Running earned Semenya two Olympic gold medals and three World Championships in women's races—first in 2009 at the age of 18, and again in 2016 and 2017. After the 2009 race, during which Semenya was timed more than two seconds faster than the nearest competitor, fellow athletes objected to the winner being allowed to compete because in their eyes Semenya was a man—displaying a toned, heavily muscled body, broad shoulders, a prominent Adam's apple, low waist, and a deep masculine voice. A *New Yorker* reporter described a "torso like the chest plate on a suit of armor" and "a build that slides straight from her ribs to her hips"—very narrow hips—along with "a strong jawline" that conveyed typical distinct masculinity. So many people found it difficult to see this person as a woman that Semenya "became accustomed to visiting the bathroom with a member of a competing team so that they could look at her private parts and then get on with the race."[57]

After Semenya's 2009 win, the International Association of Athletics Federations (IAAF), which governs rules for track and field events, conducted sex verification tests. "They thought I had a dick, probably," Semenya told an interviewer years later. "I told them: 'It's fine. I'm a female, I don't care. If you want to see I'm a woman, I will show you my vagina. All right?'"[58] Some time later, results that were supposed to be confidential were leaked by *Daily Telegraph*, an Australian newspaper. In addition to having what appeared to be an external vagina, Semenya possessed internal male gonads that produced testosterone at a level three times higher than that of most women. Furthermore, that level was capable of conferring a performance boost of between 10 and 13 percent.[59]

Despite Semenya's many supporters, there was plenty of resentment from track and field competitors. They were accused of racism, as Semenya is black and most of the other runners are white. No matter how much the white athletes insisted that their objections were due to sex rather than race, they were often disbelieved. One female athlete who spoke against Semenya's being allowed to race even received death threats.

In 2011, the IAAF ruled that all female athletes with hyperandrogenism, as the organization called it, must take testosterone-lowering medication if they wanted to compete. "It made me sick, made me gain weight, panic attacks, I don't know if I was ever going to have a heart attack," Semenya recounted. "It's like stabbing yourself with a knife every day. But I had no choice. I'm 18, I want to run, I want to make it to [the] Olympics."[60]

We now know that Semenya was born with a DSD (Divergence of Sexual Development) known as 46,XY—one of the very few, rare intersex conditions. Even though Semenya's testicles never descended from their initial location in the abdominal cavity, the testosterone they secreted was plentiful, thus creating a heavily masculinized body. As with some other 46,XY individuals, Semenya possesses what appears to be a vagina, but lacks ovaries and a uterus. The external vaginal structure appears to be the sole reason for Semenya's identification as female. In view of the athlete's heavily masculine appearance, it's surprising that no one ever brought Caster to a doctor for a medical exam—especially after the child went through puberty—to see what was going on hormonally.

After the IAAF stated that women with high testosterone levels would have to lower them to a range below that of men (a reasonable enough rule), in 2015 the Court of Arbitration for Sport (CAS) reversed that IAAF rule. Despite the vast amount of literature proving the benefits of testosterone on athletic performance, CAS wrote that it "was unable to conclude that hyperandrogenic female athletes may benefit from such a significant performance advantage that it is necessary to exclude them from competing in the female category." In other words, such athletes could enjoy unlimited, abnormally high testosterone levels and still be regarded as female.[61]

Then in the spring of 2019, CAS reversed its position. It upheld the rule requiring Semenya and other similarly endowed athletes to lower their testosterone levels in order to be eligible to compete as women in certain elite races. Arguing gender discrimination, Semenya challenged CAS but lost. Then in March 2023, World Athletics (formerly the IAAF) ruled that anyone who had gone through "male puberty"—which is any transgender MtF athlete thus far—was not allowed to compete in track and field events. Women with DSD who showed testosterone levels above a certain limit were not allowed to compete either, unless they took drugs to lower testosterone levels to below 2.5 nanomoles per liter of blood (nmol/L) for six months before competing.[62] It should be noted that 2.5 nanomoles per liter is considerably higher—*over three times more*—than what the average female athlete naturally produces, which is about 0.8 nanomoles per liter of testosterone.[63] If a female athlete tested 2.5 nmol/L of testosterone, she would have been accused of doping.

Semenya's supporters objected to CAS's decision. They said the ruling was unfair because it targeted intersex people while failing to address females with elevated testosterone due to other causes (such as congenital adrenal hyperplasia, or CAH). But a woman with CAH still has a lower testosterone level than someone whose body contains working testes. I'll elaborate in a moment.

One supporter, a professor who objected to the forced lowering of testosterone, declared that it was "impossible to quantify" the effects of the hormone. "Semenya's best time is only 2% faster than her competitors. It is not possible to determine how much of this 2% is due to testosterone, and how much [is] due to other factors....[We don't know] how much it [testosterone] ought to be reduced to achieve a supposedly fair outcome," he wrote.[64] But the professor conveniently ignored that Semenya had gone through a typical masculinizing puberty. He suggested, quite seriously, that because some of the other contestants were very likely doping (how would he know?), why not allow *all* of the women to take a little testosterone—not too much, just "within the normal physiological range"[65]—to give every female a similar advantage? The ludicrousness of his proposal aside, he overlooked the fact that Semenya's testosterone levels weren't "within the normal physiological range," so the whole argument falls apart.

Everyone, it seems, had something to say about Semenya. Photos comparing Caster in 2009 and 2012 show subtle but noticeable change in appearance. Whereas in 2009 a *New Yorker* writer had called Semenya "breathtakingly butch,"[66] after the testosterone-lowering drugs another reporter described Semenya as having a "fit, feminine body. Relaxed, poised and, it must be said, pretty, the young woman with an irresistible smile is almost unrecognizable from photographs taken during the height of the controversy."[67] Still another reporter agreed that Semenya's "face has gotten rounder, hair longer and figure curvier."[68] Some critics, however, argued that forcing genetic testing on Semenya was due to cultural prejudice concerning how "feminine" women are supposed to look, and the policies were unfair because they indicated "policing femininity." Canadian sports policy advisor Bruce Kidd is quoted as saying, "It's still the old patriarchal fear, or doubt, that women can do outstanding athletic performances. If they do, they can't be real women. It's that clear, it's that prejudicial....At some point we're faced with the intrusiveness and degradation of privacy...and that doesn't seem right."[69]

While the critics were correct that cultural stereotypes place unfair pressure on women to appear a certain way, and medical exams and testing can be (and usually are) invasive, the demand that Semenya take estrogen may not have been due to prejudice about feminine appearance. It may have been based on a body that produced ample testosterone and not much estrogen—and the key to knowing this, and the reason for the medical testing, was Semenya's appearance. This is an important distinction. While Semenya's feminized exterior may have been more pleasing to some, perhaps the testosterone-lowering requirement was somewhat sincere, to help level the playing field for the other competitors.

Nevertheless, one cannot dismiss the possibility that Semenya was targeted as an intersexual—because the sexually ambiguous athlete was treated quite harshly, compared to the male-bodied self-identified women or MtFs who have been intruding into women's sports. We cannot know the intent of the sports officials, but one thing is clear: Semenya behaved honorably. Unlike biological males who "identify" as women to seize money and trophies, or MtF transgenders who have undergone puberty but insist they have no advantage over natal female competitors, it was never Semenya's intention to deceive or take advantage of others. It doesn't seem fair that the intersex athlete was put through such an ordeal while male competitors have been enjoying special privileges.

Still, taking drugs in the hope that they will nullify any competitive inequities is a poor solution for *anyone*. Cross-sex hormones—not to mention additional drugs that suppress natural levels of natal hormones—cause health problems no matter who you are. As discussed in Chapter 3, there are severe consequences of interfering with the body's natural hormone production and assimilation. Almost all drugs have considerable "side" effects, damage which Semenya experienced firsthand. One must question if Semenya's system was intended to accommodate such vastly lowered testosterone levels or unnaturally heightened estrogen levels. When Semenya was taking those drugs, several seconds were added to the total running time. For an elite athlete, even a small increase in running time can make the difference between winning and losing.

Most importantly, no matter how many testosterone-suppressing drugs Semenya might ingest, because the hormone had been introduced *in utero*, the athlete still had improved oxygen-carrying capacity, muscular strength, and a stronger, denser male skeletal structure—just like that of any biological man. As we have seen, lowering testosterone levels in an adult does not, and cannot, change the basic structure of the body.

There's yet another issue, a highly charged one, that mainstream media did not address. Because of Semenya's testosterone-producing male gonads—and *especially* considering the lack of ovaries—in "important biological ways,"

Matthew Brealey writes in a detailed analysis, "Caster Semenya is male."[70] High school classmates often mistook Semenya for a boy. So did the woman who decided to marry Caster anyway, even after discovering her lover's configuration. The entire Semenya family assumed that the child was female based on a structure that appeared to be a vagina—but *if we view Semenya as a biological male with incompletely formed male genitalia*, an entirely different story emerges.

Is Semenya really a male? Her supporters say no, because 46,XY intersexuals can fall anywhere on the masculinity-femininity spectrum, with bodies that differ greatly in structure, function, and appearance. There can be huge variations in how much of a given hormone a 46,XY body produces, the sensitivity and number of receptor sites to that hormone, and which reproductive structures are present or absent. But Brealey makes an astute and compelling point:

> It's very clear that testosterone benefits women, and men, in all sports, but we haven't had the courage to say that the difference between men and women's sport is not so much about some arbitrary hormone level, *but about having testes vs. ovaries*. Women whose ovaries produce too much testosterone exist (PCOS) [polycystic ovary syndrome], but they don't dominate in sport. They are simply women with slightly higher T[estosterone] (2–5 nmol/L typically, versus 20 nmol/L for men). *This is not at all the same thing as a person who was raised and is legally female simply because of a severely undervirilized penis.* [emphasis added][71]

Brealey ascribes ulterior motives to the IAAF and the International Olympic Committee when they devised rules in 2010 that at best, indicate an inexcusably (and unlikely) poor knowledge of biology and at worst, constitute a deliberate manipulation of language. The organizations used the term *hyperandrogenism*—which, Brealey writes, "previously applied to a woman who is suffering from excess testosterone due to a cause such as ovarian tumours, adrenal cancer, [and] PCOS [polycystic ovary syndrome], a medical condition leading to acne, hirsutism [excess hair growth on the body and face], and other problems in women." Using the term "hyperandrogenism" in their rules was a diversion. "The IAAF went to great lengths to include irrelevant conditions…only applying to women with ovaries, in order to obscure the fact that they had 46,XY individuals *with full functioning testes competing in women's sport*."[72] Compared to Semenya, 46,XY individuals who don't produce large amounts of testosterone, or who may have weak receptor sites for it—thus appearing distinctly feminine—might be less likely to compete in professional athletics. So Brealey's contention is worth considering.

> You cannot believe what you might have read or understood from the media that "Caster Semenya is a woman"…[G]enitals are private and in general shouldn't be a matter for public discussion, however in cases such as this, Caster Semenya's privacy conflicts with the rights of women (black, white and Asian) who have been denied

medals, prizes, sponsorship, and so on, because of the presence of an athlete with male gonads and male testosterone levels in women's sport. Since we have accepted that male-to-female transgender athletes should, at a minimum, be subject to testosterone restrictions to compete in women's sport, because they have the advantage of possessing male gonads and male testosterone levels, there doesn't seem to be any logical reason why Caster Semenya should be exempt from these rules.[73]

As it turned out, with the latest rulings Semenya was no longer exempt. A regulation was made that to compete at the 2024 Olympics, the athlete would have to take testosterone-suppressing drugs for six months prior. Understandably, Semenya does not want to do this again. Other DSD athletes born with variations in their genetic and hormonal makeup—including Francine Niyonsaba of Burundi and Christine Mboma of Namibia—have also refused to go on drugs that would suppress testosterone levels to below 5 nanomoles per liter of blood for at least six months before competing.[74]

******

Another reported intersexual, Edinanci Fernandes da Silva, may be less well known, but his participation in women's sports is worth noting. Born on August 23, 1976 in Brazil, Da Silva possessed both male and female sex organs. However, it was his testes, along with high testosterone levels, that had clearly predominated. Possessing a masculine physique, he was raised as male. After his sexual "reassignment" surgery in the mid-1990s—during which he had his male reproductive organs removed—he lived as a woman and was permitted to compete in women's sports. Da Silva won the gold medal in the half heavyweight division at the Pan American Games. To an unbiased observer, his square angular jaw, wide shoulders, testosterone-infused skeleton, narrow hips, low waist below the navel, and testosterone-powered muscles are those of a typical male. He also wore clothing designed for men and chose to wear his hair in a very short cut typical of most men. One must wonder if da Silva allowed his male organs to be removed for the sole purpose of competing and winning in women's sports. His Wikipedia page, updated in July 2023, does not list any championships or games later than 2008.[75] The athlete is now coaching others.

******

The inclusion of intersexuals in athletic competitions, especially women's sports, raises many complex and difficult issues. Matthew Brealey's guideline—"If a person has testes or did have testes at some point, he shouldn't be allowed to compete against women"—seems reasonable at first. But what if the testes didn't work, or aren't working? And what if the receptor sites for androgen hormones are malfunctioning to such a degree that they cannot absorb or process those hormones? I would amend Brealey's guideline to indicate "working testes and functional receptor sites" in conjunction with a certain minimal level of testosterone.

It would be unfair to deny intersex people the pleasures of competing in athletic events. All events, including at the professional level, should include an "open" category that does not require a disclosure of "gender identity" or the sex of the athlete. This way, people's privacy could be respected while they are playing the sports that they love.

The Future of Sports

Lawsuits

In most high schools and colleges, if a male merely declares that he's transgender, he is allowed to participate in an athletic event intended for females. The motives—a desire to win and be noticed, along with callousness or outright hostility toward women—seem obvious. As a result, female athletes in high schools, colleges and universities have begun fighting back through the legal system, although not always successfully.

In the spring of 2018, track and field athlete Selina Soule, a student at Glastonbury High School in Connecticut, ran a race. Soule ranked sixth among her biological female competitors, but because two biological men who said they were trans were allowed to participate, Soule finished eighth. In this race, only the top six athletes were allowed to advance to the next round, thus eliminating Soule. So in February 2020, Soule—along with two other female athletes, Chelsea Mitchell and Alanna Smith (who attended different high schools)—filed a federal suit against the Connecticut Association of Schools, the Connecticut Interscholastic Athletic Conference, and the boards of education in Bloomfied, Cromwell, Glastonbury, Canton, and Danbury. The three athletes rightly argued that the policy allowing trans athletes to compete violates Title IX by failing to provide female athletes with equal treatment. "Mentally and physically, we know the outcome before the race even starts," said one of the students. "That biological unfairness doesn't go away because of what someone believes about gender identity. All girls deserve the chance to compete on a level playing field."[76] Their court papers read, "They trained hard to shave fractions of seconds off their race times so they could compete in state and regional meets, stand atop the winners' podium, and perhaps even secure college athletic scholarships and gainful employment beyond. Yet those dreams were dashed, as the policy forced them to compete—and lose—to biological males."[77] The state of Connecticut—which has no rules that restrict trans people from competing—argued untruthfully that the female athletes did not suffer any actual harm, and three years later the U.S. District Court judge dismissed the lawsuit. The two self-identified trans athletes who had beat Selina Soule had graduated; and because there were no other trans athletes whom the young women could identify, there was no longer a dispute that needed resolving. However, the judge did leave open the possibility of another challenge if MtF athletes competed the following year. Significantly, the two trans athletes who had won the races against the natal females said that "they are still in the process of transitioning, but…declined to provide details."[78] With Connecticut's "no restrictions" policy, it's highly doubtful that the usurpers had done anything at all except declare their convenient trans identity.

"Just two athletes took so many opportunities away from biological females," Chelsea Mitchell told a reporter. "Even though there were only two of them, they took 15 state championships away from other girls—and there were 85 girls that were directly impacted from them being in the races."[79] In 2021, Mitchell (now graduated from high school) published an op-ed piece in *USA Today* about how it felt to be disrespected as a female athlete. Four days after the piece appeared, the editor apologized for Mitchell's original "hurtful language" and provided an updated version that Mitchell never approved. The change? Chelsea Mitchell had used the word "male" to describe the biological males against whom she'd been forced to compete. In the newspaper's altered version, "male" was changed to "transgender."[80] "I was the fastest girl in Connecticut," the title of the modified article read. "But transgender athletes made it an unfair fight."[81] Readers who never saw the original piece as Mitchell wrote it must wonder if the headline was intended to read, "I was the fastest girl in Connecticut. But male athletes made it an unfair fight." Fortunately, the poignant caption beneath the header was kept: "When I raced transgender athletes on the track, colleges didn't see the fastest female in Connecticut. They saw a second- or third-place runner."[82] Mitchell eventually did win a state championship race against one of the self-proclaimed transgenders. However, just one or two biological males now hold a minimum of ten state records that at least nine different females had previously won.

Self-declared MtF trans athletes are using the legal system as well. In states that expressly forbid or limit transgender participation on women's teams, lawsuits have been filed that accuse schools and athletics organizations of prejudice.

Quitting

Not all female athletes have the fortitude or finances to engage in grueling and costly legal battles. Some are leaving sports entirely. In 2023, after having lost to transgender competitors, 35-time cyclocross winner Hannah Arensman announced that she would retire at the young age of 25. "I came in 4th place, flanked on either side by male riders awarded 3rd and 5th places." She believed that she'd lost the opportunity to be considered for an international team due to those men. "It has become increasingly discouraging to train as hard as I do, only to have to lose to a man…[who has] an obvious advantage over me, no matter how hard I train….I have felt deeply angered, disappointed, overlooked, and humiliated that the rule makers of women's sports do not feel it is necessary to protect women's sports to ensure fair competition for women anymore."[83]

Rules That Don't Apply to Everyone

The presence of transgenders in women's and men's sports has been made easy by the majority of sports organizations and educational institutions, although some sports groups are less welcoming of such athletes than they were in the past. The World Athletics Council, the governing body for international track and field, has taken a firm stand to help protect natal female athletes and their sport by no longer allowing MtF athletes who transitioned after puberty to compete against biological women. Intersexuals will be also affected by this rule, because the Council is halving the amount of testosterone athletes can have in their bodies.[84] The World Swimming and World Rugby federations have also banned MtF transgenders from competing against females. All three organizations based their decisions, *The Guardian* reported, on scientific articles—many of them discussed in this book—showing that MtFs retain "significant advantages in strength, power, lung capacity and other indicators of physical performance after transitioning."[85]

The USA Powerlifting Transgender Participation Policy was instituted to rightly exclude FtM and MtF transgenders from participating. The organization stated that it wasn't discriminating against transgenders per se, but was trying to "provide a level playing field....Take sports such as curling, equestrian, shooting and archery, these sports are more sport of skill, whereas powerlifting is a sport of strength. Men naturally have a larger bone structure, high bone density, stronger connective tissue and higher muscle density than women. These traits, even with reduced levels of testosterone, do not go away. While MtF[s] may be weaker and less muscle[d] than they once were, the biological benefits given them at birth still remain over...a female." The organization also recognized that participants who were taking androgen hormones for "therapeutic" purposes—that would be FtM individuals—were also not contributing to a level playing field.[86] Despite these clear guidelines, in March 2023 a court ruled in favor of JayCee Cooper, a biological male who claimed he was really a woman. Cooper had filed a discrimination case against the federation in 2001 after being denied entry into the USAPL's female-only competitions. Part of the judge's ruling stated:

> The harm [that Cooper cited] is in making a person pretend to be something different, the implicit message being that who they are is less than....The USAPL's evidence of competitive advantage does not take into account any competitive disadvantage a transgender athlete might face from, for example, increased risk of depression and suicide, lack of access to coaching and practice facilities, or other performance suppression common to transgender persons.[87]

Even when a sports organization such as USA Powerlifting sincerely tries to make athletic competitions fair, an unjust verdict handed down by an irrational (or bribed) judge can obliterate its best efforts. While over a dozen states in the U.S. have banned transgenders from playing on teams, it seems that the numbers—and demands—of trans-identified individuals have risen. Complicating the issue is the existence of thousands of teams—local, regional, national, and worldwide—devoted to the same sport. Each sport has its own governing body. Any group's regulations can change, which they often do. And some of the local governing groups answer to international groups, which also keep changing their demands. Therefore it's difficult to keep track of all the rules. Below is a general summary of possible regulations. The inconsistencies clearly indicate that their rules are politically motivated rather than science-based.

- Biological males and MtF transgenders are forbidden to compete against women (best case scenario). One exception is if the teams are now stated to be mixed-sex.
- Biological females and FtM transgenders are forbidden to compete against men (best case scenario). One exception is if the teams are now stated to be mixed-sex.
- Males who claim they "identify as women" are allowed to compete against women as long as they have taken cross-sex hormones and/or testosterone-suppressing drugs (usually both). They must submit proof that their testosterone levels have been below a certain level for a specified period of time before the first competition. However, the maximum levels of testosterone are subject to change. And the amount of time required for the person to be on testosterone-lowering drugs may change as well (it could be as brief as four months). High schools may require a year and professional sports teams may require two years—but again, this can change. Most important, these men are allowed to keep their natal male genitalia.
- Males who claim that they "identify as women" are allowed to compete against women, even if they have not taken cross-sex hormones or testosterone-suppressing drugs, or had surgery. The so-called transgender athletes may be asked to provide a signed, written document stating that their gender identity is female, but this is not always required.
- FtM transgenders are allowed to compete on men's teams without restriction. The so-called transgender athletes may be asked to provide a signed, written document stating that their gender identity is male, but this is not always required.

Although some policies for admitting trans athletes have become slightly more stringent, many have remained exceedingly lax. In 2019, the International Olympic Committee (IOC) allowed MtF trans individuals to compete in women's divisions if, among other criteria, their testosterone levels were below 10 nanomoles per liter—an amount significantly higher than that of natal women.[88] However, now there are even more drastic changes in IOC rules, which have been renamed "guidelines." Sex "reassignment" surgery is no longer required for trans athletes, and there are no limits for testosterone levels![89] How could this have possibly happened?

In November 2021, the IOC issued a document, *IOC Framework on Fairness, Inclusion and Non-Discrimination on the Basis of Gender Identity and Sex*

Variations. The document—loaded with great-sounding phrases such as "health, safety, and dignity," "level playing field," and "respecting human rights"— also states, "Measures should be put in place with a view to making sporting environments and facilities *welcoming to people of all gender identities*.... Mechanisms to prevent harassment and abuse in sport should be further developed by taking into account *the particular needs and vulnerabilities of transgender people* and people with sex variations." [emphasis added][90] There is no mention of the particular needs and increasing vulnerabilities of the majority. The IOC document further advises, "Where sports organizations elect to issue eligibility criteria for men's and women's categories for a given competition, they should do so with a view to: Providing confidence that *no athlete within a category has an unfair and disproportionate competitive advantage (namely an advantage gained by altering one's body or one that disproportionately exceeds other advantages that exist at elite-level competition)*." [emphasis added][91] This sounds equitable and encouraging—until you read a contradiction a little later: There should be "no presumption of advantage. *Until evidence...determines otherwise, athletes should not be deemed to have an unfair or disproportionate competitive advantage due to their sex variations, physical appearance and/or transgender status*." [emphasis added][92]

In other words, in the IOC universe, all the scientific evidence we have amassed thus far—not to mention common sense, which is now clearly dead and buried—doesn't count. No matter how many platitudes the Committee spouts, biology doesn't matter. And science isn't evidence, no matter how many studies are conducted or how many papers make it to publication. Also, athletes must be given "accessible, legitimate, safe and predictable avenues to raise concerns and grievances connected to gender-based eligibility."[93] If you oppose the prospect of competing against the opposite sex, you're not being "inclusive," another word bandied about in the document.

Another portion of the IOC document reads, "Athletes should never be pressured by an International Federation, sports organization, or any other party... to undergo medically unnecessary procedures or treatment to meet eligibility criteria. Criteria to determine eligibility for a gender category should not include gynaecological examinations or similar forms of invasive physical examinations, aimed at determining an athlete's sex, sex variations or gender."[94] Protecting intersex athletes from invasive medical exams is respectful; but in this paradigm, "invasive" could also apply to an assessment of whether a natal man who claims to be a woman has kept his penis. A rapid visual assessment would be sufficient without involving an "invasive physical examination." After laboriously plowing through the incredible amount of double-talk, the reader is left with only one possible interpretation: Transgenders—and people who claim to be "truly trans," whether they are or not—are now a protected class with rights and privileges that far exceed the rights of the majority. The IOC might still claim that there are men's sports and women's sports, but these categories have now been rendered meaningless.

One interesting aspect of the IOC document is that its coercive demands are presented as guidelines and not legally binding rules. Apparently it's up to each sports division to follow the guidelines. Therefore, should a natal athlete wish to legally challenge the "gender identification" of another athlete, he or she might have to sue the sports organization of his or her competition category instead of the IOC. Did the IOC set up the "guidelines" in this manner to protect itself from lawsuits?

Another interesting feature of the IOC document is that it mentions unnamed "stakeholders" in several places. Not only athletes, but *stakeholders* must also be given "accessible, legitimate, safe and predictable avenues to raise concerns and grievances connected to gender-based eligibility." [emphasis added][95] Stakeholders wouldn't have such grievances if they weren't intimately connected to the trans agenda. It appears that the sources funding trans activists are strongly linked with the sources that fund professional sports. The finances behind the transgender movement was addressed in Chapter 7.

Where to Go From Here

Science can teach us a great deal. But while I am grateful for all of the well-conceived studies from honest researchers devoted to discovering the truth, one important point is rarely discussed: the need for common sense. You don't need a university degree to know that as a group, males have greater muscular force than females and thus tend to excel at physical activities that require extra strength. Yet common sense, crucial for our survival as a species, is being more than merely circumvented. It's clear that trans activists and their allies are making active attempts to obliterate it.

Being "open-minded," "inclusive," and "tolerant" is being used as a weapon by a tiny minority against the majority. Men who are allowed to compete in women's sports are being praised for their "courage" by some. But it's cowardice, not courage, when someone with an inborn athletic advantage competes against an entire class of people who were born with different biology and physiology. Not too long ago, the girls' basketball team of the Collegiate Charter School in Lowell, Massachusetts, played against another school whose team included a 6-foot-tall, bearded biological male who "identified" as a female. After three girls were injured during the game, the Collegiate Charter coach forfeited the game during timeout, stating that he didn't want to see any more of the girls get hurt. The teammates of the injured girls, expressing concern about their own safety, said they wanted to make sure they'd be well enough to participate in the playoffs. What is most troubling is that the Massachusetts Interscholastic Athletic Association (MIAA), whose guidelines emphasize "inclusion," is more concerned about accommodating biological males than ensuring the safety of the females who play against them.

A Gallup poll released in June 2023 revealed that 69% of Americans say that biological males—no matter how they identify themselves—should only be allowed to play on sports teams whose members consist solely of other biological males.[96] Entire teams of women are now starting to walk off the playing field when told they must compete against MtF transgenders (or males who claim they are). Not only are athletes protesting, but trans-promoting sports organizations and educational institutions are starting to receive negative feedback from the public.

Nevertheless, I would be remiss if I failed to mention that there can be repercussions for protesting. In February 2023, the Mid Vermont Christian School girls' basketball team withdrew from a tournament after learning that a member of the opposing team was a biological male—again, who "identified" as a female. The head of the school said that competing against a "biological male jeopardizes the fairness of the game and the safety of our players....Allowing biological males to participate in women's sports sets a bad precedent for the future of women's sports in general."[97] The coach, Chris Goodwin, offered a valuable perspective. "I've got four daughters. I've coached them all at one point in their careers playing high school basketball....I've also filled in for the boys' coach when he can't make a practice, and I run those practices, and boys just play at a different speed, a different force...than the girls play. It's a different game." He added that males playing against females would be "irresponsible" and "asking for an injury" to the smaller female athletes.[98] Because Goodwin tried to protect the girls under his care, the Vermont Principals' Association forbade the team to play in any future activities and tournaments. The school filed a lawsuit.

The backlash against women under the guise of "respect for transgenders" is serious and growing. Men's sports are also becoming contaminated, although it's still too early to tell what all the repercussions will be of allowing testosterone-enhanced nonmales to play against actual ones. A good guess, however, is that the extremely high levels of androgen hormones that FtMs are allowed to take will be enough to damage men's sports as more FtMs start entering and winning competitions for males.

At this point, two things are certain. Now that identity politics has overthrown the reality of biology, athletic competitions are no longer the same games. Also, the common theme of sports is now the legitimized use of dangerous exogenous substances—drugs—to substitute for natural talent, dedication, training, and hard work. *This is part of the agenda to create artificial humans.*

It's going to be a fight to keep our humanity. The athletic field is one venue in which the battle is taking place.

Notes

Introduction

1. Online Etymology Dictionary, https://www.etymonline.com/word/trans- (July 7, 2023).

Chapter 1. Male and Female Development

1. Theresa M. Wizemann and Mary-Lou Pardue, Ed., *Exploring the Biological Contributions to Human Health: Does Sex Matter?* (Washington, D.C.: National Academy Press: 2001), p. 46.
2. Cordelia Fine, *Testosterone Rex: Myths of Sex, Science, and Society* (New York: W.W. Norton & Company, 2017), p. 86.
3. Bonnie Auyeung, Michael V. Lombardo, and Simon Baron-Cohen, "Prenatal and postnatal hormone effects on the human brain and cognition." *European Journal of Physiology* (2013).
4. A common mistake is to refer to a woman's *labia majora* (Latin for "major lips") and the sometimes much more hidden *labia minora* (Latin for "minor lips") as the vagina. Actually, both lips comprise the *vulva*. The *vagina* is the muscular, tube-like inner passage that starts just below the urethral opening (which is for urination) and ends at the uterus.
5. Despite the biologically determined difference in fat content, the standards of beauty for women nowadays are much more suited to a man's lean straight body than a woman's curvy one. Thin, with no fat, is regarded as the feminine ideal. As a result, many women experience intense social pressure to be something that they are not, and never can be. Although plump females were promoted as the ideal during certain periods in history, this was never for their benefit. Women's increased weight indicated that their husbands could afford to feed them; therefore, women were considered a positive reflection of the men's status.
6. Andrew Langford, "Sex Differences, Gender, and Competitive Sport." Quillette, April 5, 2019. https://quillette.com/2019/04/05/sex-differences-gender-and-competitive-sport (July 14, 2020).
7. J.W. Nieves, C. Formica, J. Ruffing, et al, "Males have larger skeletal size and bone mass than females, despite comparable body size." *Journal of Bone and Mineral Research* 2005, 20(3), 529–535.
8. Daniel J. Levitin, *This is Your Brain on Music* (Dutton, 2006).
9. Lise Eliot, *Pink Brain Blue Brain* (New York: Houghton Mifflin Harcourt Publishing Company, 2009), pp. 6.
10. C. De Lacoste, R.L. Holloway, and D.J. Woodward, "Sex differences in the fetal human corpus callosum." *Human Neurobiology* 1986; 5(2): 93–96. Cited in Anne Fausto-Sterling, *Sexing the Body: Gender Politics and the Construction of Sexuality* (New York: Basic Books, 2020), pp. 120, 121.
11. Phil Donahue, *The Human Animal* (New York: Simon & Schuster, 1986), p. 119.
12. Bean, R.B., "Some racial peculiarities of the negro brain." *American Journal of Anatomy* 5, September 1, 1906: 353–415.
13. Anne Fausto-Sterling, *Sexing the Body: Gender Politics and the Construction of Sexuality* (New York: Basic Books, 2020), p. 124.
14. Lise Eliot, *Pink Brain Blue Brain* (New York: Houghton Mifflin Harcourt Publishing Company, 2009), p. 8.

I quoted Dr. Eliot's conclusion; but for a more thorough picture, read her entire work. I am obliged to mention here that when informed of my manuscript pre-publication, she wrote: "[If] you are using evidence of gender similarity to make the case that there is no need for children to undergo gender-affirming medical and psychiatric care...I cannot endorse this position and would appreciate you stating that this is not my view. Although I do have concerns about the extent of these practices, I also see the benefit for some children and believe it should be left up to individual families and their health care providers. I also feel that we need more research in this area to better understand the costs and benefits of such therapy." [Personal email received December 31, 2023.] This book clearly states the "costs and benefits" of such so-called therapy.

15. Bonnie Auyeung, Michael V. Lombardo and Simon Baron-Cohen, "Prenatal and postnatal hormone effects on the human brain and cognition." *European Journal of Physiology* (2013), pp. 465, 557.

16. Ivanka Savic, Alicia Garcia-Falgueras, and Dick F. Swaab, "Sexual differentiation of the human brain in relation to gender identity and sexual orientation." *Progress in Brain Research*, Volume 186, 2010.

17. In the current climate, the "nature versus nurture" debate has become transformed into something else entirely. Some scientists and academics claim that there's no such thing as "gender" (biological sex), and being male or female is related solely to culture. This position completely negates the biological basis for determining sex (a male's testes and a female's ovaries). I will discuss this unscientific paradigm in later chapters.

18. For more information, see Cordelia Fine, *Testosterone Rex: Myths of Sex, Science, and Society* (New York: W.W. Norton & Company, 2017).

19. Ibid, pp. 137–138.

20. Ibid, p. 95.

21. Ibid, pp. 94, 95.

22. Daphna Joel, Zohar Berman, Ido Tavor, et al, "Sex beyond the genitalia: The human brain mosaic." *Proceedings of the National Academy of Sciences*, December 2015, 112(50): 15468–15473, p. 15468.

23. Daphna Joel, Ariel Persico, Moshe Salhov, et al, "Analysis of Human Brain Structure Reveals that the Brain 'Types' Typical of Males Are Also Typical of Females, and Vice Versa." *Frontiers in Human Neuroscience*, Volume 12, Article 399, October 18, 2018.

24. Cordelia Fine, *Testosterone Rex: Myths of Sex, Science, and Society* (New York: W.W. Norton & Company, 2017), p. 105.

25. Ibid, pp. 141, 142.

26. Lise Eliot, *Pink Brain Blue Brain* (New York: Houghton Mifflin Harcourt Publishing Company, 2009), pp. 9–10 .

27. Ibid.

28. Leonard Sax, *Why Gender Matters: What Parents and Teachers Need to Know about the Emerging Science of Sex Differences* (New York: Harmony Books, 2005), p. 75.

29. R. Guinsburg, C. de Araujo Peres, M.F. Branco de Almeida, et al, "Differences in pain expression between male and female newborn infants." *Pain*, March 2000; 85(1–2): 127–133.

30. Marco Bartocci, Lena L. Bergqvist, Hugo Lagercrantz, and K.J.S. Anand, "Pain activates cortical areas in the preterm newborn brain." *Pain*, May 2006; 122(1–2): 109–117.

31. Lise Eliot, *Pink Brain Blue Brain* (New York: Houghton Mifflin Harcourt Publishing Company, 2009), pp. 94, 100.

32. A. Servin, G. Bohlin, and L. Berlin, "Sex differences in 1-, 3-, and 5-year-olds' toy-choice in a structured play-session." *Scandinavian Journal of Psychology*, March 1999; 40(1):43–48.

    As might be expected, the behavior of children from families that do not subscribe to gender roles is less stereotyped than the behavior of children whose parents do invest in such roles. Also, having an older sibling of the opposite sex influences a child to play with less gender-traditional toys—which makes sense, as it's a matter of exposure. Many younger children idolize their older sisters and brothers and want to become involved in what their sibling is doing. Incidentally, researchers have discovered that the amount of physical activity a child engages in (running, climbing, etc.) is more influenced by the type of toy being played with than the sex of the child, which makes sense. See Lise Eliot, *Pink Brain Blue Brain* (New York: Houghton Mifflin Harcourt Publishing Company, 2009), pp. 136, 137.

33. Marilyn R. Bradbard, Carol Lynn Martin, Richard C. Endsley, et al, "Influence of Sex Stereotypes on Children's Exploration and Memory. A Competence Versus Performance Distinction." *Developmental Psychology*, July 1, 1986, 481–486.

34. Marilyn R. Bradbard and Richard C. Endsley, "The effects of sex-typed labeling on preschool children's information-seeking and retention." *Sex Roles* 9, February 1983, 247–260.

35. Meagan M. Patterson and Rebecca S. Bigler, "Preschool Children's Attention to Environmental Messages About Groups: Social Categorization and the Origins of Intergroup Bias." *Child Development*, Volume 77, Issue 4, July 25, 2006, 847–860.

36. Sandra Bem, *An Unconventional Family* (New Haven, Connecticut: Yale University Press, 1998).

37. I am reminded of the very talented jazz musician and entertainer Billy Tipton, born Dorothy Lucille Tipton (1914–1989). After futilely trying for years to get a job as a musician and consistently being refused due to prejudice (women were considered unfit to perform on the stage), Tipton cut her hair and bound her breasts, and eventually began passing as a man. Her acting was so good—she displayed all the conventional masculine mannerisms expected of males during that time period—that she convinced the vast majority of people around her that she was male. She even had five committed long-term "marriage" relationships with women, the last four of whom believed that she was a man. It was only after Tipton died, and her secret was disclosed by a medical examiner, that the world knew the truth. Even then, people with whom Tipton had interacted still saw her as a male. Tipton's biographer, Diane Wood Middlebrook, wrote that despite the irrefutable medical proof that Billy Tipton appeared to be a normal female, most of Billy's friends and colleagues "rejected the claim that Billy was a woman acting the part of a man....[because] Billy's conduct was not only stereotypically masculine (smoking cigars and so forth) but also honorable, truthful to a cultural ideal we label 'manly.'" One young woman whom Billy had befriended "did not permit the revelation of Billy's biological sex to influence her assessment of his [masculine] character." [Diane Woods Middlebrook, *Suits Me: The Double Life of Billy Tipton* (Boston & New York: Houghton Mifflin Company, 1998), p. 174.]

38. The toys that children like are influenced by many more factors than one might think. For instance, studies of twins suggest that there's a strong genetic component to choosing toys. Also, the birth order of the child plays a role. Girls with older brothers tend to be more interested in toys that boys tend to choose.

39. The linking of testosterone to competitiveness is a throwback to an antiquated hypothesis from evolutionary biologists that males are competitive (courtesy of that hormone) in order to sow their seed in all those waiting and receptive females. Newer studies—conducted without the bias of previous researchers, and with the benefit of modern DNA testing—prove that female animals are just as promiscuous as males; they are simply sneakier about it. Therefore, the animal studies used to bolster the argument that human females are by nature less interested in sex than males, are

invalid. For more information on the actual sex lives of female humans and animals, see Cordelia Fine, *Testosterone Rex: Myths of Sex, Science, and Society* (New York: W.W. Norton & Company, 2017).

40. M. Healy, J. Gibney, C. Pentecost, et al, "Endocrine profiles in 693 elite athletes in the postcompetition setting." *Clinical Endocrinology*, 2014, 81(2), 294–305.

41. Cordelia Fine, *Testosterone Rex: Myths of Sex, Science, and Society* (New York: W.W. Norton & Company, 2017), p. 115, 121.

42. Wen Shan, Jin Shenghua, Hunter Morgan Davis, et al, "Mating strategies in Chinese culture: female risk avoiding vs. male risk taking." *Evolution and Human Behavior*, Volume 22, Issue 2, May 2012, 182–192; p. 182.

43. Cordelia Fine, *Testosterone Rex: Myths of Sex, Science, and Society* (New York: W.W. Norton & Company, 2017), p. 121.

44. Lise Eliot, *Pink Brain Blue Brain* (New York: Houghton Mifflin Harcourt Publishing Company, 2009), p. 99.

45. Ibid. p. 18.

46. Cordelia Fine, *Testosterone Rex: Myths of Sex, Science, and Society* (New York: W.W. Norton & Company, 2017), pp. 89–90.

47. Cordelia Fine, *Delusions of Gender: how our minds, society, and neurosexism create difference* (New York: W.W. Norton & Company, 2010), pp. 236, 237.

48. According to popular mainstream medicine, serotonin maintains mood, along with regulating appetite and digestion, promoting sleep, and enhancing memory. Too low a level is said to cause irritability, depression, obsessiveness, and even low self-esteem. The rationale for giving a depressed or anxious person a selective serotonin reuptake inhibitor (SSRI) drug is that it prevents some of the serotonin produced by the body from being reabsorbed by the nerves, which naturally occurs during a process known as *reuptake*. In theory, inhibiting reuptake is beneficial because then more serotonin can be available to the brain. But people on SSRIs often experience negative physical and emotional "side" effects, including insomnia, hostility, hallucinations, even more depression, and paradoxically, an often outright blunting of emotions. Sometimes people on these drugs engage in suicidal and homicidal acts. Thus serotonin's reputation as the "happy" hormone appears to be unwarranted.

Designating serotonin "happy" presents additional problems. As far back as 2002, it was known that *higher*, rather than lower, brain levels of serotonin were more likely to cause depression in some individuals. [P.J. Cowen, "Cortisol, serotonin and depression: all stressed out?" in *The British Journal of Psychiatry*, 2002.] It's also known that SSRI drugs desensitize the body's serotonin receptor sites, which—because they're no longer being used—eventually deteriorate. Medical science even has a term for their loss of function: *downregulation*. A 2002 study showed that it takes only fifteen days for an SSRI drug to deactivate 80% of the body's serotonin receptor sites. [S. Benmansour, W.A. Owens, M. Cecchi, et al, "Serotonin clearance in vivo is altered to a greater extent by antidepressant-induced downregulation of the serotonin transporter than by acute blockade of this transporter." *The Journal of Neuroscience*, August 1, 2002 (15):6766–6672.] The value of SSRI drugs (and the function of serotonin) is further disputed by the fact that some medications used to combat anxiety are selective serotonin reuptake *enhancers* (SSREs), which have the exact opposite effect of SSRIs. Also, normal serotonin blood levels are impossible to establish because those levels are constantly fluctuating, due to many factors including diet (only the body can make serotonin).

Perhaps the most revealing disclaimer for the desirability of high serotonin levels is found in misleading reports from mainstream media. Some reports correlate low serotonin to the onset and proliferation of dementia—which appears to justify the need to raise serotonin levels. But the original studies cited measured the amounts of the serotonin *transporter* SERT (5-HTT), not serotonin itself. SERT transports serotonin across neurons. The SERT transporters and receptors are located in the central, peripheral, and enteric (gut) nervous systems. When SERT—which is responsible for the uptake and deactivation of serotonin—*decreases*, serotonin quantities *rise*, not fall. "Press articles," states Dr. Georgi Dinkov, "state the exact opposite—that lower levels of…serotonin were associated with dementia…most likely due to an attempt to preserve the status of serotonin as the 'happy hormone,' as well as to delay/prevent the avalanche of lawsuit for iatrogenic [doctor-caused] dementia from all people taking SSRI and other serotonergic drugs." [Georgi Dinkov, quoted in Joseph Mercola, "Media Twists Findings of Study Linking High Serotonin to Dementia," March 6, 2024. https://www.sgtreport.com/2024/03/media-twists-findings-of-study-linking-high-serotonin-to-dementia (April 13, 2024).]

Yet another problem with positively typecasting serotonin is that no hormone operates in a vacuum. All hormones and neurotransmitters are required, but they need to be present in the proper balance—and in a complex feedback loop, biochemicals are designed to keep a check on other biochemicals. Via a few steps, serotonin induces the release of cortisol, a widely recognized stress hormone secreted by the adrenal glands that in excess causes *more*, not less, anxiety. (See Chapter 9 for details about stress and hormones.) Most importantly, the *antagonist* of serotonin, or that which has the *opposite* effect, is the amino acid *GABA* (short for *gamma-aminobutyric acid*). People high in GABA are low in serotonin (because GABA increases the rate of serotonin degradation); and higher serotonin levels mean lower GABA levels (serotonin blocks the cell receptors for GABA). GABA's calming effects on the brain and nervous system have been proven and widely recognized since 1950. Known as an inhibitory neurotransmitter, GABA reduces the amount of excitation in the neurons, which enables them to process and organize information being transmitted from the senses in a balanced and systematic manner. People with insomnia, anxiety, Parkinson's disease, epilepsy, schizophrenia, autism, Tourette's syndrome, and depression, have abnormally low or wildly fluctuating levels of GABA. Yet instead of recommending supplementation of this simple amino acid whose absence causes mental and emotional symptoms, pharmaceutical companies claim that oral GABA supplements don't work. But GABA supplementation has proven very safe and effective; even 100 mg can significantly lower anxiety. Taken with the amino acid L-theanine, the effects are amplified. GABA is also an *agonist* of progesterone. This means that they can both bind to the same receptor sites: One augments the effects of the other. If more GABA is ingested than what the body can immediately use, the GABA converts to succinic acid, which helps support the mitochondria (the fuel-burning units of a cell). Patented, expensive drugs such as Valium and Librium may deliver a calming effect—they bind to the same neuronal receptors as GABA—but Valium alone can also cause some very negative symptoms including depression, panic, confusion, hallucinations, insomnia, shallow breathing, nausea, double or blurred vision, muscle weakness, shortness of breath, fever, and headache, among other symptoms [https://www.rxlist.com/valium-drug.htm (April 15, 2024)]. Librium causes similar health issues. Because at least 20 percent of the American population is taking some form of mood-altering drug, pharmaceutical companies are understandably reluctant to disclose the dangers of those drugs, and cannot be expected to disclose or admit that there are safer alternatives.

Given all these considerations, there is every reason to presume that the personality type Fisher ascribes to serotonin is actually due to GABA. However, Fisher is not the only scientist or medical professional to misrepresent serotonin studies—especially if researchers withhold and outright lie about critical data. So with this one caveat, Fisher's classification of personality types appears very valid.

For more information on the alarmingly high occurrence of falsified and outright fabricated research, see Chapter 2.

49. Helen Fisher, *Why Him? Why Her?* (New York: Henry Holt and Company, 2009), p. 5.
50. Ibid. pp. 7, 8.

51. Colin Wright, "Sex Chromosome Variants Are Not Their Own Unique Sexes." Reality's Last Stand, December 1, 2020. https://www.realityslaststand.com/p/sex-chromosome-variants-are-not-their (August 18, 2023).
52. MedlinePlus, "Intersex," August 10, 2021. https://medlineplus.gov/ency/article/001669.htm (August 18, 2023).
53. "What's intersex?" Planned Parenthood, 2023. https://www.plannedparenthood.org/learn/gender-identity/sex-gender-identity/whats-intersex (August 18, 2023).
54. "Intersex population figures," 2013. Intersex Human Rights Australia, https://ihra.org.au/16601/intersex-numbers/ (August 19, 2023).
55. Colin Wright, "Intersex Is Not as Common as Red Hair." Reality's Last Stand, December 7, 2020. https://www.realityslaststand.com/p/intersex-is-not-as-common-as-red (August 18, 2023).
56. Robert Preidt, "About 1 in 1,000 Babies Born 'Intersex,' Study Finds." WebMD, May 3, 2019. www.webmd.com/parenting/baby/news/20190503/study-about-1-in-1000-babies-born-intersex (September 3, 2020).
57. Dainis Graveris, "How Common Is Intersex: 2023 Intersex Population Figures & Facts." https://sexualalpha.com/how-common-is-intersex/, February 8, 2023 (August 2, 2023).
58. Counting the number of intersex people can be tricky because the percentage of reported intersexuals can vary greatly between countries. In certain cultures, the less ambiguously intersexed infants are assumed at birth to be male. China, India, and some countries in Europe do not permit an ambiguous identification at birth, which likely accounts for a low percentage of reported intersex births. [Data is from "Intersex People by Country 2023," World Population Review, https://worldpopulationreview.com/country-rankings/intersex-people-by-country (June 14, 2023).] Then, too, many of the variations are not obvious—either to the individuals themselves, or to the doctors or midwives who deliver them. The organ variations might be internal and inaccessible. If there are departures, they don't manifest until the child reaches puberty, when he or she starts to exhibit signs of sexual maturation that are characteristic of the opposite sex, rather than the sex in which the child had been raised.
59. Hida, "How Common is Intersex? An Explanation of the Stats." Intersex Campaign for Equality, April 1, 2015. www.intersexequality.com/how-common-is-intersex-in-humans/ (September 3, 2020).
60. Melanie Blackless, Anthony Charuvastra, Amanda Derryck, et al, "How Sexually Dimorphic Are We? Review and Synthesis." *American Journal of Human Biology*, March 2000, 12(2):151–166.
61. Colin Wright, "Intersex Is Not as Common as Red Hair." Reality's Last Stand, December 7, 2020. https://www.realityslaststand.com/p/intersex-is-not-as-common-as-red (August 18, 2023).
62. Ibid.
63. Sufficient protein intake is key to helping cells regenerate. Intermittent fasting—eating between five and eight hours a day, and then drinking just water the rest of the time—gives the body a chance to rest when it's not digesting food. The rest cycle lowers inflammation and helps the system eliminate toxins so cells have a chance to regenerate. Sometimes this helps boost circulating levels of testosterone. See Tatiana Moro, Grant Tinsley, Antonino Bianco, et al., "Effects of eight weeks of time-restricted feeding (16/8) on basal metabolism, maximal strength, body composition, inflammation, and cardiovascular risk factors in resistance-trained males." *Journal of Translational Medicine* 2016; 14: 290. https://www.ncbi.nlm.nih.gov/pmc/articles/PMC5064803/ (May 30, 2024).

Vitamin D deficiency has been implicated in hormone imbalance and reduced sensitivity to androgen receptors. See Ningjian Wang, Bing Han, Qin Li, et al., "Vitamin D is associated with testosterone and hypogonadism in Chinese men: Results from a cross-sectional SPECT-China study." *Reproductive Biology and Endocrinology*, 2015; 13: 74. https://www.ncbi.nlm.nih.gov/pmc/articles/PMC4504177/ (May 30, 2024).

Finally, resistance training in the form of quick sessions of heavy weight lifting may stimulate a release of testosterone and increase androgen receptor function. See Lawrence D. Hayes, Peter Herbert, Nicholas F. Sculthorpe, and Fergal M. Grace, "Exercise training improves free testosterone in lifelong sedentary aging men." Endocrine Connections, July 2017; 6(5): 306–310. https://www.ncbi.nlm.nih.gov/pmc/articles/PMC5510446/ (May 30, 2024). Also see Thomas D. Cardaci, Steven B. Machek, Dylan T. Wilburn, et al., "High-Load Resistance Exercise Augments Androgen Receptor–DNA Binding and Wnt/β-Catenin Signaling without Increases in Serum/Muscle Androgens or Androgen Receptor Content." *Nutrients*, December 2020, 12(12): 3829. https://www.ncbi.nlm.nih.gov/pmc/articles/PMC7765240/ (May 30, 2024).

64. "Congenital adrenal hyperplasia," Mayo Clinic, 2020. www.mayoclinic.org/diseases-conditions/congenital-adrenal-hyperplasia/symptoms-causes/syc-20355205 (August 19, 2020).

65. "What are the symptoms of congenital adrenal hyperplasia (CAH)?" US Department of Health and Human Services, December 1, 2016. www.nichd.nih.gov/health/topics/cah/conditioninfo/symptoms (August 19, 2020).

66. "Congenital Adrenal Hyperplasia," Cleveland Clinic, 2020. https://my.clevelandclinic.org/health/diseases/17817-congenital-adrenal-hyperplasia (August 19, 2020).

67. "What are the symptoms of congenital adrenal hyperplasia (CAH)?" US Department of Health and Human Services, December 1, 2016. www.nichd.nih.gov/health/topics/cah/conditioninfo/symptoms (August 19, 2020).

68. Anne Fausto-Sterling, *Sexing the Body: Gender Politics and the Construction of Sexuality* (New York: Basic Books, 2020), p. 11.

69. Kristina Turner and Ori Turner, "Intersex is Awesome," TEDxWWU, July 25, 2018. https://www.youtube.com/watch?v=kRzbVxQVJWA (June 14, 2023).

70. "Corrective" surgery for girls with ambiguous genitalia is a version of *female genital mutilation (FGM)*—albeit less severe, and under sterile, rather than life-threatening conditions. Female genital mutilation is a cruel, violent, sadistic procedure that is sometimes called "female circumcision" to make it appear less drastic than it actually is. Practiced mainly by a certain sect of Muslims in India, Pakistan, Yemen and East Africa, it has no medical justification but is performed to control women. During FGM the clitoris is completely or partially cut off, and in one-tenth of cases, the inner and outer labia are as well. This ritual cutting is done with a razor, scissors or piece of sharp bamboo—and without any anesthetic. If the opening to the vagina is sewn or stapled shut, a small hole is left to allow menstrual blood and urine to pass through. The hole is opened to allow for sexual intercourse and childbirth.

The terrified, screaming girls who are forcibly restrained to undergo this extremely painful, traumatic procedure are usually between four and 12 years old. It's equivalent to either cutting off a man's testes and penis, or just the testes. Immediate negative physical effects from FGM include horrible pain, extensive bleeding, burning and pain on urination, and infection that often causes fever and shock and—if left untreated—death. Long-term physical repercussions include severe pain during sexual intercourse or complete loss of sensitivity, the inability to feel pleasure, infertility, and complications for both mother and baby during childbirth. Lifelong emotional effects include the loss of safety, lack of trust, and the inability to enjoy one's body.

I bring up FGM because in some ways its physical and emotional effects are similar to those when an infant girl's clitoris is surgically "corrected" for being "too" large. Although of course FGM is substantially more dangerous than clitoral surgery (which is performed with anesthesia in a sterile environment), and more psychologically traumatic (the girls are awake and the atmosphere is one of being overtly assaulted), the similarities between the two are nonetheless striking. It's ironic that many doctors in the presumably civilized West who are shocked and appalled by FGM think it's fine to cut and alter the exquisitely sensitive sexual tissue of a female infant.

The common practice of *circumcision*, the surgical removal of the foreskin from a penis, belongs in a similar category. Circumcision is generally not recognized for what it actually is—the sexual mutilation of infant boys. In the United States, about 80 percent of boys are circumcised at birth. In many African countries and the Middle East, the rate of circumcision is 100 percent. In Australia, it's about 50 percent. The rate is practically zero in Europe, Asia, and South America ["Circumcision by Country 2023," https://worldpopulationreview.com/country-rankings/circumcision-by-country (August 23, 2023)]. This practice is widespread among Jews and Muslims, who cite religious doctrine ("God wants this") to justify the genital mutilation of a male. Claims of health benefits are not rational because it's a simple task to regularly keep the penis clean to prevent the buildup of smegma (oils and skin cells) that can sometimes cause adhesions between the glans penis and the foreskin. The assumed psychological benefit ("I want my boy to fit in with other circumcised boys; otherwise he'll feel strange") is also indefensible. Abundant scientific evidence shows that circumcision is not only unnecessary, but harmful because it interferes with men's sexual pleasure. It also lessens the enjoyment of their female partners: Women report experiencing more pleasure during intercourse with intact men. Most importantly, MRI data from Dr. Paul Tinari shows that circumcision changes the structure of the amygdala, the frontal lobe, and the temporal lobe of the brain (which is associated with reasoning, perception and emotions). Tinari's research team was threatened with legal action and a loss of their jobs if they published their study. [Tinari, Paul D. "Circumcision Permanently Alters the Brain," undated. https://circumcision.org/circumcision-permanently-alters-the-brain/ (May 8, 2018).] Circumcision is almost always done without anesthesia—another assault on the infant. Although a man might not consciously remember the trauma, the pain and fear remain imprinted in the body's tissues unless they can be released.

The research of Dr. Tinari very likely also applies to infant girls on whom "corrective" genital surgery is performed, even though they are anesthetized. And some aspect of Tintari's research must also certainly pertain to girls subjected to FGM.

71. "Congenital Adrenal Hyperplasia (CAH) Effects on Girls and Boys." Michigan Medicine, May 2011. www.med.umich.edu/yourchild/topics/caheffects.htm (August 18, 2020).
72. Hans Lindahl and Stephani Lohman, "Congenital Adrenal Hyperplasia Surgery: A Mom and Nurse Busts 5 Myths." InterAct, July 8, 2020. https://interactadvocates.org/genital-surgery-and-congenital-adrenal-hyperplasia/ (September 4, 2020).
73. Cheryl Chase, "Genital Surgery On Intersexed Children." Letter to a judge in Columbia, South America, February 7, 1998. https://www.healthyplace.com/gender/inside-intersexuality/genital-surgery-on-intersexed-children (August 10, 2023).
74. Morgan Holmes, "Medical politics and cultural imperatives: Intersexuality beyond pathology and erasure." Master's Thesis, Interdisciplinary Studies, York University, 1994.
75. Hans Lindahl and Stephani Lohman, "Congenital Adrenal Hyperplasia Surgery: A Mom and Nurse Busts 5 Myths." InterAct, July 8, 2020. https://interactadvocates.org/genital-surgery-and-congenital-adrenal-hyperplasia/ (September 4, 2020).
76. The psychologist reported to have introduced the concept of gender roles is John Money, who (mis)used a legitimate principle to advance his own warped agenda. Money's philosophy—eerily prescient of the dark objectives of today's trans activists—was that girls and boys were not born, but made; and with the appropriate human intervention, young children could be molded into one sex or the other. He had the chance to prove his theory when he found identical twin boys on whom to experiment. The tragic case of the boy who was eventually revealed to be David Reimer demonstrates the consequences of interfering with children's bodies and disrespecting their emotional well-being.

David Reimer (original name, Bruce) and his identical twin brother Brian were born in Canada in 1965. Early in infancy when the twins were circumcised, the electrical equipment—which used an unconventional method called electrocauterization—malfunctioned; and David's penis was burned and shriveled beyond repair. Two years later, David's parents brought him to Johns Hopkins Hospital in Baltimore, Maryland, to see psychologist John Money (who decades later was discovered to have conducted scientific fraud and abused children). Money convinced the Reimer parents to allow the child to undergo numerous surgeries that would remove his testicles and give him a pseudo-vagina. In addition, the growing child would receive estrogen, and be raised as a girl named "Brenda." The opportunity to work with identical twins was too much for Money to resist: Here was a built-in DNA control for his "nature versus nurture" experiment.

Money skyrocketed to fame after publishing accounts of what he called the "John/Joan" case in medical journals. He claimed that Brenda had acclimated well to behaving as a girl and was very different from "her" brother Brian. But the truth was exactly the opposite. Not only was it disclosed three decades later that the experiment was a spectacular failure, but Money was finally unmasked as a pedophile. During his regular follow-up visits to the Reimer household, Money insisted on being alone with the boys and on occasion would force them to undress, perform sexual acts with each other, and touch him sexually. Money justified these acts as a rehearsal for later adult sexual activities. Ultimately, the boys refused to cooperate and Money was no longer welcome in the Reimer household—but not before a great deal of damage had been inflicted.

Both boys were scarred by not only the sexual abuse, but also the secrecy that constantly hung over the Reimer household. "Brenda" suffered the additional loss of parts of his anatomy and the justified feeling that something was not right. Not surprisingly, the child grew up angry and restless, depressed and suicidal. Repeatedly telling his parents that he felt like a boy, he tore off the frilly dresses he was forced to wear and put on jeans and shirts. He misbehaved in school and beat up his brother in frustration. "Brenda" was ostracized and bullied by his peers for the masculine tendencies that in his case could not be eradicated by even the estrogen he was forced to take. It was only after a psychologist convinced "Brenda's" parents to tell him the truth that he transitioned back to living as a male at around age 15. He underwent a double mastectomy (his estrogen treatments had caused the growth of breasts), and began testosterone injections. He assumed the name "David" and eventually married, becoming an adoptive father to his partner's children. However, David's life was tortured. He could never possess a functional penis, and the many betrayals in his past weighed heavily on him. His twin brother Brian died of an overdose of antidepressants in 2002. In May of 2004, two days after his wife told him she wanted to separate, David committed suicide by shooting himself.

There are several valuable lessons to be learned from David Reimer's sad life. David's parents—who thought doctors knew best—failed to honor David's natural inclinations; and as a result, he was miserably unhappy. Certain inclinations, preferences, and affinities are hardwired into the human brain, some of which we associate with sex role stereotypes/gender roles. Although David naturally gravitated to what we regard as typically masculine tendencies, not every male does. Some are considered quite feminine (effeminate), while others straddle the line between masculine and feminine. The moral of this story—and a worthwhile goal—is to allow people to express themselves authentically without feeling that in order to do so, they have to undergo a transgender transition protocol.

A relaxation of sex role expectations would also have made it much easier for David growing up and reduced the amount of intense bullying he endured. Because he did not exhibit any conventionally feminine traits (no matter how frilly his dresses were), he was mercilessly tormented by his classmates, who called him "cavewoman." It's also worth noting that even though David was given estrogen very early in life—which gave him, as an adult, a smaller and more delicate skeletal frame than that of his identical twin brother—his inherent maleness was evident anyway (even though his bullying classmates might not have been able to verbalize what exactly it was that made David so undesirably different). Not everyone who undergoes sexual reassignment surgery has the desired outcome of being able to pass; and in fact, many cannot. This is covered in more detail in Part III, in the discussion of male-to-female transgenders.

The tragedy of David Reimer also points to the importance of telling children the truth, especially if their behavior indicates deep-seated anger, anxiety, and stress. It's clear that David was acting out because he was frustrated and living in an atmosphere of lies, and who he was—indeed, his very existence—was constantly disrespected and denied.

For details of David Reimer's life, read John Colapinto's definitive biography *As Nature Made Him: The Boy Who Was Raised as a Girl* (HarperCollins, 2001).

77. Sarah Creighton, "Surgery for intersex." *Journal of the Royal Society of Medicine*, May 2001, 94(5): 218–220. https://www.ncbi.nlm.nih.gov/pmc/articles/PMC1281452/ (June 18, 2023).

78. Kurt Newman, Judson Randolph, and Kathryn Anderson, "The Surgical Management of Infants and Children With Ambiguous Genitalia." *Annals of Surgery*, June 1992, 215(6): 644–653, pp. 646, 651.

79. "A Gender Variance Who's Who: Christiane Völling," May 30, 2008. https://zagria.blogspot.com/2008/05/christiane-vlling-1960-nurse.html (June 22, 2023).

80. Nils Muižnieks, *Human Rights and Intersex People*, April 1, 2015, p. 9. Available at https://intersexrights.org/coe/issue-paper-human-rights-and-intersex-people/ (June 22, 2023).

81. There's an astonishing variety in how women's genitals look, much more so than men's. *I'll Show You Mine* (www.showoffbooks.com) contains dozens of photos of women's genitalia with accounts of the owners. And in Betty Dodson's *Sex for One*, illustrated by the author, Dodson viewed other women's vaginas and faithfully rendered them in pen and ink to indicate the variation in women's genitals. The general belief in just a few variations of a "normal" vagina and clitoris is not based in fact.

With the widespread use of airbrushing and Photoshop—not to mention the influence of pornography—women have been made to feel ashamed of how their genitals look. Women who are not even intersex choose cosmetic surgery to alter the size or shape of different parts of their genitals because they mistakenly think that they aren't normal. The surgery, called labiaplasty, may reduce the size or shape of the inner labia or lips (labia minora) of the vagina if the woman thinks they are too large or assymetrical or hang "too far" outside the outer labia. Sometimes the size of the clitoral hood is reduced. Females may even have their genitals altered due to pigment variations in the tissue, which they perceive as discoloration.

Some articles on the benefits of labiaplasty mention that "excess" tissue can harbor bacteria, which may cause urinary tract infections. But this same argument is used as a justification for circumcising males. In most cases, careful attention to hygiene will lessen or eliminate the risk of infection.

To be fair, there are some instances in which a labiaplasty is warranted. Occasionally the inner labia of some girls are so naturally large that they protrude and rub against clothing, causing pain. Or, after childbirth, the labia minora might stretch and cause discomfort due to friction during exercise or sexual intercourse. In these cases, surgery is not merely or primarily cosmetic, but a necessity. That said, most women undergo this elective surgery because they feel self-conscious about how they look, based on a totally unrealistic standard. Furthermore, many women are not warned about the complications of such surgery. According to the articles on the website of The American College of Obstetricians and Gynecologists (https://www.acog.org/search#q=labiaplasty&sort=relevancy), these complications may include bleeding, adhesions, scarring, infection, altered and reduced sensation, or (at the other extreme) painful sexual intercourse.

If more women saw the great variety in female genitalia, there would be fewer customers for labiaplasty.

82. Colin Wright, "What is a Woman? Debunking Myths About the Biology of Sex." ICONS [Independent Council on Women's Sports] Conference, June 27, 2022, Las Vegas, Nevada. https://www.youtube.com/watch?v=5-rhLH5lYi4&t=805s (July 3, 2023).

83. Although Anne Fausto-Sterling, in my opinion, sometimes sacrifices data accuracy in favor of a political agenda, I still think that she's an excellent researcher. She offers interesting historical insight into how different cultures in various time periods viewed people who were different.

The ancient Greeks and Romans, early Jews, and citizenry in Europe's Middle Ages all posited often elaborate theories as to how and why intersex people were born the way they were. These theories ranged from the temperature of various bodily organs to the dominance and interaction of energies on either side of the uterus. Elaborate laws were drawn up as to whether or not, or when, intersexuals could marry, inherit property, own land, dress in a certain manner, or vote. There was no uniform viewpoint on intersex people. "Different countries and different legal and religious systems viewed intersexuality in different ways. The Italians seemed relatively nonplussed by the blurring of gender borders, the French rigidly regulated it, while the English, although finding it distasteful, worried more about class transgressions" [Anne Fausto-Sterling, *Sexing the Body: Gender Politics and the Construction of Sexuality* (New York: Basic Books, 2020), 38]. Tales abound of various intersex individuals who lived as men or women, and then as the opposite sex, depending on the circumstances. In 1601 in Piedra, Italy, a half-man, half-woman soldier named Daniel Burghammer—who had been christened as a male and served as a blacksmith—gave birth to a healthy girl. His wife later divorced him.

84. *Merriam-Webster's Collegiate Dictionary*, tenth edition 1993, p. 69.

85. Ibid. p. 180.

86. Some animals not only exhibit behaviors normally attributed to the opposite sex, but they can actually transform into their sexual opposites. For example, the bearded dragon (a type of lizard) can change its sex from male to female in incubation temperatures above 89.6 degrees Fahrenheit (32° Celsius). [Sarah L. Whiteley, Clare E. Holleley, Susan Wagner, et al, "Two transcriptionally distinct pathways drive female development in a reptile with both genetic and temperature dependent sex determination." *Plos Genetics*, April 15, 2021. https://journals.plos.org/plosgenetics/article?id=10.1371/journal.pgen.1009465 (June 15, 2023).] Green sea turtles can also change their sex from male to female, but only prior to birth, as temperatures increase. Many frog species, including common reed frogs, cricket frogs and African clawed frogs, can change their sex. This is in unpolluted environments, not polluted locations laden with synthetic plastics and pesticides, which can trigger estrogenic effects (discussed in Chapter 5). [Douglas Main, "Healthy frogs can mysteriously reverse their sex." *National Geographic*, March 21, 2019. https://www.nationalgeographic.com/animals/article/frogs-reverse-sex-more-often-than-thought (June 15, 2023).]

Almost five hundred species of fish can reverse their sex. For some, the trigger is temperature. For others, it's based on the reproductive needs of their populations. For instance, social groups of the clownfish are headed not by a dominant male but by a dominant female, who is the largest of all the fish. If that female dies or leaves the group, the dominant male will eat more to gain weight and he'll become the largest of the group. Then, through a process called "sequential hermaphroditism," he will become female and take the previous female's place. This is not as difficult as it might sound, because clownfish possess both male and female organs. [See Patricia Wuest, "What Happens to a Clownfish When It Changes Sex?" *Sport Diver*, September 2, 2019. https://www.sportdiver.com/what-happens-to-clownfish-when-it-changes-sex (June 15, 2023).] Even some plants can change their sex, depending on which sets of genes are activated. [See Angela J. McDonnell, Heather B. Wetreich, Jason T. Cantley, et al, "Solanum plastisexum, an enigmatic new bush tomato from the Australian Monsoon Tropics exhibiting breeding system fluidity." *PhytoKeys*, June 18, 2019, 124: 39–55. https://phytokeys.pensoft.net/article/33526 (June 15, 2023).]

Another celebrated example of a fish changing sex is the bluehead wrasse in New Zealand. It can do this quickly if there's an appropriate visual trigger. Each established social group contains a single dominant male (which has a blue head) that protects many females (which are completely yellow). If the male is removed from the group, the largest female becomes male. Her behavior can change in mere hours, although it takes between eight and ten days for physical changes to occur. The fish's ovary becomes a testis, and then starts producing sperm. Geneticist Jenny Graves, who was awarded the Prime Minister's Prize for Science in 2017, remarked: "How sex can reverse so spectacularly has been a mystery for decades. The genes haven't changed, so it must be the signals that turn them off and on." ["Secrets of a sex changing fish revealed," La Trobe University, July 2019. ttps://www.latrobe.edu.au/news/articles/2019/release/secrets-of-a-sex-changing-fish-revealed (June 15, 2023).]

Another paper by these researchers stated:

> In most organisms, a fundamental dichotomy [that is, the state of being binary] is established in early embryonic development; individuals become either female or male and maintain these fates throughout life. However, some plant and animal species exhibit remarkably diverse and plastic sexual developmental patterns, and some even retain the ability to change sex in adulthood...[S]ex change involves distinct epigenetic reprogramming. [Erica V. Todd, Oscar Ortega-Recalde, Hui Liu, et al, "Stress, novel sex genes, and epigenetic reprogramming orchestrate socially controlled sex change." *Science Advances* 2019; Vol 5, No 7. https://www.science.org/doi/10.1126/sciadv.aaw7006 (June 15, 2023).]

Chapter 2. Sex Role Stereotypes

1. "Gender," Online Etymology Dictionary, https://www.etymonline.com/word/gender (June 20, 2023).
2. See Chapter 1, Note 76, for more information on John Money's famous and very cruel experiment.
3. Ann Oakley, *Sex, Gender, and Society* (U.S. and UK: Routledge, 2015). This is a reissue of the original book, with an updated introduction.
4. David Haig, "The Inexorable Rise of Gender and the Decline of Sex: Social Change in Academic Titles, 1945–2001." *Archives of Sexual Behavior* 33, 87–96, April 2004.
5. Theresa M. Wizemann and Mary-Lou Pardue, Ed., *Exploring the Biological Contributions to Human Health: Does Sex Matter?* (Washington, D.C.: National Academy Press: 2001), pp. 174, 175, 176.
6. "Answers to Your Questions About Transgender People, Gender Identity and Gender Expression," American Psychological Association pamphlet. http://www.apa.org/topics/lgbt/transgender.pdf.
7. "Gender stereotyping," Office of the High Commissioner of Human Rights, 2023. https://www.ohchr.org/en/women/gender-stereotyping (August 2, 2023).
8. Chu Kim-Prieto, Lizabeth A. Goldstein, and Blake Kirschner, "Effect of Exposure to an American Indian Mascot on the Tendency to Stereotype a Different Minority Group." *Journal of Applied Social Psychology*, 2010, 40; p. 535.
9. "Gender," Online Etymology Dictionary, https://www.etymonline.com/word/gender (June 20, 2023).

10. Miriam Grossman, *Lost in Trans Nation: A Child Psychiatrist's Guide Out of the Madness* (New York, NY: Skyhorse Publishing, 2023), p. 21.
11. Angell, Marcia. "Drug Companies and Doctors: A Story of Corruption." *The New York Review of Books*, January 15, 2009. nybooks.com/articles/archives/2009/jan/15 (July 2, 2015).
12. John P.A. Ioannidis, "Why Most Published Research Findings Are False." *Plos Medicine*, August 30, 2005. journals.plos.org/plosmedicine/article?id=10.1371/journal.pmed.0020124 (July 2, 2015).
13. Richard Horton, "Offline: What is medicine's 5 sigma?" *Lancet*, April 11, 2015, Volume 385, p. 1380.
14. Cordelia Fine, *Delusions of Gender: how our minds, society, and neurosexism create difference* (New York: W.W. Norton & Company, 2010).
15. Ibid. pp. 163, 164.
16. Mark Liberman, Language Log, "Blinding Us With Science," June 19, 2007. itre.cis.upenn.edu/~myl/languagelog/archives/004618.html (November 2, 2023).
17. The color pink was not always associated with girls and blue was not always associated with boys. Jo B. Paoletti explains that if pink and blue did represent concepts, those meanings were often inconsistent. Moreover, when there were gender-linked meanings they often changed, depending on the time period and even the countries in which the baby clothes were made. The "pink is for girls and blue is for boys" associations in the United States were created through advertising and marketing trends that did not become firmly cemented until the 1950s. Before then, pink was often considered primarily a boy's color because it was viewed as vibrant and intense, while blue was viewed as more muted and dainty. Paoletti gives one possible explanation why "pink-blue gender coding" did not become "dominant until the 1950s in most parts of the United States and [was] not universal until a generation later....Not everyone was comfortable with the notion of accelerating gender identity, after generations of seeing babies as sexless cherubs." [Jo Paoletti, *Pink and Blue: Telling the Girls From the Boys in America* (Bloomington and Indianapolis: Indiana University Press, 2012), p. 89.] This hypothesis seems correct, considering that for hundreds of years before the 19th century, and even in many places until World War II, Europeans and Americans dressed both female and male babies—and even toddlers up to age 6—in identical white dresses or gowns. Long white unisex dresses were easy for mothers to sew, they made diapering easy, and they were easy to keep clean as they could be repeatedly bleached with no damage to the fabric.

    The hair of boys was allowed to grow. When in a dress, often a little boy would be mistaken for a girl. A famous 1884 photo shows American president Franklin Delano Roosevelt at age two-and-a-half wearing a white skirt and patent leather party shoes, hair flowing down to his shoulders.
18. Anne M. Koenig, "Comparing Prescriptive and Descriptive Gender Stereotypes About Children, Adults, and the Elderly." *Frontiers in Psychology*, June 2018, Volume 9, Article 1086, p. 1 (reprint).
19. Ibid.
20. David Smith, Judith Rosenstein, Margaret C. Nikolov, and Darby A. Chaney, "The Power of Language: Gender, Status, and Agency in Performance Evaluations." *Sex Roles* 2019, 80, pp. 159–171.
21. "Women are beautiful, men rational." *Neuroscience News*, August 27, 2019. https://neurosciencenews.com/male-female-adjectives-14804/ (August 1, 2023).
22. Cecilia L. Ridgeway and Shelley J. Correll, "Unpacking the Gender System: A Theoretical Perspective on Gender Beliefs and Social Relations." *Gender & Society*, Volume 18, Number 4, August 2004, 510–531, p.513.
23. "Myth," www.dictionary.com/browse/myth (September 18, 2020).

24. Cordelia Fine, *Testosterone Rex: Myths of Sex, Science, and Society* (New York: W.W. Norton & Company, 2017), p. 101.
25. The "brain" of the cell is not in the nucleus, as was previously thought, but in the membrane, which interfaces with the world outside the cell. Many substances not only cause a given DNA strand to switch on and off, they can also mutate DNA. Just a few examples are some pesticides, certain drugs, radiation used to treat cancer, and 4G and (even worse) 5G wireless signals. For an in-depth discussion of 4G and 5G, see Arthur Firstenberg, *The Invisible Rainbow: A History of Electricity and Life* (Hartford, Vermont: Chelsea Green Publishing, 2020) and B. Blake Levitt, *Electromagnetic Fields: A Consumer's Guide to the Issues and How to Protect Ourselves* (San Diego, California: Harcourt Brace & Company, 1995). I discuss studies linking pesticides and plastics to DNA damage in Chapter 5. This has particular relevance for young boys.

    Stem cell biologist Bruce Lipton made groundbreaking discoveries that pioneered the field of epigenetics. For more information, read his seminal book *The Biology of Belief* (Carlsbad, California: Hay House Inc: 2015).
26. Michelle N. Edelmann and Anthony P. Auger, "Epigenetic impact of simulated maternal grooming on estrogen receptor alpha within the developing amygdala." *Brain, Behavior and Immunity*, October 2011; 25(7): 1299–1304.
27. Laura R. Cortes, Carla D. Cisternas, and Nancy G. Forger, "Does Gender Leave an Epigenetic Imprint on the Brain?" *Frontiers in Neuroscience*, Volume 13, Article 173, February 26, 2019.
28. Anna Varela, "Society's Gender Expectations Alter Brain Cells." Futurity, April 17, 2019. www.futurity.org/gender-identity-brains-2037992 (July 15, 2020).
29. On February 18, 2021, Assembly Bill No. 1084 was introduced into the California state legislature that would ban retail stores with over 500 employees from having a separate boy's and girl's sections for toys. It's a huge overreach for the government to stipulate how a merchant labels and markets products. However, the idea of an entire toy section that's not labeled by gender stereotyping makes sense. How many boys would feel comfortable buying toys—or asking their parents to buy toys—that belong to the "girl's" section? Or vice-versa? Thankfully, from a political freedoms perspective the bill did not pass. However, a similar bill was passed, effective January 1, 2024. Bill AB 1084 requires large department stores to have a gender-neutral or "unisex" toy section, with non-compliance exponentially incurring fines. From a political standpoint, the law is a failure because this one also constitutes government overreach. And from social and psychological perspectives the law is a failure, because the original problem remains—there are still aisles of toys thought to belong to the realm of either males or females. A troubling question arises: Who makes the decision about which toys are appropriate for which sex? It would be much more productive if merchants voluntarily assigned their toy subsections by category and/or age: "dolls and action figurines," "stuffed animals," "sports equipment," "puzzles," "art supplies," "toys for infants" (such as mobiles and other toys that must follow legal anti-choking criteria), "science experiments," "for older children," etc.
30. Cordelia Fine, *Delusions of Gender: how our minds, society, and neurosexism create difference* (New York: W.W. Norton & Company, 2010), p. 224.
31. Emily R. Mondschein, Karen Adolph, and Catherine S. Tamis-LeMonda, "Gender Bias in Mothers' Expectations about Infant Crawling." *Journal of Experimental Child Psychology*, December 2000, 77(4), p. 304.
32. Tara M. Chaplin, Pamela M. Cole, and Carolyn Zahn-Waxler, "Parental Socialization of Emotion Expression: Gender Differences and Relations to Child Adjustment." *Emotion*, March 2005, Volume 5(1), 80–88.
33. Jennifer S. Mascaro, Kelly E. Rentscher, Patrick D. Hackett, et al. "Child gender influences paternal behavior, language, and brain function." *Behavioral Neuroscience*, June 2017, Volume 131(3), 262–273.

34. Elizabeth A. Gunderson, Sarah J. Gripshover, Carissa Romero, et al, "Parent Praise to 1-3 Year-Olds Predicts Children's Motivational Frameworks 5 Years Later." *Child Development*, September 2913, 84(5): 1526–1541. www.ncbi.nlm.nih.gov/pmc/articles/PMC3655123/ (September 29, 2020).
35. Jan Morris, *Conundrum* (Harmondsworth, Middlesex: Penguin Books, 1987), p. 140.
36. Lucy Pasha-Robinson, "Children feel they are treated differently because of their gender, finds survey." *Independent*, January 18, 2018. www.independent.co.uk/news/uk/home-news/gender-difference-children-education-teachers-parents-family-survey-a8164321.html (September 29, 2020).
37. Soraya Chemaly, "All Teachers Should Be Trained To Overcome Their Hidden Biases." *Time*, February 12, 2015. https://time.com/3705454/teachers-biases-girls-education (July 15, 2020).
38. Ben A. Barres, "Does Gender Matter?" Cited in *The Autobiography of a Transgender Scientist* (Cambridge, Massachusetts: The MIT Press, 2018), p. 110.
39. Joanna Moorhead, "Boys will be boys? How schools can be guilty of gender bias." *The Guardian*, April 23, 2019. www.theguardian.com/education/2019/apr/23/school-guilty-bias-against-boys-gender-gap-education (July 15, 2020).
40. Ibid.
41. Ibid.
42. Janice McCabe, Emily Fairchild, Liz Grauerholz, and Daniel Tope, "Gender in Twentieth-Century Children's Books: Patterns of Disparity in Titles and Central Characters." *Sociologists for Women in Society*, Volume 25, Issue 2, January 1, 2011.
43. Lenore J. Weitzman, Deborah Eifler, Elizabeth Hokada, and Catherine J. Ross, "Sex-role socialization in picture books for preschool children." *American Journal of Sociology*, 1972, 77(6), 1125–1150, p. 1141.
44. Kennedy Casey, Kylee Novick, and Stella F. Lourenco, "Sixty years of gender representation in children's books: Conditions associated with overrepresentation of male versus female protagonists." *Plos One* 16(12), December 15, 2021.
45. Stephen Beech, "Children's books still dominated by male characters, study finds." *Independent*, December 15, 2021. https://www.independent.co.uk/news/uk/children-s-books-still-dominated-by-male-characters-b1976537.html (July 24, 2023).
46. Cordelia Fine, *Delusions of Gender: how our minds, society, and neurosexism create difference* (New York: W.W. Norton & Company, 2010), p. 223.
47. Some more recent critics of the gender imbalance in literature are saying that in addition to girls, "non-binary" and transgender people should be promoted as main characters in children's books. I see this as a dangerous precedent. If girls were represented proportionately and fairly in books, and shown as empowered, intelligent, charismatic leaders, there would be no "need" for "non-binary" or transgender characters.
48. Sarah Shaffi, "Four times more male characters in literature than female, research suggests." *The Guardian*, April 12, 2022. https://www.theguardian.com/books/2022/apr/27/four-times-more-male-characters-in-literature-than-female-research-suggests (July 24, 2023).
49. Joanna Moorhead, "Boys will be boys? How schools can be guilty of gender bias." *The Guardian*, April 23, 2019. www.theguardian.com/education/2019/apr/23/school-guilty-bias-against-boys-gender-gap-education (July 15, 2020).
50. Armand Chatard, Serge Guimond, and Leila Selimbegovic, "'How good are you in math?' The effect of gender stereotypes on students' recollection of their school marks." *Journal of Experimental Social Psychology* 2007, Number 43, 1017–1024.
51. Cordelia Fine, *Delusions of Gender: how our minds, society, and neurosexism create difference* (New York: W.W. Norton & Company, 2010), p. 8.

52. Shelley J. Correll, "Gender and the Career Choice Process: The Role of Biased Self-Assessments." *American Journal of Sociology*, May 2001, Volume 106, Number 6, pp. 1724, 1696.

53. Catherine Good, Joshua Aronson and Jayne Ann Harder. "Problems in the pipeline: Stereotype threat and women's achievement in high-level math courses." *Journal of Applied and Developmental Psychology*, Volume 29, Number 1, January 2008, 17–28.
    See also Katie J. Van Loo and Robert J. Rydell, "On the experience of feeling powerful: perceived power moderates the effect of stereotype threat on women's math performance." *Personality and Social Psychology Bulletin*, March 2013; 39(3): 387–400.

54. Paul Davies, Steven Spencer, Diane M. Quinn, and Rebecca Gerhardstein Nader, "Consuming Images: How Television Commercials That Elicit Stereotype Threat Can Restrain Women Academically and Professionally." *Journal of Personality and Social Psychology*, December 2002. 28(12): 1615–1628.
    Paul Davies led another, similar study—this one, to test women's motivation to be in positions of leadership after being exposed to gender-stereotyped TV commercials. As one might expect, women chose "nonthreatening subordinate roles" after viewing stereotyped commercials." [Paul Davies, Steven Spencer, and Claude Steele, "Clearing the Air: Identity Safety Moderates the Effects of Stereotype Threat on Women's Leadership Aspirations." *Journal of Personality and Social Psychology*, 88(2), 276–287.]

55. Dustin B. Thoman, H. White, Niwako Yamawaki, and Hirofumi Koishi, "Variations of Gender-math Stereotype Content Affect Women's Vulnerability to Stereotype Threat." *Sex Roles* 58, February 14, 2008, 702–712.

56. David M. Marx and Jasmin S. Roman, "Female Role Models: Protecting Women's Math Test Performance." *Personality and Social Psychology Bulletin*, Volume 28, Number 9, September 2002, 1183–1193.

57. Ibid, p. 1192.

58. Soraya Chemaly, "All Teachers Should Be Trained To Overcome Their Hidden Biases." *Time*, February 12, 2015. https://time.com/3705454/teachers-biases-girls-education (July 15, 2020).

59. Yasemin Copur-Gencturk, Joseph R. Cimpian, Sarah Theule Lubienski, and Ian Thacker, "Teachers' Bias Against the Mathematical Ability of Female, Black, and Hispanic Students." *Sage Journals*, December 5, 2019.

60. Bruce Goldman, "Two minds: The cognitive differences between men and women." *Stanford Medicine Magazine*, Spring 2017. https://stanmed.stanford.edu/2017spring/how-mens-and-womens-brains-are-different.html (July 15, 2020).

61. Although the brains of males of all ages are about 9 percent larger than those of females, it would be difficult to draw a definitive conclusion from the data. See Cordelia Fine's analysis in Chapter 1 of how the subtle differences in male and female brains may be the result of adaptations to testosterone). Eliot analogizes this to the larger kidney size of prepubertal boys, compared to prepubertal girls of the same height and weight: Although boys possess larger kidneys, they are not assumed to have better urinary tract function.
    However, there may be a simple explanation for the larger kidneys (and also urinary bladders) of males. Women possess more internal organs—among them a uterus, which needs room to expand when a baby grows. This reproductive equipment may necessitate the reduction in size of organs devoted to urinary function.

62. Mark Liberman, Language Log, "Leonard Sax on Hearing," August 22, 2006. http://itre.cis.upenn.edu/%7Emyl/languagelog/archives/003487.html (November 2, 2023).

63. Christopher Karpowitz, Tali Mendelbert and Lee Shaker, "Gender Inequality in Deliberative Participation." *American Political Science Review*, August 2012, Volume 106, Issue 3, pp. 533–547.

64. Campbell Leaper and Melanie M. Ayres, "A meta-analytic review of gender variations in adults' language use: talkativeness, affiliative speech, and assertive speech." *Personality and Social Psychology Review*, November 2007, 11(4): 328–363.
65. Maryam Pakzadian and Arezoo Ashoori Tootkaboni, "The role of gender in conversational dominance: A study of EFL learners." *Cogent Education*, 2018, Volume 5, Issue 1.
66. Lise Eliot, *Pink Brain Blue Brain* (New York: Houghton Mifflin Harcourt Publishing Company, 2009), p. 173.
67. Madhura Ingalhalikar, Alex Smith, Drew Parker, et al, "Sex differences in the structural connectome of the human brain." *Proceedings of the National Academy of Sciences of the United States of America*, January 14, 2014; 111(2): 823–828, p. 823.
68. Cordelia Fine, *Delusions of Gender how our minds, society, and neurosexism create difference* (New York: W.W. Norton & Company, 2010), p. 27.
69. Ibid. p. 28.
70. Isabelle D. Cherney, "Mom, Let Me Play More Computer Games: They Improve My Mental Rotation Skills." *Sex Roles* 59, 2008, 776–786.
71. Sheila Brownlow, Amanda J. Janas, Kathleen A. Blake, et al, "Getting by with a Little Help from My Friends: Mental Rotation Ability after Tacit Peer Encouragement." *Psychology*, Volume 2, Number 4, July 2011, 363–370.
72. Susan C. Levine, Marina Vasilyeva, Stella F. Lourenco, et al, "Socioeconomic status modifies the sex difference in spatial skill." *Psychological Science*, November 2005; 16(11): 841–845.
73. John W. Berry, "Temne and Eskimo Perceptual Skills." *International Journal of Psychology*, October 1966, Volume 1, Issue 3, pp. 207–229.
74. Sandra Newman, "Man, weeping." Aeon, September 9, 2015. https://aeon.co/essays/whatever-happened-to-the-noble-art-of-the-manly-weep (July 28, 2023).
75. Ibid.
76. Ibid.
77. Dhruv Marwha, Meha Halari, and Lise Eliot, "Meta-analysis reveals a lack of sexual dimorphism in human amygdala volume." *NeuroImage*, Volume 147, February 15, 2017, 282–294.
78. "Mounting challenge to brain sex differences," *Science Daily* press release, January 17, 2017, from Rosalind Franklin University of Medicine and Science. https://www.sciencedaily.com/releases/2017/01/170117135943.htm (July 28, 2023).
79. Testosterone levels rise as a result of achieving social dominance. [A. Mazur and A. Booth, "Testosterone and dominance in men." *The Behavioral and Brain Sciences*, June 1998; 21(3): 353–363.] Levels even rise in those *connected* with the ones who have achieved social dominance, such as men who watch their favorite sports team win on the field. In a domino effect, aggressive behavior raises testosterone levels—and this is in both sexes (although levels are less in women, who start out with a lower baseline level of the hormone than men). Put another way, the more that males behave in ways corresponding to their socialization, the more they will become like stereotypical males—and the more difficult it may be for them to stop behaving like that. There is always a social corollary to the biological, and it's often difficult to separate them.

The extreme of high-testosterone behavior may be found in violent offenders. "There is evidence," reports M.L. Batrinos, "that testosterone levels are higher in individuals with aggressive behavior, such as prisoners who have committed violent crimes. Several field studies have also shown that testosterone levels increase during the aggressive phases of sports games." [Menelaos L. Batrinos, "Testosterone and Aggressive Behavior in Man." *International Journal of Endocrinology and Metabolism,* Summer 2012, 10(3): 563–568; p 563.]

80. Sean Haldane, *Emotional First Aid* (New York: Irvington Publishers, 1984), p. 122.
81. Matthew Jakupcak, Matthew T. Tull, and Lizabeth Roemer, "Masculinity, Shame, and Fear of Emotions as predictors of Men's Expressions of Anger and Hostility." *Psychology of Men and Masculinity*, October 2005.
82. Henry A. Montero, "Depression in Men: The Cycle of Toxic Masculinity." Psycom, June 8, 2022. https://www.psycom.net/depression/depression-in-men/toxic-masculinity (July 28, 2023).
83. Melissa Dahl, "Why Do Women Cry More Than Men?" *New York Magazine*, January 7, 2015. Accessed at https://www.thecut.com/2015/01/why-do-women-cry-more-than-men.html (September 23, 2023).
84. Matthew Oransky and Jeanne Marecek, "'I'm Not Going to Be a Girl': Masculinity and Emotions in Boys' Friendships and Peer Groups." *Journal of Adolescent Research*, January 2009, 24(2): 218–241.
85. Sean Haldane, *Emotional First Aid* (New York: Irvington Publishers, 1984), pp. 121, 122.
86. Billy Doidge Kilgore, "The key to letting boys actually be boys? See them as the emotional beings they are." *The Washington Post*, November 12, 2019. https://www.washingtonpost.com/lifestyle/2019/11/12/key-letting-boys-be-boys-see-them-emotional-beings-they-are/ (July 28, 2023).
87. Benjamin P. Chapman, Kevin Fiscella, Ichiro Kawachi, et al, "Emotion Suppression and Mortality Risk Over a 12-Year Follow-up." *Journal for Psychosomatic Research*, October 2013, 75(4): 381–385.
88. Jainish Patel and Prittesh Patel, "Consequences of Repression of Emotion: Physical Health, Mental Health and General Well Being." *International Journal of Psychotherapy Practice and Research*, Volume 1, Issue 3, February 12, 2019, 16–21.
89. Lise Eliot, *Pink Brain Blue Brain* (New York: Houghton Mifflin Harcourt Publishing Company, 2009), p. 76.
90. Ilona Jerabek and Deborah Muoio, "The Lost Boys: Young Men Struggle Emotionally and Socially." PsychTests AIM Inc., August 2018.
91. Lin Bian, Sarah-Jane Leslie, and Andrei Cimpian, "Gender stereotypes about intellectual ability emerge early and influence children's interests." *Science*, Volume 244, Number 6323, 389–391, January 27, 2017.
92. "Teacher Bias: The Elephant in the Classroom," Marco Learning, August 27, 2018. www.thegraidenetwork.com/blog-all/2018/8/1/teacher-bias-the-elephant-in-the-classroom/#download-teacher-bias (July 15, 2020).
93. Sylvia Ann Hewlett, Carolyn Buck Luce, Lisa J. Servon, et al, "The Athena Factor: Reversing the Brain Drain in Science, Engineering, and Technology." *Harvard Business Review Research Report*, June 2008.
94. Ben A. Barres, *The Autobiography of a Transgender Scientist* (Cambridge, Massachusetts: The MIT Press, 2018), pp. 112, 113.
95. Sara Rigbgy, "22 pioneering women in science history you really should know about." Science Focus, March 8, 2023. https://www.sciencefocus.com/science/10-amazing-women-in-science-history-you-really-should-know-about/ (May 11, 2023).
96. Ibid.
97. "Were the bathrooms at NASA segregated?" https://moviecultists.com/were-the-bathrooms-at-nasa-segregated (May 11, 2023).
98. Anne Fausto-Sterling, *Sexing the Body: Gender Politics and the Construction of Sexuality* (New York: Basic Books, 2020), pp. 350, 351.

99. Hasmik Gharibyan, "Gender Gap in Computer Science: Studying Its Absence in One Former Soviet Republic." *2007 American Society for Engineering Education Conference Proceedings*, Honolulu, Hawaii; pp. 2, 4, 5.

100. Becky Little, "When Computer Coding Was a 'Woman's' Job." History, February 9, 2021. https://www.history.com/news/coding-used-to-be-a-womans-job-so-it-was-paid-less-and-undervalued (October 29, 2023).

101. Brynn Holland, "Human Computers: The Early Women of NASA." History, September 28, 2023. https://www.history.com/news/human-computers-women-at-nasa (October 29, 2023).

102. Becky Little, "When Computer Coding Was a 'Woman's' Job." History, February 9, 2021. https://www.history.com/news/coding-used-to-be-a-womans-job-so-it-was-paid-less-and-undervalued (October 29, 2023).

103. Carina Box, "New resources on the gender gap in computer science," April 30, 2021. https://blog.google/outreach-initiatives/code-with-google/gender-gap-computer-science/ (July 17, 2023).

104. Laurie A. Rudman and Peter Glick, "Feminized Management and Backlash Toward Agentic Women: The Hidden Costs to Women of a Kinder, Gentler Image of Middle Managers." *Journal of Personality and Social Psychology* 1999, Volume 77, Number 5, 1004–1010.

105. Ibid.

106. Kathy Caprino, "Gender Bias Is Real: Women's Perceived Competency Drops Significantly When Judged As Being Forceful." *Forbes*, August 25, 2015. https://www.forbes.com/sites/kathycaprino/2015/08/25/gender-bias-is-real-womens-perceived-competency-drops-significantly-when-judged-as-being-forceful/?sh=7f68601e2d85 (August 1, 2023).

107. Naznin Tabassum and Bhabani Shankar Nayak, "Gender stereotyping is considered to be a significant issue obstructing the career progressions of women in management." *IIM Kozhikode Society & Management Review*, February 10, 2021, Volume 10, Issue 2, 192–208, p. 192.

108. Cordelia Fine, *Delusions of Gender: how our minds, society, and neurosexism create difference* (New York: W.W. Norton & Company, 2010), pp. 62–63.

109. Julia B. Bear and Peter Glick, "Breadwinner Bonus and Caregiver Penalty in Workplace Rewards for Men and Women." *Social Psychological and Personality Science*, December 14, 2016.

110. Leonardo Christov-Moore, Elizabeth A. Simpson, et al, "Empathy: Gender effects in brain and behavior." *Neuroscience and Biobehavioral Reviews* 46 (2014), 604–627.

111. Erik Gustafsson, Florence Levréro, David Reby, and Nicolas Mathevon, "Fathers are just as good as mothers at recognizing the cries of their baby." *Nature Communications* 2013, Volume 4, Article number 1698.

112. Eyal Ibrahim and Ruth Feldman, "Oxytocin and Fathering," June 7, 2018. The Good Men Project, https://goodmenproject.com/featured-content/oxytocin-and-fathering-sjbn/ (September 26, 2020).

113. Cordelia Fine, *Delusions of Gender: how our minds, society, and neurosexism create difference* (New York: W.W. Norton & Company, 2010), p. 88.

114. F. Hashemian, F. Shafigh, and E. Roohi, "Regulatory role of prolactin in paternal behavior in male parents: A narrative review." *Journal of Postgraduate Medicine*, July-September 2016; 62(3): 182–187.

115. Eyal Ibrahim and Ruth Feldman, "Oxytocin and Fathering." The Good Men Project, June 7, 2018. https://goodmenproject.com/featured-content/oxytocin-and-fathering-sjbn/ (September 26, 2020).

116. Colleen Sharkey, "New study first to define link between testosterone and father' social roles outside the family." Medical Xpress, September 24, 2020. https://medicalxpress.com/news/2020-09-link-testosterone-fathers-social-roles.html (September 26, 2020).
117. Ibid.
118. Leonardo Christov-Moore, Elizabeth A. Simpson, Gino Coudé, et al, "Empathy: Gender Effects in Brain and Behavior." *Neuroscience and Biobehavioral Reviews* 46 (2014), 604–627.
119. Nancy Eisenberg and Randy Lennon, "Sex Differences in Empathy and Related Capacities." *Psychological Bulletin* 1983, Volume 94, No. 1, 100–131.
120. Ibid.
121. William Ickes, discussed in Cordelia Fine, *Delusions of Gender: how our minds, society, and neurosexism create difference* (New York: W.W. Norton & Company, 2010), pp. 20, 21.
122. Cordelia Fine, *Delusions of Gender: how our minds, society, and neurosexism create difference* (New York: W.W. Norton & Company, 2010), p. 21.
123. Lise Eliot, *Pink Brain Blue Brain* (New York: Houghton Mifflin Harcourt Publishing Company, 2009), p. 116 .
124. Lorena Castillo, "Must-Know Makeup Statistics." Gitnux Market Data Report 2023, December 16, 2023. https://gitnux.org/makeup-statistics/ (January 3, 2024).

    According to this website's data, the United States is the largest beauty products market. In 2020, 89.4 billion dollars was spent on cosmetics. It may not be a coincidence that as of this writing, the U.S. is also the country that pushes the hardest to transition children.
125. Diederik F. Janssen, "Homosexual/Heterosexual: First Print uses of the Terms by Daniel von Kászony (1868–1871)." *Journal of Homosexuality*, December 6, 2021; 68(14): 2574–2579.
126. "Homosexuality," *Britannica*, October 17, 2023. https://www.britannica.com/topic/homosexuality (October 22, 2023).
127. James H. Jones, *Alfred C. Kinsey: A Public/Private Life* (New York: W.W. Norton & Company, 1997), p. 296.
128. Anne Fausto-Sterling, *Sexing the Body: Gender Politics and the Construction of Sexuality* (New York: Basic Books, 2020), p. 15.

    Homosexual activity is regarded differently depending on the culture. In certain African tribes, the shaman is homosexual, thought to be imbued with special powers. At least two dozen Native American traditions honor the *Berdache* (usually a male) who assumes the dress, role, and social status of the opposite sex. In the 1990s, the term *two-spirit* was substituted for *Berdache*. What makes these people unique is their lack of being classified as men or women. The Navajo Indians of the United States have their own version of *Berdache*, which they call *nádleehí*. They do not perceive such persons in terms of gender transgression. Nor do they describe a man with women's mannerisms as "feminine" because, in their world view, male and female characteristics are always present in everyone, in fluctuating amounts and intensities.
129. Stephen Whittle, "A brief history of transgender issues." *The Guardian*, June 2, 2010. https://www.theguardian.com/lifeandstyle/2010/jun/02/brief-history-transgender-issues (October 22, 2023).
130. Christine Jorgensen, *Christine Jorgensen: A Personal Autobiography.* (New York: Bantam Books, 1967), p. 105.
131. Sheila Jeffreys, *Gender Hurts* (London and New York: Routledge, 2014), p. 22.
132. Jacob Poushter and Nicholas Kent, "The Global Divide on Homosexuality Persists." Pew Research Center, June 25, 2020. https://www.pewresearch.org/global/2020/06/25/global-divide-on-homosexuality-persists/ (August 11, 2023).

Chapter 3. Becoming Transgender

1. Louise Perry, "What Is Autogynephilia? An Interview with Dr Ray Blanchard," November 6, 2019. https://quillette.com/2019/11/06/what-is-autogynephilia-an-interview-with-dr-ray-blanchard/ (May 1, 2023).
2. Ibid.
3. Abigail Shrier, *Irreversible Damage: The Transgender Craze Seducing Our Daughters* (Washington, DC: Regnery Publishing, 2020), pp. 169, 170.
4. Elie Vandenbussche, "Detransition-Related Needs and Support: A Cross-Sectional Online Survey." *Journal of Homosexuality* 2022, Volume 69, Number 9, 1602–1620.
5. Lisa Littman, "Parent reports of adolescents and young adults perceived to show signs of a rapid onset of gender dysphoria." *Plos One*, August 16, 2018, 1–44. https://journals.plos.org/plosone/article/file?id=10.1371/journal.pone.0202330&type=printable (August 9, 2023), pp. 25, 26.
6. Ibid.
7. Lisa Marchiano, "Transgenderism and the Social Construction of Diagnosis." Quillette, March 1, 2018. https://quillette.com/2018/03/01/transgenderism-social-construction-diagnosis/ (August 10, 2023).
8. Teny Sahakian, "Mental health professionals have 'abandoned' duty of care in treatment of trans youth, therapist says." Fox News, October 22, 2022. https://www.foxnews.com/health/mental-health-professionals-abandoned-duty-care-treatment-trans-youth-therapist-says (August 9, 2023).
9. All pharmaceuticals have effects, some of which are desirable and some of which are not. The medical industry introduced the phrase *side effects* to divert attention from the unwanted, usually harmful effects of drugs. Usually, the "side" effects are not only inconvenient but life-threatening, and vastly outnumber the one or two outcomes for which people are actually using the drug. I believe that if more people approached drug-taking with this mindset, fewer would be inclined to take pharmaceuticals.
10. Grace Lidinsky-Smith, "There's No Standard for Care When it Comes to Trans Medicine." *Newsweek*, June 25, 2021. https://www.newsweek.com/theres-no-standard-care-when-it-comes-trans-medicine-opinion-1603450 (August 4, 2023).
11. Lisa Marchiano, "Trans Activism's Dangerous Myth of Parental Rejection." Quillette, July 20, 2018. https://quillette.com/2018/07/20/trans-activisms-dangerous-myth-of-parental-rejection/ (August 11, 2023).
12. Ibid.
13. Ibid.
14. Miriam Grossman, *Lost in Trans Nation: A Child Psychiatrist's Guide Out of the Madness* (New York, NY: Skyhorse Publishing, 2023), pp. 224–225.
15. Lisa Marchiano, "Trans Activism's Dangerous Myth of Parental Rejection." Quillette, July 20, 2018. https://quillette.com/2018/07/20/trans-activisms-dangerous-myth-of-parental-rejection/ (August 11, 2023).
16. Miriam Grossman, *Lost in Trans Nation: A Child Psychiatrist's Guide Out of the Madness* (New York, NY: Skyhorse Publishing, 2023), p. xxxvii.
17. "9 Side Effects Of Hormone Replacement Therapy (HRT)," Curejoy Editorial, March 1, 2018. www.curejoy.com/content/side-effects-of-hormone-replacement-therapy/ (August 22, 2020).
18. Talal Alzahrani, T. Nguyen, A. Ryan, et al, "Cardiovascular Disease Risk Factors and Myocardial Infarction in the Transgender Population." *Circulation: Cardiovascular Quality and Outcomes*, April 5, 2019, Vol.12, No. 4.

19. Eva Moore, Amy Wisniewski, and Adrian Dobs, "Endocrine Treatment of Transsexual People: A Review of Treatment Regimens, Outcomes, and Adverse Effects." *The Journal of Clinical Endocrinology & Metabolism* 2003, 88(8), 3467.
20. Becky McCall, "75% of Transgender Women Fail to Suppress Testosterone." Medscape, March 1, 2018. https://www.medscape.com/viewarticle/893280?form=fpf (August 22, 2023).
21. Diane J. Persson, "Unique challenges of transgender aging: implications from the literature." *Journal of Gerontological Social Work* 2009, Number 52, 633–646.
22. H. Asscheman, L.J.G. Gooren, and P.L.E. Eklund. "Mortality and morbidity in transsexual patients with cross-gender hormone treatment. *Metabolism* 1989, Number 38 (9): 867–873.
23. Eva Moore, Amy Wisniewski, and Adrian Dobs. "Endocrine Treatment of Transsexual People: A Review of Treatment Regimens, Outcomes, and Adverse Effects." *The Journal of Clinical Endocrinology & Metabolism* 2003, 88(8), 3467–3473, p. 3469.
24. Paul McHugh, "Surgical Sex: Why We Stopped Doing Sex Change Operations." First Things, November 2004. www.firstthings.com/article/2004/11/surgical-sex (July 23, 2020).
25. "Male and Female Testosterone: the Facts," NAVA Health, 2023. https://navacenter.com/male-and-female-testosterone-the-facts/ (August 22, 2023).
26. Millicent Odunze, "Preparation and Procedures Involved in Gender Reassignment Surgery," January 2, 2020. www.verywellhealth.com/sex-reassignment-surgery-2710288 (July 16, 2020).
27. T. Alzahrani, T. Nguyen, A. Ryan, et al, "Cardiovascular Disease Risk Factors and Myocardial Infarction in the Transgender Population." *Circulation: Cardiovascular Quality and Outcomes*, April 5, 2019; Vol.12, No. 4.
28. Eva Moore, Amy Wisniewski, and Adrian Dobs, "Endocrine treatment of transsexual people: a review of treatment regimens, outcomes, and adverse effects." *The Journal of Clinical Endocrinology & Metabolism*, 2003. 88(8), 3467–3473.
29. Walter Futterweit, "Endocrine therapy of transsexualism and potential complications of long-term treatment." *Archives of Sexual Behavior*, March 31, 1998, 27(2), 209–226.
30. Alyssa Litoff and Lauren Effron, "Chaz Bono's 'Transition': Bono Talks About Gender Reassignment Surgery and What It's Done for His Sex Life." ABC News, May 9, 2011, https://abcnews.go.com/Entertainment/chaz-bonos-transition-sonny-chers-child-man-sex/story?id=13561466 (July 14, 2020).
31. Walter Futterweit, "Endocrine therapy of transsexualism and potential complications of long-term treatment." *Archives of Sexual Behavior*, March 31, 1998, 27(2), 209–226.
32. Lisa Marchiano, "Misunderstanding a New Kind of Gender Dysphoria." Quillette, October 6, 2017. https://quillette.com/2017/10/06/misunderstanding-new-kind-gender-dysphoria/ (August 10, 2023).
33. Deborah Cohen and Hannah Barnes, "Gender dysphoria in children: puberty blockers study draws further criticism." *British Medical Journal*, September 20, 2019; 366.
34. https://www.lupronpedpro.com/isi.html; https://www.luprongyn.com/lupron-for-endometriosis; https://www.lupronpedpro.com/ (July 26, 2023).
35. Alec Schemmel, "FDA warns puberty blocker may cause brain swelling, vision loss in children." ABC National Desk, July 26, 2022. https://katv.com/news/nation-world/fda-warns-puberty-blocker-may-cause-brain-swelling-vision-loss-in-children-rachel-levine (September 4, 2022).
36. Maiko A. Schneider, Poli M. Spritzer, Bianca Machado Borba Soll, et al, "Brain Maturation, Cognition and Voice Pattern in a Gender Dysphoria Case under Pubertal Suppression." *Frontiers in Human Neuroscience*, November 14, 2017, Volume 11.

37. Sarah-Jayne Blakemore, Stephanie Burnett, and Ronald E. Dahl, "The role of puberty in the developing adolescent brain." *Human Brain Mapping*, June 2010; 31(6): 926–933.
38. Hilary Cass, Letter to National Health Service England, July 19, 2022. https://cass.independent-review.uk/wp-content/uploads/2022/07/Cass-Review-Letter-to-NHSE_19-July-2022.pdf (September 2, 2023).
40. Michael K. Laidlaw, Quentin L. Van Meter, Paul W. Hruz, et al, "Letter to the Editor: 'Endocrine Treatment of Gender-Dysphoric/Gender-Incongruent Persons: An Endocrine Society Clinical Practice Guideline.'" *The Journal of Clinical Endocrinology & Metabolism* March 2019, 104(3): 686–687.
41. Susan Berry, "FDA: Thousands of Deaths Linked to Puberty Blockers." Breitbart, October 2, 2019. www.breitbart.com/politics/2019/10/02/fda-thousands-of-deaths-linked-to-puberty-blockers/ (August 26, 2020).41. Michael K. Laidlaw, Quentin L. Van Meter, et al, "Endocrine Treatment of Gender-Dysphoric/Gender-Incongruent Persons: An Endocrine Society Clinical Practice Guideline." *The Journal of Clinical Endocrinology & Metabolism*, March 2019, 104(3):686–687; pp. 686, 687.
42. Interestingly, GnRH analogs only started to be used to completely block puberty in the 1990s. Before then, in the 1980s, they were used primarily to treat precocious puberty, or puberty that occurs too early. Precocious puberty is prevented with a constant level of synthetic GnRH, which desensitizes the pituitary and leads to a decrease in the secretion of gonadotropins, which in turn causes a delay in the maturation of gonads—thus avoiding the secretion of testosterone and estrogen that would catalyze puberty. See Paul W. Hruz, Lawrence S. Mayer, and Paul R. McHugh, "Growing Pains: Problems with Puberty Suppression in Treating Gender Dysphoria." *The New Atlantis*, Spring 2017.
43. Brian Blum, "Would you give up on orgasm?," June 2, 2022. *Jerusalem Post*, https://www.jpost.com/opinion/article-708397 (May 16, 2023).
44. Ibid.
45. Michael K. Laidlaw, Quentin L. Van Meter, Paul W. Hruz, et al, "Letter to the Editor: 'Endocrine Treatment of Gender-Dysphoric/Gender-Incongruent Persons: An Endocrine Society Clinical Practice Guideline.'" *The Journal of Clinical Endocrinology & Metabolism* March 2019, 104(3): 686–687.
46. Miriam Grossman, *Lost in Trans Nation: A Child Psychiatrist's Guide Out of the Madness* (New York, NY: Skyhorse Publishing, 2023), p. 176.
47. David Batty, "Mistaken identity." *The Guardian*, July 30, 2004. www.theguardian.com/society/2004/jul/31/health.socialcare (August 21, 2020).
48. Sheila Jeffreys, *Gender Hurts* (London and New York: Routledge, 2014), pp. 70–71.
49. S. Weyers, H. Verstraelen, J. Gerris, S. Monstrey, Gdos S Santiago, B. Saerens, E. De Backer, G. Claeys, M. Vaneechoutte, R. Verhelst, "Microflora of the penile skin-lined neovagina of transsexual women." *BMC Microbiology*, May 20, 2009; 9:102, p. 180. doi: 10.1186/1471-2180-9-102. PMID: 19457233; PMCID: PMC2695466. (102).
50. S. Cristofari, B. Bertrand, S. Leuzzi, et al, "Postoperative complications of male to female sex reassignment surgery: A 10-year French retrospective study." *Annales de chirurgie plastique et esthetique* [*Annals of plastic and aesthetic surgery*], February 2019; 64(1):24-32. Abstract, https://pubmed.ncbi.nlm.nih.gov/30269882/ (March 1, 2024).
51. The Report of the 2015 *U.S. Transgender Survey*. National Center for Transgender Equality, https://transequality.org/sites/default/files/docs/usts/USTS-Full-Report-Dec17.pdf (June 15, 2023).
52. Breast binders are reminiscent of the corsets that Victorian women wore. Because their corsets were often pulled tight and the many layers of clothing trapped heat close to the body, women often suffered from breathing difficulties and sudden changes in blood pressure—which was why they often needed to lie down. "Fainting couches"

were specially constructed pieces of long, easy-to-climb-on furniture to accommodate these women and their voluminous garments that restricted their compressed, tortured bodies. It's not surprising that women who wear breast binders today suffer similar (though perhaps not quite as drastic) health problems.

53. The Report of the *2015 U.S. Transgender Survey*. National Center for Transgender Equality, https://transequality.org/sites/default/files/docs/usts/USTS-Full-Report-Dec17.pdf (June 15, 2023). Data are on p. 101.
54. M.S. Irwin, K. Childs, and A.B. Hancock, "Effects of testosterone on the transgender male voice." *Andrology*, September 19, 20167.
55. Annie M.Q. Wang, Vivian Tsang, Peter Mankowski, et al, "Outcomes Following Gender Affirming Phalloplasty: A Systematic Review and Meta-Analysis." *Sexual Medicine Reviews*, October 2022; 10(4): 499-512.
56. The Report of the 2015 *U.S. Transgender Survey*. National Center for Transgender Equality, https://transequality.org/sites/default/files/docs/usts/USTS-Full-Report-Dec17.pdf (June 15, 2023). Data are on p. 101.

Chapter 4. Gender Dysphoria and Mental Illness

1. Paul McHugh, "Transgenderism: A Pathogenic Meme." *Public Discourse*, June 10, 2015. www.thepublicdiscourse.com/2015/06/15145 (July 20, 2020).
2. Ranna Parekh, "What Is Gender Dysphoria?" American Psychiatric Association, February 2016. www.psychiatry.org/patients-families/gender-dysphoria/what-is-gender-dysphoria (July 17, 2020).
3. Psychiatrist Miriam Grossman points out that a very few people set the policy for the entire membership of the American Psychiatric Association. Nonetheless, these policies are being followed.
4. Walt Heyer, "Gender dysphoria diagnoses are too general, and they're destroying people." Life Site News, August 19, 2019. https://www.lifesitenews.com/opinion/gender-dysphoria-diagnoses-are-too-general-and-theyre-destroying-people/ (August 9, 2023).
5. Walt Heyer, "62.7% of Transgenders Have Untreated Mental Disorders," December 15, 2016. https://waltheyer.com/62-7-of-transgenders-have-untreated-mental-disorders (July 14, 2020).
6. Elie Vandenbussche, "Detransition-Related Needs and Support: A Cross-Sectional Online Survey." *Journal of Homosexuality* 2022, Volume 69, Number 9, 1602–1620.
7. E. Abbruzzese, Stephen B. Levine and Julia W. Mason, "The Myth of 'Reliable Research' in Pediatric Gender Medicine: A critical evaluation of the Dutch Studies—and research that has followed." *Journal of Sex and Marital Therapy*, January 2, 2023. https://www.tandfonline.com/doi/full/10.1080/0092623X.2022.2150346 (July 10, 2023).
8. Ibid.
9. "WPATH Gender Affirming Doctor Shows Concern for Mental Health of Minors After Transition Surgeries." Project Veritas, October 6, 2022. YouTube video, https://www.youtube.com/watch?v=9EYdzTPaguU (July 30, 2023).
10. E. Abbruzzese, Stephen B. Levine and Julia W. Mason, "The Myth of 'Reliable Research' in Pediatric Gender Medicine: A critical evaluation of the Dutch Studies—and research that has followed." *Journal of Sex and Marital Therapy*, January 2, 2023. https://www.tandfonline.com/doi/full/10.1080/0092623X.2022.2150346 (July 10, 2023), pp 21, 1, 2.
11. Ibid.

12. Daniel Shumer, Aser Abrha, Henry A. Feldman, and Jeremi Carswell, "Overrepresentation of Adopted Adolescents at a Hospital-Based Gender Dysphoria Clinic." *Transgender Health* 2017, 2(1): 76–79.
13. "Behavioral and Emotional Issues in Adopted Children." Children's Hospital of Philadelphia, 2023. https://www.chop.edu/conditions-diseases/behavioral-and-emotional-issues-adopted-and-foster-children (January 5, 2024).
14. "WPATH Gender Affirming Doctor Shows Concern For Mental Health of Minors After Transition Surgeries." Project Veritas, October 6, 2022. https://www.youtube.com/watch?v=9EYdzTPaguU (July 30, 2023).
15. *Transgender Regret*, 2018 Dutch documentary. https://www.youtube.com/watch?v=1bV8AaeYKjQ (October 1, 2023).
16. Ibid.
17. Ibid.
18. Ibid.
19. Ibid.
20. Ibid.
21. Ashley Bateman, "The Whole Transgender Industry Is Founded On Two Faulty Studies." *The Federalist*, February 1, 2023. https://thefederalist.com/2023/02/01/the-whole-transgender-industry-is-founded-on-two-faulty-studies/ (July 10, 2023).
22. Ranna Parekh, "What Is Gender Dysphoria?" American Psychiatric Association, February 2016. www.psychiatry.org/patients-families/gender-dysphoria/what-is-gender-dysphoria (July 17, 2020).
23. Kelsey Bolar and Andrea Mew, "Female student alleges she was raped in trans-inclusive bathroom at New Mexico middle school." *Post Millennial*, June 20, 2023. https://thepostmillennial.com/exclusive-female-student-alleges-she-was-raped-in-trans-inclusive-bathroom-at-new-mexico-middle-school?cfp (July 10, 2023).
24. Ibid.
25. Sheila Jeffreys, "The politics of the toilet: A feminist response to the campaign to 'degender' a women's space." *Women's Studies International Forum* 45 (2014), 42–51, p. 45.
26. Jonathon Van Maren, "Trans activist threatens to murder people who stop men from entering girls' bathrooms: 'Buy a gun.'" Life Site News, April 24, 2023. https://www.lifesitenews.com/blogs/buy-a-gun-trans-activist-threatens-to-murder-people-who-stop-males-from-using-girls-bathrooms/?utm_source=top_news&utm_campaign=usa (July 10, 2023).
27. Madeleine Kearns, "California's Transgender Prison Policy Is a Disaster for Women." *National Review*, June 26, 2019. www.nationalreview.com/2019/06/californias-transgender-prison-policy-is-a-disaster-for-women/ (August 4, 2020).
28. Chris Cameron, "Trump Presses Limits on Transgender Rights Over Supreme Court Ruling." *The New York Times*, July 24, 2020. www.nytimes.com/2020/07/24/us/politics/trump-transgender-rights-homeless.html (August 4, 2020).
29. Nico Lang, "Trump administration moves to repeal transgender protections in homeless shelters." NBC News, July 2, 2020. www.nbcnews.com/feature/nbc-out/trump-administration-moves-repeal-transgender-protections-homeless-shelters-n1232849 (August 4, 2020).
30. Madeleine Kearns, "Women-Only Rape-Relief Shelter Defunded, Then Vandalized." *National Review*, August 28, 2019. www.nationalreview.com/2019/08/women-only-rape-relief-shelter-defunded-then-vandalized/ (August 25, 2020).

31. Matt Masterson, "Lawsuit: Female Prisoner Says She Was Raped by Transgender Inmate." WTTW, February 19, 2020. https://news.wttw.com/2020/02/19/lawsuit-female-prisoner-says-she-was-raped-transgender-inmate (August 25, 2020).
32. April Roach, "Female prison officers raped by inmates who self-identify as trans, ex-Tory minister Rory Stewart claims." *The Sun*, August 11, 2020. www.thesun.co.uk/news/11381963/female-prison-officers-raped-trans-rory-stewart/ (August 25, 2020).
33. https://olympusspa.com/ (August 3, 2023).
34. Zachary Stieber, "Female-Only Spa Forced to Accept 'Transgender Women' Reveals Next Move." *The Epoch Times*, June 12, 2023. https://www.theepochtimes.com/us/female-only-spa-forced-to-accept-transgender-women-reveals-next-move-5327263?ea_med=desktop_news_health&tmp=1&ea_src=ai_recommender (August 3, 2023).
35. Lal Coveney, "Transsexuals in the women's liberation movement," 1979. Paper for the Rad/Rev Conference, Leeds, September 22–23, 1979. Lesbian Archive Collection, Glasgow Women's Library. Box no: LAIC 1/3. Quoted in Jeffreys, *Gender Hurts* (London and New York: Routledge, 2014), p. 38.
36. Brett Cooper, "My Biology Is Not Your Costume." The Comments Section with Brett Cooper, YouTube, January 31, 2023. https://www.youtube.com/watch?v=iq_1PWEEzOs&t=7s (March 21, 2023).
37. Sheila Jeffreys, *Gender Hurts* (London and New York: Routledge, 2014), p. 37.
38. Paul McHugh, "Transgenderism: A Pathogenic Meme." Public Discourse, June 10, 2015. www.thepublicdiscourse.com/2015/06/15145 (July 20, 2020).
39. Paul McHugh, "Psychiatric misadventures." *American Scholar* 61 (7):497–510, pp. 502, 503. Also at https://www.transgendermap.com/politics/psychiatry/paul-mchugh/ (November 15, 2023).
40. Paul McHugh, "Surgical Sex: Why We Stopped Doing Sex Change Operations." First Things, November 2004. www.firstthings.com/article/2004/11/surgical-sex (July 23, 2020).
41. Brandon Morse, "Data Shows that Suicide Rate of Transgender Teens is Breathtakingly high." Red State, September 12, 2018. www.redstate.com/brandon_morse/2018/09/12/data-shows-suicide-rate-transgender-students-breathtakingly-high (July 17, 2020).
42. Ibid.
43. Austen Hartke, "3 Mental Health Issues Facing Transgender People and How to Help," undated. http://thesaltcollective.org/3-mental-health-issues-facing-transgender-people-and-how-to-help (July 17, 2020).
44. Daniel Payne, "The Transgender Suicide Rate Isn't Due To Discrimination." *The Federalist*, July 7, 2016. https://thefederalist.com/2016/07/07/evidence-the-transgender-suicide-rate-isnt-due-to-discrimination (July 17, 2020).
45. "Suicide Facts and Myths," Transgender Trend, undated. www.transgendertrend.com/the-suicide-myth/ (July 18, 2020).
46. Daniel Payne, "The Transgender Suicide Rate Isn't Due To Discrimination." *The Federalist*, July 7, 2016. https://thefederalist.com/2016/07/07/evidence-the-transgender-suicide-rate-isnt-due-to-discrimination (July 17, 2020).
47. David Batty, "Mistaken identity." *The Guardian*, July 30, 2004. www.theguardian.com/society/2004/jul/31/health.socialcare (August 21, 2020).
48. Scott Newgent interview with Preston Sprinkle, "A Transman's Unexpected Thoughts on Trans-Related Issues: Scott Newgent," 2022. https://www.youtube.com/watch?v=zazsZ_HO3LM (January 20, 2024).
49. Azadeh Mazaheri Meybodi, Ahmad Hajebi, and Atefeh Ghanbari Jolfaei, "Psychiatric Axis I Comorbidities among Patients with Gender Dysphoria." *Psychiatry Journal* 2014: 971–814.

50. Cecilia Dhejne, Paul Lichtenstein, Marcus Boman, et al, "Long-Term Follow-Up of Transsexual Persons Undergoing Sex Reassignment Surgery: Cohort Study in Sweden." *Plos One*, February 2011, Volume 6, Issue 2. https://journals.plos.org/plosone/article?id=10.1371/journal.pone.0016885 (July 13, 2023).

51. Jack L. Turban, Dana King, Jeremi M. Carswell, et al, "Pubertal Suppression for Transgender Youth and Risk of Suicidal Ideation." *Pediatrics*, February 2020; 145(2).

52. Cecilia Dhejne, Paul Lichtenstein, Marcus Boman, et al, "Long-Term Follow-Up of Transsexual Persons Undergoing Sex Reassignment Surgery: Cohort Study in Sweden." *Plos One*, February 2011, Volume 6, Issue 2. https://journals.plos.org/plosone/article?id=10.1371/journal.pone.0016885 (July 13, 2023).

53. Suzanna Diaz and J. Michael Bailey, "Rapid Onset Gender Dysphoria: Parent Reports on 1655 Possible Cases." *Archives of Sexual Behavior* (March 29, 2023) 52:1031–1043. https://link.springer.com/article/10.1007/s10508-023-02576-9#change-history (July 9, 2023).

54. "Retraction Note: Rapid Onset Gender Dysphoria: Parent Reports on 1655 Possible Cases." *Archives of Sexual Behavior* (June 14, 2023) 52:1031–1043. https://link.springer.com/article/10.1007/s10508-023-02635-1 (July 9, 2023).

55. Nathan Worcester, "Journal Retracts Study of Rapid-Onset Gender Dysphoria in Youth." *The Epoch Times*, June 16, 2023. https://www.theepochtimes.com/journal-retracts-study-of-rapid-onset-gender-dysphoria-in-youth_5339026.html (July 9, 2023).

56. Ibid.

57. Kai Dallas, Paige Kuhlman, Karyn Eilber, Victoria Scott, et al, "Rates of Psychiatric Emergencies Before and After Gender Affirming Surgery." *The Journal of Urology*, Volume 206, Issue Supplement 3, September 1, 2021.

58. https://www.lupronpedpro.com/isi.html; https://www.lupronpedpro.com/; https://www.luprongyn.com/lupron-for-endometriosis (July 26, 2023).

59. Alex Bollinger, "Puberty blockers reduce suicidal thoughts in trans people. Republicans want to ban them." LGBTQ Nation, January 24, 2020. https://www.lgbtqnation.com/2020/01/puberty-blockers-reduce-suicidal-thoughts-trans-people-republicans-want-ban/ (July 26, 2023).

60. Michael Biggs, "Puberty Blockers and Suicidality in Adolescents Suffering from Gender Dysphoria." *Archives of Sexual Behavior* 2020, 49(7): 2227–2229. https://www.ncbi.nlm.nih.gov/pmc/articles/PMC8169497/ (July 26, 2023).

61. Ibid.

62. Michael Biggs, "The Dutch Protocol for Juvenile Transsexuals: Origins and Evidence." *Journal of Sex and Marital Therapy* 2023, Volume 49, Issue 4: 348–368; p. 356.

63. Yuan-Hung Pong, Yu-Chuan Lu, Vinscent F.S. Tsai, et al, "Acute manic and psychotic symptoms following subcutaneous leuprolide acetate in a male patient without prior psychiatric history: A case report and literature review." *Urological Science* 25, 2014, 22–24.

64. Ibid.

65. Roberto D'Angelo, Ema Syrulnik, Sasha Ayad, et al, "One Size Does Not Fit All: In Support of Psychotherapy for Gender Dysphoria." *Archives of Sexual Behavior* 2021, Number 50, 7–16; pp. 7, 13.

66. Tijen Butler, "What percentage of the US population is transgender?" PinkNews, April 2, 2019. www.pinknews.co.uk/2019/04/02/percentage-us-population-transgender-statistics (July 17, 2020).

67. "How Many Adults Identify as Transgender in the United States?" UCLA School of Law, Williams Institute, June 2016. https://williamsinstitute.law.ucla.edu/publications/trans-adults-united-states/ (July 23, 2020).

Chapter 5. Why Someone Might Transition

1. *Diagnostic and Statistical Manual of Mental Disorders*, 4th Edition, text revision (DSM-IV-TR) (Washington, D.C.: American Psychiatric Association, 2000).
2. *Diagnostic and Statistical Manual of Mental Disorders*, 5th Edition, text revision (DSM-IV-TR) (Washington, D.C.: American Psychiatric Association, 2013).
3. M. Goodman and R. Nash, *Examining Health Outcomes for People Who Are Transgender* (Washington, D.D.: Patient-Centered Outcomes Research Institute, 2019). www.pcori.org/sites/default/files/Goodman076-Final-Research-Report.pdf.
4. T. Steensma, P. Cohen-Ketenis, and K. Zucker, "Evidence for a Change in the Sex Ratio of Children Referred for Gender Dysphoria: Data from the Center of Expertise on Gender Dysphoria in Amsterdam (1988–2016)." *Journal of Sex & Marital Therapy* 44, Number 7 (2018): 713–715.
5. Parents with Inconvenient Truths about Trans (PITT). "Learning from the Detransitioners," April 29, 2022. https://pitt.substack.com/p/learning-from-the-detransitioners (August 3, 2023).
6. Ewa Matuszczak, Marta Diana Komarowska, Wojciech Debek, and Adam Hermanowicz, "The Impact of Bisphenol A on Fertility, Reproductive System, and Development: A Review of the Literature." *International Journal of Endocrinology*, Volume 2019, Article ID 4068717, https://doi.org/10.1155/2019/4068717.
7. Shirin A. Hafezi and Wael M. Abdel-Rahman, "The Endocrine Disruptor Bisphenol A (BPA) Exerts a Wide Range of Effects in Carcinogenesis and Response to Therapy." *Current Molecular Pharmacology*, August 2019; 12(3): 230–238.
8. Lanlan Li, Qianqian Wang, Yan Zhang, et al, "The Molecular Mechanism of Bisphenol A (BPA) as an Endocrine Disruptor by Interacting with Nuclear Receptors: Insights from Molecular Dynamics (MD) Simulations." *Plos One*, March 23, 2015.
9. Alex Formuzis, "Landmark BPA Study Finds Troubling Health Effects at FDA's 'Safe' Levels." Environmental Working Group, September 14, 2018. www.ewg.org/release/first-us-bpa-lab-study-humans-finds-troubling-health-effects-levels-deemed-safe-fda-epa (July 23, 2020).
10. Susan M. Duty, Narendra P. Singh, Manori J. Silva, et. al., "The relationship between environmental exposures to phthalates and DNA damage in human sperm using the neutral comet assay." *Environmental Health Perspectives* July 2003; 111(9):1164–1169.
11. Xiaona Huo, Dan Chen, Yonghua He, et al, "Bisphenol-A and Female Infertility: A Possible Role of Gene-Environment Interactions." *International Journal of Environmental Research and Public Health* September 2015; 12(9): 11101–11116. www.ncbi.nlm.nih.gov/pmc/articles/PMC4586663/ (July 23, 2020).
12. Jennifer T. Wolstenholme, Zuzana Drobná, Anne D. Henriksen, et al, "Transgenerational Bisphenol A Causes Deficits in Social Recognition and Alters Postsynaptic Density Genes in Mice." *Endocrinology* 160, 2019: 1854–1867.
13. "Bisphenol A (BPA): Use in Food Contact Application." U.S. Food & Drug Administration Website, November 2014. https://www.fda.gov/food/food-packaging-other-substances-come-contact-food-information-consumers/bisphenol-bpa-use-food-contact-application#summary (November 11, 2023). Also see Department of Health & Human Services Memorandum dated June 17, 2014, at https://www.fda.gov/media/90124/download (November 11, 2023).
14. Valérie S. Langlois and Isabelle Plante, "Science shows that BPA and other endocrine disruptors are harmful to human health, which should incite tighter regulations." The Conversation, March 30, 2022. https://theconversation.com/science-shows-that-bpa-and-other-endocrine-disruptors-are-harmful-to-human-health-which-should-incite-tighter-regulations-178872 (November 11, 2023).

15. Phillippe Grandjean and Phillip Landrigan, "Neurobehavioural effects of developmental toxicity." *Lancet Neurology* 214, February 15, 2014; 13:330–338.

16. BPA has also not only been linked to asthma, it also negatively affects genes, impairing the body's natural ability to reduce and remove high levels of chloride from the central nervous system. BPA significantly changes how glucose affects insulin levels, thus setting the stage for obesity and diabetes. See Richard W. Stahlhut, John Peterson Myers, Julia A. Taylor, et al, "Experimental BPA Exposure and Glucose-Stimulated Insulin Response in Adult Men and Women." *Journal of the Endocrine Society*, Volume 2, Issue 10, October 2018, 1173–1187.

    Research has also linked even low-dose BPA exposure to cardiovascular problems, including heart attacks, high blood pressure and angina; and wheezing and other asthma-like symptoms. See Susan M. Duty, Narendra P. Singh, Manori J. Silva, et. al., "The relationship between environmental exposures to phthalates and DNA damage in human sperm using the neutral comet assay." *Environmental Health Perspectives* July 2003; 111(9):1164–1169.

    Due to the estrogenic effects of BPA and similar plastics, their effect on endocrine glands can lead to metabolic syndrome and obesity. See Lanlan Li, Qianqian Wang, Yan Zhang, et al, "The Molecular Mechanism of Bisphenol A (BPA) as an Endocrine Disruptor by Interacting with Nuclear Receptors: Insights from Molecular Dynamics (MD) Simulations." *Plos One*, March 23, 2015.

    These plastics also cause immune impairment, an increased risk of cancer, and an increase in metabolic disorders including diabetes. See Elizabeth G. Radke, Audrey Galizia, Kristina A.Thayer, and Glinda S.Cooper, "Phthalate exposure and metabolic effects: a systematic review of the human epidemiological evidence." *Environmental International* Volume 132, November 2019.

17. Tyrone B. Hayes, Vicky Khoury, Anne Narayan, et al, "Atrazine induces complete feminization and chemical castration in male African clawed frogs (Xenopus laevis)." *Proceedings of the Natural Academy of Sciences USA*, March 9, 2010; 107(10):4612–4617. https://pubmed.ncbi.nlm.nih.gov/20194757/ (June 21, 2023).

18. Canadian Paediatric Society, "Concerns for the use of soy-based formulas in infant nutrition." *Paediatrics Child Health*, February 2009, 14(2): 109–113.

19. Hideyuki Imai, Hiroto Nishikawa, et al, "Secondary Hypogonadism due to Excessive Ingestion of Isoflavone in a Man." *Internal Medicine*, October 1, 2022; 61(19), 2899-2903.

20. The increasing number of males who are experiencing radical hormonal alteration means that the population of healthy, strong, adult men is decreasing. The very hormonal development that helps give men physical strength and stamina is being eradicated. This makes them poor protectors, unfit for military service in times of crisis.

21. Stefania D'Angelo, Marika Scafuro, and Rosaria Meccariello, "BPA and Nutraceuticals, Simultaneous Effects on Endocrine Functions." *Endocrine, Metabolic & Immune Disorders - Drug Targets*, August 2019; 19(5): 594–604.

22. Jazz Jennings, "Being Jazz: My Life as a (Transgender) Teen." *Time*, May 31, 2016. https://time.com/4350574/jazz-jennings-transgender/ (August 20, 2023).

23. Malcolm Clark, "The tragedy of Jazz Jennings." Spiked, August 20, 2023. https://www.spiked-online.com/2023/08/20/the-tragedy-of-jazz-jennings (September 18, 2023).

24. Ibid.

25. *20:20 My Secret Self* complete documentary with Barbara Walters, March 15, 2016. https://www.youtube.com/watch?v=eJ_BHY5RolA&t=1202s (September 18, 2023).

26. Lily Hayes, "Watch: Trans Child Celebrity Admits They Never Feel Like Themselves Despite Gender-Confirming Surgeries." Louder with Crowder, February 28, 2023. https://www.louderwithcrowder.com/jazz-jennings-themselves (August 11, 2023).

27. Malcolm Clark, "The tragedy of Jazz Jennings." Spiked, August 20, 2023. https://www.spiked-online.com/2023/08/20/the-tragedy-of-jazz-jennings (September 18, 2023).
28. *20:20 My Secret Self* complete documentary with Barbara Walters, March 15, 2016. https://www.youtube.com/watch?v=eJ_BHY5RolA&t=1202s (September 18, 2023).
29. Miriam Grossman, *Lost in Trans Nation: A Child Psychiatrist's Guide Out of the Madness* (New York, NY: Skyhorse Publishing, 2023), p. 188.
30. Abigail Shrier, *Irreversible Damage: The Transgender Craze Seducing Our Daughters* (Washington, DC: Regnery Publishing, 2020), p. 26.
31. Jonathan Kay, "An Interview With Lisa Littman, Who Coined the Term 'Rapid Onset Gender Dysphoria.'" Quillette, March 19, 2019. https://quillette.com/2019/03/19/an-interview-with-lisa-littman-who-coined-the-term-rapid-onset-gender-dysphoria/ (August 9, 2023).
32. Jonathon Van Maren, "Even some LGBT activists are disturbed by the devastating impact transgender mania has on children." Life Site News, November 11, 2022. https://www.lifesitenews.com/blogs/even-some-lgbt-activists-are-disturbed-by-the-devastating-impact-transgender-mania-has-on-children/?utm_source=top_news&utm_campaign=usa (August 9, 2023).
33. Erin Brewer, *Detransitioners: Stories of Medical Child Abuse, Part 1.* YouTube, February 6, 2020. https://www.youtube.com/watch?v=r7TM6BA0JEY (August 25, 2020).
34. Denise Witmer, "The Media and Your Teen's Body Image." Very Well Mind, April 4, 2020. https://www.verywellmind.com/body-image-issues-teens-and-the-media-2609236#citation-1 (August 2, 2023).
35. Matthew Lapierre, Frances Fleming-Milici, Esther Rozendaal, et al, "The Effect of Advertising on Children and Adolescents." *Pediatrics*, November 1, 2017, Volume 140, Supplement 2, S152–S156.
36. L.C. Soares Filho, R.F.L. Batista, V.C. Cardoso, et al, "Body image dissatisfaction and symptoms of depression disorder in adolescents." *Brazilian Journal of Medical and Biological Research*, 2021, Volume 54 (1).
37. Fiorela Flores-Cornego, Mayumi Kamego-Tome, Mariana A. Zapata-Pachas, and German F. Alvarado, "Association between body image dissatisfaction and depressive symptoms in adolescents." *Brazilian Journal of Psychiatry*, October–December 2017, 39 (4).
38. Jacinthe Dion, Marie-Eve Blackburn, Julie Auclair, et al, "Development and aetiology of body dissatisfaction in adolescent boys and girls." *International Journal of Adolescence and Youth*, April 3, 2015, 20(2): 151–166.
39. Siân McLean, Rachel F. Rodgers, Amy Slater, et al, "Clinically significant body dissatisfaction: prevalence and association with depressive symptoms in adolescent boys and girls." *European Child & Adolescent Psychiatry*, December 2022; 31(12): 1921–1932.
40. L.C. Soares Filho, R.F.L. Batista, V.C. Cardoso, et al, "Body image dissatisfaction and symptoms of depression disorder in adolescents." *Brazilian Journal of Medical and Biological Research*, 2021, Volume 54 (1).
41. Y. Efrati, "Problematic and Non-problematic Pornography Use and Compulsive Sexual Behaviors Among Understudied Populations: Children and Adolescents." *Current Addiction Reports* 7, January 13, 2020, 68–75.
42. Abigail Shrier, *Irreversible Damage: The Transgender Craze Seducing Our Daughters* (Washington, DC: Regnery Publishing, 2020), p. 154.
43. Whitney Rostad, Daniel Gittins-Stone, Charlie Huntington, et al, "The Association Between Exposure to Violent Pornography and Teen Dating Violence in Grade 10 High School Students." *Archives of Sexual Behavior* 48, July 15, 2019, 2137–2147.

44. National Center for Transgender Equality, The Report of the 2015 *U.S. Transgender Survey.* https://transequality.org/sites/default/files/docs/usts/USTS-Full-Report-Dec17.pdf (June 15, 2023). Data are on p. 101.
45. Lisa Marchiano, "The Ranks of Gender Detransitioners Are Growing. We Need to Understand Why." Quillette, January 2, 2020. https://quillette.com/2020/01/02/the-ranks-of-gender-detransitioners-are-growing-we-need-to-understand-why/ (August 9, 2023).
46. Lisa Marchiano, "Transgenderism and the Social Construction of Diagnosis." Quillette, March 1, 2018. https://quillette.com/2018/03/01/transgenderism-social-construction-diagnosis/ (August 10, 2023).
47. Abigail Shrier, *Irreversible Damage: The Transgender Craze Seducing Our Daughters* (Washington, DC: Regnery Publishing, 2020), p. 70.
48. Ibid. p. 73.
49. "Understanding How Testosterone Can Affect Your Emotions During Transition." Plume, July 26, 2022. https://getplume.co/blog/understanding-how-testosterone-can-affect-your-emotions-during-transition/ (August 2, 2022).
50. Connor Grannis, Scott F. Leibowitz, Shane Gahn, et al, "Testosterone treatment, internalizing symptoms, and body image dissatisfaction in transgender boys." *Psychoneuroendocrinology*, October 2021, Volume 132.
51. Abigail Shrier, *Irreversible Damage: The Transgender Craze Seducing Our Daughters* (Washington, DC: Regnery Publishing, 2020), p. 8.
52. Sarah Creighton, "Surgery for intersex." *Journal of the Royal Society of Medicine*, May 2001, 94(5): 218–220; pp. 219, 220.
53. Interfering with the function of healthy genitals is a hostile, anti-pleasure, life-negating act. It is my hope that both the medical establishment and the general public make the connection between the damaging effects of genital surgery for intersex children and the still-common practice of circumcising infant males—not to mention the barbaric practice of female genital mutilation or FGM, which is inflicted on older females who are completely conscious. See Chapter 1, Note 70, for more details.
54. Virginia Erhardt, Editor, *Head Over Heels: Wives Who Stay With Cross-Dressers and Transsexuals* (New York: Routledge, 2007), p. 193.
55. "Autognephilia," Wiktionary. https://en.wiktionary.org/wiki/autogynephilia (August 21, 2023).
56. Ray Blanchard, "The concept of autogynephilia and the typology of male gender dysphoria." *The Journal of Nervous and Mental Disease* 1989, Number 177, 616–623.
57. Louise Perry, "What Is Autogynephilia? An Interview with Dr Ray Blanchard," November 6, 2019. https://quillette.com/2019/11/06/what-is-autogynephilia-an-interview-with-dr-ray-blanchard/ (May 1, 2023).
58. Ibid.
59. "Autognephilia," LGBT Project Wiki. https://lgbt.wikia.org/wiki/Autogynephilia (August 21, 2020).
60. "How My Journey in Autogynephilia Began," Friday, April 20, 2012. https://how-my-journey-began.blogspot.com/2012/04/how-my-journey-in-autogynephilia.html (August 21, 2020).
61. Walt Heyer, "Hormones, surgery, regret: I was a transgender woman for 8 years—time I can't get back." *USA Today*, February 11, 2019. https://www.usatoday.com/story/opinion/voices/2019/02/11/transgender-debate-transitioning-sex-gender-column/1894076002/ (August 4, 2023).
62. Kristen Schilt, "Just One of the Guys?: How Transmen Make Gender Visible at Work." *Gender and Society* 2006, 20 (4):465–490.

63. James St. James, "These 25 Examples of Male Privilege from a Trans Guy's Perspective Really Prove the Point." Everyday Feminism, May 30, 2015. https://everydayfeminism.com/2015/05/male-privilege-trans-men/ (January 14, 2021).
64. Ibid.
65. James St. James, "25 (More) Examples of Male Privilege as Experienced By a Trans Man." Everyday Feminism, June 21, 2015. https://everydayfeminism.com/2015/06/more-male-privilege-trans-man/ (April 25, 2022).
66. "The State of the Gender Pay Gap 2020," www.payscale.com/data/gender-pay-gap (August 24, 2020).
67. Katherine Haan, "Gender Pay Gap Statistics in 2023." *Forbes Advisor*, February 27, 2023. https://www.forbes.com/advisor/business/gender-pay-gap-statistics/ (November 12, 2023).
68. Carey, *Detransitioned*, 2018. https://vimeo.com/276349075
69. Dorothy Cummings McLean, "At world's first gender 'detransition' conference, women express regret over drugs, mutilation." Life Site News, December 2, 2019. www.lifesitenews.com/news/at-worlds-first-gender-detransition-conference-women-express-regret-over-drugs-mutilation (August 25, 2020).
70. James Barnes, "I'm a Trans Man. I Didn't Realize How Broken Men Are." *Newsweek*, August 6, 2023. https://www.newsweek.com/trans-man-broken-men-1817169 (January 7, 2024).
71. Marc Freeman, "Ben Barres: neuroscience pioneer, gender champion." *Nature*, October 22, 2018. www.nature.com/articles/d41586-018-07109-2 (August 24, 2020).
72. Ben A. Barres, "Does gender matter?" *Nature*, July 13, 2006, Volume 442, p. 134.
73. Ibid. p. 135.
74. Ben A. Barres, *The Autobiography of a Transgender Scientist* (Cambridge, Massachusetts: The MIT Press, 2018), pp. 10, 11.
75. Ibid. pp. 57, 58.
76. Scott Newgent interview with Preston Sprinkle, "A Transman's Unexpected Thoughts on Trans-Related Issues: Scott Newgent," 2022. https://www.youtube.com/watch?v=zazsZ_HO3LM (January 20, 2024).

Chapter 6. Trans Regret and Detransitioners

1. Albert Eisenberg, "The Plight of the Detransitioners." *National Review Magazine*, May 29, 2023. https://www.nationalreview.com/magazine/2023/05/29/the-plight-of-the-detransitioners/ (August 4, 2023).
2. Syb, "Purification Rites." Substack, April 26, 2022. https://sybmantics.substack.com/p/purification-rites?s=r (August 3, 2023).
3. Scott Newgent interview with Preston Sprinkle, "A Transman's Unexpected Thoughts on Trans-Related Issues: Scott Newgent," 2022. https://www.youtube.com/watch?v=zazsZ_HO3LM (January 20, 2024).
4. Skye Davies, Stephen McIntyre, and Craig Rypma, "Detransition rates in a national UK Gender Identity Clinic, April 11, 2019." 3rd Biennial EPATH Conference Inside Matters. On Law, Ethics and Religion, April 11–13, 2019, p. 118. https://epath.eu/wp-content/uploads/2019/04/Boof-of-abstracts-EPATH2019.pdf.
5. "Detransition Facts and Statistics 2022: Exploding the Myths Around Detransitioning," June 21, 2021. https://www.gendergp.com/detransition-facts/ (August 4, 2023).
6. Valerie Richardson, "Ex-transgender 'detransitioners' raise red flags about 'gender-affirming care.'" *The Washington Times*, March 14, 2023. https://www.

NOTES 337

washingtontimes.com/news/2023/mar/14/ex-transgender-detransitioners-raise-red-flags-abo/ (August 4, 2023).

7. Michael S. Irwig, "Detransition Among Transgender and Gender-Diverse People—An Increasing and Increasingly Complex Phenomenon." *The Journal of Clinical Endocrinology & Metabolism*, Volume 107, Issue 10, October 2022, e4261–e4262.

8. J.L.Turban, S.S. Loo, A.N. Almazan, and A.S. Keuroghlian, "Factors Leading to 'Detransition' Among Transgender and Gender Diverse People in the United States: A Mixed-Methods Analysis." LGBT Health, 2020, 8(4): 273–280.

9. Lisa Littman, "Individuals Treated for Gender Dysphoria with Medical and/or Surgical Transition Who Subsequently Detransitioned: A Survey of 100 Detransitioners." *Archives of Sexual Behavior* 2021, Number 50, 3353–3369.

10. Ibid.

11. Elie Vandenbussche, "Detransition-Related Needs and Support: A Cross-Sectional Online Survey." *Journal of Homosexuality* 2022, Volume 69, Number 9, 1602–1620; pp. 1602, 1611.

12. Ibid, p. 1611.

13. Ibid, p. 1612.

14. Ibid, p. 1612.

15. Lisa Marchiano, "The Ranks of Gender Detransitioners Are Growing. We Need to Understand Why." Quillette, January 2, 2020. https://quillette.com/2020/01/02/the-ranks-of-gender-detransitioners-are-growing-we-need-to-understand-why/ (July 21, 2020).

16. Sophia Lee, "Walt's story." *World Magazine*, March 30, 2017. https://world.wng.org/2017/03/walt_s_story (August 21 2020).

17. Ibid.

18. Tullip R's account, June 15, 2022. https://threadreaderapp.com/thread/1536422533230206976.html (June 30, 2022)

19. Syb, "Purification Rites." Substack, April 26, 2022. https://sybmantics.substack.com/p/purification-rites?s=r (August 3, 2023).

20. Ibid.

21. Ibid.

22. Mary Zwicker, "Ex-trans teen Chloe Cole to sue doctors who removed her breasts when she was just 15 years old." LifeSite News, November 11, 2022. https://www.lifesitenews.com/news/eighteen-year-old-girl-to-sue-doctors-who-removed-her-breasts/ (August 9, 2023).

23. Ramon Tomey, "Former trans teens express regret over gender reassignment procedures." Transhumanism.News, July 15, 2022. https://transhumanism.news/2022-07-15-former-trans-teens-express-regret-gender-reassignment.html# (August 9, 2023).

24. "Ninety Day Notice of Intent to Sue Pursuant to C.C.P. § 364," November 9, 2022, Limandri & Jonna LLP. https://www.dhillonlaw.com/wp-content/uploads/2022/11/Letter-of-Intent-Chloe-Cole.pdf, p. 2.

25. Ibid, pp. 2, 3.

26. Chloe Cole, "Detransitioner Chloe Cole's full testimony to Congress is a 'final warning' to stop gender surgery. *New York Post*, August 9, 2023. https://nypost.com/2023/07/28/detransitioner-chloe-coles-full-testimony-to-congress-is-a-final-warning-to-stop-gender-surgery/ (August 9, 2023).

27. Ibid.

28. Ibid.

29. Zachary Stieber, "Girl Sues Hospital for Removing Her Breasts at Age 13." *The Epoch Times*, June 15, 2023. https://www.theepochtimes.com/us/girl-sues-hospital-for-removing-her-breasts-at-age-13-post-5335492?welcomeuser=1 (August 9, 2023).
30. Ibid.
31. Ramon Tomey, "Former trans teens express regret over gender reassignment procedures." Transhumanism.News, July 15, 2022. https://transhumanism.news/2022-07-15-former-trans-teens-express-regret-gender-reassignment.html# (August 9, 2023).
32. Helena Kerschner, interview with Ben Shapiro, "Former Transgender Teenager Shares Powerful Story About Going In and Out of Transition." You Tube, April 28, 2022. https://www.youtube.com/watch?v=HwVyozpWWAU&t=872s (August 11, 2023).
33. Ibid.
34. Ibid.
35. Ramon Tomey, "Former trans teens express regret over gender reassignment procedures." Transhumanism.News, July 15, 2022. https://transhumanism.news/2022-07-15-former-trans-teens-express-regret-gender-reassignment.html# (August 9, 2023).
36. "Interview: Scott Newgent," Gender Dysphoria Alliance, December 18, 2021. https://www.genderdysphoriaalliance.com/post/meet-scott-newgent (August 9, 2023).
37. Scott Newgent, "We Need Balance When It Comes To Gender Dysphoric Kids. I Would Know." *Newsweek*, February 9, 2021. https://www.newsweek.com/we-need-balance-when-it-comes-gender-dysphoric-kids-i-would-know-opinion-1567277 (August 9, 2021).
38. Wesley Yang, "Every forward step in my transition at first brought elation, but it was ephemeral. As the joy faded, I was encouraged to take the next step. I was not only a cash cow, I was a willing disciple." Quoting Scott Newgent's speech, November 13, 2022. https://wesleyyang.substack.com/p/every-forward-step-in-my-transition (August 9, 2023).
39. "I'm Transgender, and I Oppose the Medical Transition of Children." The Center for Bioethics and Culture Network, April 2, 2020. https://cbc-network.org/2020/04/im-transgender-and-i-oppose-the-medical-transition-of-children/ (October 2, 2023).
40. "Scott Newgent Unboxing | Becoming Trans Ruined My Life," undated. https://thestoryboxpodcast.com/podcast/scott-newgent-unboxing-becoming-trans-ruined-my-life/ (August 10, 2023).
41. Sheila Jeffreys, *Gender Hurts* (London and New York: Routledge, 2014), p. 79.

Chapter 7. Who's Behind the Trans Agenda

1. Elle Bradford, "You Won't Believe How Much It Costs to Be Transgender in America." *Teen Vogue*, November 24, 2015. www.teenvogue.com/story/transgender-operations-hormone-therapy-costs (July 20, 2020).
2. "How Much Does Transgender Surgery Cost," CostAide, undated. https://costaide.com/transgender-surgery-cost/ (July 20, 2020).
3. Alyssa Wright, "Trans-Tech Is A Budding Industry: So Why Is No One Investing In It?" *Forbes*, December 8, 2020. https://www.forbes.com/sites/alyssawright/2020/12/08/trans-tech-is-a-budding-industry-so-why-is-no-one-investing/?sh=36e9955e3c3a (July 30, 2023).
4. https://www.scottnewgent.com/ (August 9, 2023).
5. Scott Newgent interview with Preston Sprinkle, "A Transman's Unexpected Thoughts on Trans-Related Issues: Scott Newgent," 2022. https://www.youtube.com/watch?v=zazsZ_HO3LM (January 20, 2024).

6. "Sex Reassignment Surgery Market to hit USD 1.5 Bn by 2026: Global Market Insights, Inc.," March 31, 2020. https://www.globenewswire.com/news-release/2020/03/31/2009112/0/en/Sex-Reassignment-Surgery-Market-to-hit-USD-1-5-Bn-by-2026-Global-Market-Insights-Inc.html (July 30, 2023).
7. Miriam Grossman, *Lost in Trans Nation: A Child Psychiatrist's Guide Out of the Madness* (New York, NY: Skyhorse Publishing, 2023), pp. 187, 188.
8. Seth Fiegerman, "Apple, Microsoft, PayPal join legal fight for transgender rights." CNN Business, February 24, 2017. https://money.cnn.com/2017/02/24/technology/tech-transgender-amicus-brief/index.html (July 29, 2023).
9. Jennifer Bilek, "The Billionaire Family Pushing Synthetic Sex identities (SSI)." *Tablet*, June 14, 2022. https://www.tabletmag.com/sections/news/articles/billionaire-family-pushing-synthetic-sex-identities-ssi-pritzkers (May 8, 2023).
10. Abigail Shrier, *Irreversible Damage: The Transgender Craze Seducing Our Daughters* (Washington, DC: Regnery Publishing, 2020), pp. 45, 44.
11. Asia Grace, "TikTok brainwashed me into being transgender—now I'm detransitioning." *New York Post*, July 7, 2023. https://nypost.com/2023/07/07/teens-says-tiktok-influenced-her-to-identify-as-transgender/ (July 8, 2023).
12. Drag Story Hour website, https://www.dragstoryhour.org/ (July 8, 2023).
13. Christopher F. Rufo, "The Real Story Behind Drag Queen Story Hour." *City Journal*, Autumn 2022. https://www.city-journal.org/article/the-real-story-behind-drag-queen-story-hour (July 11, 2023).
14. Ibid.
15. Ibid.
16. Corinne Murdock, "Tucson High School Counselor Behind Teen Drag Show Arrested for Relationship With Minor." *AZ Free News*, May 17, 2022. https://azfreenews.com/2022/05/tucson-high-school-counselor-behind-teen-drag-show-arrested-for-relationship-with-minor/ (July 11, 2023).
17. Reduxx Team, "Drag Queen Charged With 25 Counts of Felony Child Sexual Abuse Material Possession," June 24, 2022. https://reduxx.info/drag-queen-charged-with-25-counts-of-felony-child-sexual-abuse-material-possession/ (July 11, 2023).
18. Steve Warren, "Second 'Drag Queen Story Hour' Reader in Houston Exposed as a Convicted Child Sex Offender." CBN, April 30, 2019. https://www2.cbn.com/news/us/second-drag-queen-story-hour-reader-houston-exposed-convicted-child-sex-offender (July 11, 2023).
19. "Houston Public Library Admits Registered Child Sex Offender red to kids in Drag Queen Storytime." NewsWest9, March 16, 2019. https://www.newswest9.com/article/news/houston-public-library-admits-registered-child-sex-offender-read-to-kids-in-drag-queen-storytime/513-4f95a6fd-67af-4fbe-8774-738c69c2b741 (July 8, 2023).
20. Katy Faust and Stacy Manning, "Drag Queen Story Hour Activist Arrested For Child Porn, Still Living With His Adopted Kids." *The Federalist*, March 25, 2021. https://thefederalist.com/2021/03/25/for-some-leftists-the-well-being-of-children-only-matters-when-they-can-be-used-as-political-props/ (July 11, 2023).
21. Aaron Keller, "Former Wisconsin Children's Court Judge Sentenced to Federal Prison for Distributing Child Pornography from County Courthouse." Law & Crime, December 23 2021. https://lawandcrime.com/judiciary/former-wisconsin-childrens-court-judge-sentenced-to-federal-prison-for-distributing-child-pornography-from-county-courthouse/ (July 11, 2023).
22. Tweet, September 24, 2022. https://twitter.com/robbystarbuck/status/1573868662393561089 (July 8, 2023).

23. Andrea Marks, "Drag Queen Story Hour Isn't Going Anywhere—But It's Getting Serious About Safety." *Rolling Stone*, June 6, 2022. https://www.rollingstone.com/culture/culture-news/drag-queen-story-hour-proud-boy-safety-1368900/ (July 8, 2023).
24. See Amanda Grossman-Scott, "8 Ways A Predator Might Groom Your Child," undated. https://educateempowerkids.org/8-ways-predator-might-groom-child/ (July 8, 2023). Also see Michael Welner, "Child Sexual Abuse: 6 Stages of Grooming," October 18, 2010. https://www.oprah.com/oprahshow/child-sexual-abuse-6-stages-of-grooming/all (July 8, 2023).
25. Gays Against Groomers, https://www.gaysagainstgroomers.com/about (July 8, 2023).
26. JD Heyes, "Biden regime turning military into a freak show as Navy uses 'non-binary' sailor who performs as a drag queen in recruitment campaign," May 7, 2023. https://www.gender.news/2023-05-07-biden-regime-turning-military-into-a-freak-show-drag-queen.html# (July 8, 2023).
27. "Target stores donating $100,000 to promote gay lifestyle to school children," May 24, 2019. https://www.afa.net/activism/action-alerts/2019/target-stores-donating-100-000-to-promote-gay-lifestyle-to-school-children/ (July 8, 2023).
28. Ethan Huff, "The North Face unleashes trans-pushing commercial with adult drag queen demanding that children 'come out!'" Natural News, May 25, 2023. https://www.naturalnews.com/2023-05-25-north-face-trans-drag-queen-children-lgbt.html (July 8, 2023).
29. "2023 Bud Light Boycott," https://en.wikipedia.org/wiki/2023_Bud_Light_boycott (July 8, 2023).
30. "Bud Lights out: Anheuser-Busch contractor shuts down, lays off hundreds," July 2, 2023. https://www.wnd.com/2023/07/bud-lights-anheuser-busch-contractor-shuts-lays-off-hundreds/ (July 10, 2023).
31. "An Essential Legal Right for Trans People." Open Society Foundations, May 2019. https://www.opensocietyfoundations.org/explainers/essential-legal-right-trans-people (September 22, 2023).
32. Michael Biggs, "The Open Society Foundations and the transgender movement." 4th Wave Now, May 25, 2018. https://4thwavenow.com/2018/05/25/the-open-society-foundations-the-transgender-movement/ (September 22, 2023).
33. Ibid.
34. Eva Kurilova, "BLM Funds Trans Organizations?" *The Gays Against Groomers Times*, Volume 1, Issue 1 (undated), 2022–2023.
35. Candace Owens, *The Greatest Lie Ever Sold*, documentary, October 2020.
36. Jennifer Bilek, "The Billionaire Family Pushing Synthetic Sex identities (SSI)." *Tablet*, June 14, 2022. https://www.tabletmag.com/sections/news/articles/billionaire-family-pushing-synthetic-sex-identities-ssi-pritzkers (May 8, 2023).
37. Ibid.
38. Ibid.
39. *National Sex Education Standards Core Content and Skills*, K-12, Second Edition (Future of Sex Education Initiative: 2020), p. 26. https://advocatesforyouth.org/wp-content/uploads/2020/03/NSES-2020-web.pdf.
40. Ibid.
41. Jennifer Bilek, "The Billionaire Family Pushing Synthetic Sex identities (SSI)." *Tablet*, June 14, 2022. https://www.tabletmag.com/sections/news/articles/billionaire-family-pushing-synthetic-sex-identities-ssi-pritzkers (May 8, 2023).
42. "What is Transhumanism?" https://whatistranshumanism.org (July 7, 2023).
43. "What is Transhumanism?" https://whatistranshumanism.org/#isnt-this-tampering-with-nature (July 7, 2023).

NOTES 341

44. Robin McKie, "No death and an enhanced life: Is the future transhuman?" *The Guardian*, May 6, 2018. https://www.theguardian.com/technology/2018/may/06/no-death-and-an-enhanced-life-is-the-future-transhuman (July 7, 2023).
45. "Trans-," Online Etymology Dictionary, https://www.etymonline.com/word/trans- (July 7, 2023).
46. American Humanist Association, https://americanhumanist.org/what-is-humanism/definition-of-humanism/(January 26, 2024).
47. Jennifer Bilek, "The Billionaire Family Pushing Synthetic Sex identities (SSI)." *Tablet*, June 14, 2022. https://www.tabletmag.com/sections/news/articles/billionaire-family-pushing-synthetic-sex-identities-ssi-pritzkers (May 8, 2023).
48. Sigal Samuel, "Elon Musk reveals his plan to link your brain to your smartphone. Vox, July 17, 2019. https://www.vox.com/future-perfect/2019/7/17/20697812/elon-musk-neuralink-ai-brain-implant-thread-robot (October 16, 2023).
49. Robert Hart, "Elon Musk Teases First Neuralink Products After Company Implants First Brain Chip In Human." *Forbes*, January 20, 2024. https://www.forbes.com/sites/roberthart/2024/01/30/elon-musk-teases-first-neuralink-products-after-company-implants-first-brain-chip-in-human/?sh=b146aa52ac39 (February 1, 2024).

    There are reports that Musk misled investors about the safety of the technology. Test monkeys suffered "paralysis, seizures and brain swelling" from the implants, and at least 12 healthy monkeys had to be euthanized as a result. [Marisa Taylor, "US lawmakers ask SEC to scrutinize Musk comments on Neuralink." Reuters, November 22, 2023, https://www.reuters.com/technology/us-lawmakers-ask-sec-scrutinize-musk-comments-neuralink-2023-11-22/ (February 1, 2024).]
50. Jessica Roy, "The Rapture of the Nerds." *Time*, April 17, 2014. https://time.com/66536/terasem-trascendence-religion-technology/ (July 7, 2023).
51. Brandon Withrow, "The New Religions Obsessed with A.I." *Daily Beast*, October 29, 2017. https://www.thedailybeast.com/the-new-religions-obsessed-with-ai (July 7, 2023).
52. Laura Aboli, "Transhumanism: The End Game," November 14, 2023. https://twitter.com/Yolo304741/status/1724556707097932054 (November 15, 2023). A longer version can be found on YouTube, June 20, 2023. https://www.youtube.com/watch?v=FCh6auCKYS0&t=5s (November 15, 2023).

Chapter 8. Stifling Dissent

1. Gays Against Groomers, "Frequently Asked Questions." https://www.gaysagainstgroomers.com/faq (July 8, 2023).
2. MIT Online Application Tips, Advice, & Clarifications." https://web.mit.edu/admissions/application/identity.html (October 8, 2023).
3. Rikki Schlott, "Ivy League LGBTQ+ numbers soar and students point to identity politics." *New York Post*, July 20, 2023. https://nypost.com/2023/07/20/ivy-league-lgbtq-numbers-soar-harvard-numbers-triple/ (July 21, 2023).
4. Jacob Kohlhepp, "California students now given six 'gender identity' choices on college admissions applications. *The College Fix*, July 27, 2015. www.thecollegefix.com/calif-students-now-given-six-gender-identity-choices-on-college-admissions-applications (July 17, 2020).
5. *Merriam-Webster Dictionary* online, https://www.merriam-webster.com/words-at-play/cisgender-meaning (June 21, 2023).
6. Jonathan Jarry, "The Word 'Cisgender' Has Scientific Roots." McGill Office for Science and Society, November 13, 2021. https://www.mcgill.ca/oss/article/history-general-science/word-cisgender-has-scientific-roots (June 21, 2023).

7. The German-language title of the journal is *Zeitschrift für Sexualforschung (Stuttgart)* and the German-language title of the article is "Die Transsexuellen und unser nosomorpher Blick" or (translated) "Transsexuals and our nosomorphic view." An internet search, conducted June 21, 2023, yielded no translation for the term "nosomorphic." The reader may recall that transgenders used to be called "transsexuals." Publications in different languages often use different terminology.

8. Genevieve Gluck, "'Cis' Coined by 'Pedosexual' Apologist," January 7, 2022. https://genevievegluck.substack.com/p/cis-coined-by-pedosexual-apologist (June 21, 2023).
   In 2010, Sigusch wrote that there is no such thing as sexual trauma, abuse, or even an abuser. He did not consider pedophilia—sexual activity between adults and children—wrong, because in his view, an adult was giving the child love and attention that the child was otherwise lacking. Claiming that children were pleased by being "loved" in that manner, Sigusch believed that people's objections to pedophilia were due to unwarranted restraints in a culture that was hostile to sensuality. He also believed that adult-child sexual activity was only a problem if the adult was exploiting the child due to a power imbalance. Of course Sigusch's claim that it's possible to avoid a power imbalance between a grown adult and a still-developing, dependent child is not only ridiculous, it's a dangerous lie. Pedophilia is always exploitive. See Volkmar Sigusch, "Sexual scientific theses on the abuse debate" ("Sexualwissenschaftliche Thesen zur Missbrauchsdebatte") in *Magazine for Sex Research* (*Zeitschrift für Sexualforschung*) 2010; 23(3): 247–257. https://www.thieme-connect.com/products/ejournals/abstract/10.1055/s-0030-1262531 (June 21, 2023).

9. Sheila Jeffreys, *Gender Hurts* (London and New York: Routledge, 2014), pp. 50–51.

10. Elon Musk, who owns the social media company Twitter (renamed X), announced on June 20, 2023 that the words "cis" and "cisgender" are "considered slurs on this platform," and that "repeated, targeted harassment against any account will cause the harassing accounts to receive, at minimum, temporary suspensions." It is unclear, however, whose account was subsequently closed for using those terms. [https://twitter.com/elonmusk/status/1671370284102819841?s=20 (June 21, 2023).]

11. Sheila Jeffreys, *Gender Hurts* (London and New York: Routledge, 2014), 51.

12. Julia Serano, "MtF trans bored over woman-centric feminism." Scum-o-rama, March 29, 2012. http://scumorama.wordpress.com/2012/03/29/mtf-trans-bored-over-reproductive-rights-centered-feminism/ (August 23, 2020).

13. Sheila Jeffreys, *Gender Hurts* (London and New York: Routledge, 2014), p. 52.

14. Nick Mordowanec, "Biden Official Praising Clinic Calling Moms 'Egg Producers' Sparks Outrage." *Newsweek*, August 17, 2023. https://www.newsweek.com/biden-official-praising-clinic-calling-moms-egg-producers-sparks-outrage-1820629 (October 8, 2023).

15. Melissa Bartick, Elizabeth K. Stehel, Sarah L. Calhoun, et al, "Academy of Breastfeeding Medicine Position Statement and Guideline: Infant Feeding and Lactation-Related Language and Gender." *Breastfeeding Medicine* Volume 16, Number 8, 2021. https://www.bfmed.org/assets/Gender%20Inclusive%20Statement.pdf (July 7, 2023).

16. Academy of Breastfeeding Medicine, Position Statements. https://www.bfmed.org/position-statements (November 26, 2023).

17. Caroline J. Chantry, Anne Eglash, and Miriam Labbok, "ABM Position on Breastfeeding—Revised 2015." *Breastfeeding Medicine* Volume 10, Number 9, 2015; p. 408. Available at https://www.bfmed.org/assets/DOCUMENTS/abm-position-breastfeeding.pdf (November 26, 2023).

18. Abigail Shrier, *Irreversible Damage: The Transgender Craze Seducing Our Daughters* (Washington, DC: Regnery Publishing, 2020), pp. 152–153.

19. Brodigan, "Woke Professor Forced to Undergo Free Speech Training After Failing Student Who Said 'Biological Women.'" Louder with Crowder, July 1, 2023. https://www.louderwithcrowder.com/melanie-rose-nipper-free-speech (July 11, 2023).
20. Richard Pollina, "University of Cincinnati student alleges professor failed her for using the term 'biological women.'" *New York Post*, July 11, 2023. https://nypost.com/2023/06/05/university-of-cincinnati-student-alleges-professor-failed-her-project-for-using-the-term-biological-women/ (July 11, 2023).
21. Zurie Pope, "'A lot to handle': Cincinnati professor at center of 'biological women' TikTok controversy speaks out." *USA Today*, June 14, 2023. https://www.usatoday.com/story/news/nation/2023/06/14/melanie-rose-nipper-cincinnati-professor-olivia-krolczyk-assignment/70322020007/ (July 11, 2023).
22. Brittany Bernstein, "University Repeals Reprimand against Professor Who Failed Student for Saying 'Biological Women.'" *National Review*, July 8, 2023. https://www.nationalreview.com/news/university-repeals-reprimand-against-professor-who-failed-student-for-saying-biological-women/ (July 11, 2023).
23. "Singular 'They': Though singular 'they' is old, 'they' as a nonbinary pronoun is new—and useful." *Merriam-Webster*, September 2019. www.merriam-webster.com/words-at-play/singular-nonbinary-they (July 20, 2020).
24. Sheila Jeffreys, Gender Hurts (London and New York: Routledge, 2014), pp. 6, 9, 7.
25. "Megyn Kelly blasts Biden's trans health secretary over bizarre gender clinic demand: 'He's a man!'" GB News, August 22, 2023. https://www.youtube.com/watch?v=zRPPBKboXz4 (August 29, 2023).
26. David Batty, "Mistaken identity." *The Guardian*, July 30, 2004. www.theguardian.com/society/2004/jul/31/health.socialcare (August 21, 2020).
27. Abigail Shrier, *Irreversible Damage: The Transgender Craze Seducing Our Daughters* (Washington, DC: Regnery Publishing, 2020), p. 63.
28. Sheryle Cruse, "'Naturally Twiggy?' Confronting the Toxic Nature of Body Shaming." Elephant, September 25, 2019. https://www.elephantjournal.com/2019/09/naturally-twiggy-confronts-the-toxic-nature-of-body-image-shaming/ (July 5, 2023).3
29. Paul McHugh, "Transgenderism: A Pathogenic Meme." *Public Discourse*, June 10, 2015. www.thepublicdiscourse.com/2015/06/15145 (July 23, 2020).
30. Raheem Suleman, "A Brief History of Electroconvulsive Therapy. *The American Journal of Psychiatry Residents' Journal*, September 10, 2020. Also at: https://psychiatryonline.org/doi/10.1176/appi.ajp-rj.2020.160103 (October 10, 2023).
31. "ECT Quick Facts," Citizens Commission on Human Rights, 2023. https://www.cchr.org/ban-ect/?utm_campaign=redirecttherapy-or-torture-the-truth-about-electroshock.html&utm_medium=direct&utm_source=watch (October 10, 2023).
32. Ibid.
33. "Therapy or Torture? The Truth About Electroshock: A Supplement to the Documentary." Citizens Commission on Human Rights, 2019. Available for download at https://www.cchr.org/ban-ect/?utm_campaign=redirecttherapy-or-torture-the-truth-about-electroshock.html&utm_medium=direct&utm_source=watch (October 10, 2023).
34. "Skin Burns and Fire Risks From Electroshock Treatment Device, Report Warns." Cision PR Newswire, August 29, 2018. https://www.prnewswire.com/news-releases/skin-burns-and-fire-risks-from-electroshock-treatment-device-report-warns-300703894.html (October 10, 2023).
35. "Sex researcher's article pulled from feminist website because it's not 'inclusive.'" *The College Fix*, June 3, 2016. www.thecollegefix.com/sex-researchers-article-pulled-feminist-website-not-inclusive (July 19, 2020).

36. Madeleine Kearns, "Dr. Zucker Defied Trans Orthodoxy. Now He's Vindicated." *National Review*, October 25, 2018. www.nationalreview.com/2018/10/transgender-orthodoxy-kenneth-zucker-vindicated/ (August 8, 2020).

37. David Walter Banks, "What Lia Thomas Could Mean for Women's Elite Sports." *The New York Times*, June 15, 2022. https://www.nytimes.com/2022/05/29/us/lia-thomas-women-sports.html (July 11, 2023).

38. "Mayo Clinic Disciplinary Letter to Michael J. Joyner, March 5, 2023." FIRE (Foundation for Individual Rights and Expression), https://www.thefire.org/research-learn/mayo-clinic-disciplinary-letter-michael-j-joyner-march-5-2023 (July 11, 2023).

39. The production of antibodies, which allows the body to mount a defense against a pathogen, is precisely what we are told vaccines are for. Therefore, there is no logical reason why any responsible medical personnel should object to convalescent plasma therapy, which by giving the person already-made antibodies has the same goal as vaccines—but without any of the "side" effects.

    All consequences of vaccines are "effects." The phrase "side effects" was created to divert attention from unwanted reactions, which can be dangerous, permanent, and sometimes life-threatening. The reactions are many, and can include itchy skin, heart problems, and even acquiring the very disease against which one is being vaccinated. Many of these "side" effects are the result of a hyper-vigilant immune reaction due to the heavy metals, DNA from aborted fetuses and animal tissue, and other bizarre substances that are routinely included in the vaccine cocktail. The insistence by the National Institutes of Health, Food and Drug Administration, American Medical Association, World Health Organization, and other agencies that everyone receive vaccines reveals their agenda. Not surprisingly, convalescent plasma therapy has a vastly better success rate than vaccines, without any of the undesirable effects.

40. Jonathon W. Senefeld, Massimo Franchini, Carlo Mengoli, et al, "COVID-19 Convalescent Plasma for the Treatment of Immunocompromised Patients: A Systematic Review and Meta-analysis." *JAMA Network Open*, January 12, 2023. https://jamanetwork.com/journals/jamanetworkopen/fullarticle/2800275?utm_source=For_The_Media&utm_medium=referral&utm_campaign=ftm_links&utm_term=011223 (July 11, 2023).

41. "Mayo Clinic Disciplinary Letter to Michael J. Joyner, March 5, 2023." FIRE (Foundation for Individual Rights and Expression), https://www.thefire.org/research-learn/mayo-clinic-disciplinary-letter-michael-j-joyner-march-5-2023 (July 11, 2023).

42. Elizabeth Cohen, "Study shows convalescent plasma works for immune-compromimsed Covid-19 patients, but it can be hard to find." CNN, January 12, 2023. https://www.cnn.com/2023/01/12/health/convalescent-plasma-immune-compromised-covid/index.html (July 11, 2023).

43. Cassie B., "Trans Militants Strike Again: Police believe vandalism at state senator's home was retaliation for sponsoring bill banning transgender surgery for minors." Gender News, April 26, 2023. https://www.gender.news/2023-04-26-vandalism-senators-home-retaliation-transgender-surgery-ban.html# (July 11, 2023).

44. Tony Kinnett, "State Senator Tells Parents to Flee His Own State Amid Bill That Would Take Kids Away From Non-'Affirming' Parents." *The Daily Signal*, June 13, 2023. https://www.dailysignal.com/2023/06/13/state-senator-tells-parents-flee-own-state-law-take-kids-away-non-affirming-parents/ (July 9, 2023).

45. Matt James, "React vs. Respond: What's the Difference?" *Psychology Today*, September 1, 2016. www.psychologytoday.com/us/blog/focus-forgiveness/201609/react-vs-respond (July 14, 2020).

46. There's good reason why Apple founder Steve Jobs didn't allow his own children to have iPads, and why Microsoft founder Bill Gates didn't give his children smart phones until they were in high school. The men wanted to wait until their children's brains had more time to develop. Another factor is the harmful electromagnetic

radiation emitted by computers and smart phones. For more information, see Paul Brodeur, *Currents of Death: Power Lines, Computer Terminals, and the Attempt to Cover Up Their Threat to Your Health* (New York: Simon and Schuster, 1989), B. Blake Levitt, *Electromagnetic Fields: A Consumer's Guide to the Issues and How to Protect Ourselves* (San Diego, California: Harcourt Brace & Company, 1995), and Arthur Firstenberg, *The Invisible Rainbow: A History of Electricity and Life* (Hartford, Vermont: Chelsea Green Publishing, 2020).

47. Alyssa N. Saiphoo, Lilach Dahoah Halevi, and Zahra Vahedi, "Social networking site use and self-esteem: A meta-analytic review." *Personality and Individual Differences* Volume 153, January 15, 2020.

48. Carly A. McComb, Eric J. Vanman, and Stephanie J. Tobin, "A Meta-Analysis of the Effects of Social Media Exposure to Upward Comparison Targets on Self-Evaluations and Emotions." *Media Psychology*, February 23, 2023.

49. Eric W. Dolan, "Upward comparison on social media harms body image, self-esteem, and psychological well-being, *PsyPost*, March 30, 2023. https://www.psypost.org/2023/03/upward-comparison-on-social-media-harms-body-image-self-esteem-and-psychological-well-being-74424 (July 12, 2023).

50. Mahreen Kyan, Amirali Minbashian, and Carolyn MacCann, "College students in the western world are becoming less emotionally intelligent: A cross-temporal meta-analysis of trait emotional intelligence." *Journal of Personality*, December 2021, Volume 89, Issue 6, 1176–1190.

51. Jean M. Twenge, "Have Smartphones Destroyed a Generation?" *The Atlantic*, September 2017.

52. Greg Lukianoff and Jonathan Haidt, "The Coddling of the American Mind." *The Atlantic*, September 2015. https://www.theatlantic.com/magazine/archive/2015/09/the-coddling-of-the-american-mind/399356/ (July 13, 2023).

The statement, in our current paradigm of political correctness, that it's "a microaggression to ask an Asian American or Latino American 'Where were you born?' because this implies that he or she is not a real American," misses a key point. If someone is a "real" American—that is, born in the United States—then he or she is simply "American." If one uses the terms "Asian American," "Latino American" or "African American," then in this paradigm there should also be a "European American," "Eastern European American," "British American," or other type of American (to acknowledge those who came over on the Mayflower). But no such terminology exists. Why should the descendents of Asians, Latinos or Africans be honored with their own designation, but not Europeans? This highlights the ludicrousness of any such designations. The identical, blue-eyed twin brothers Keith and Kevin Hodge—whose ancestry is largely black—have said on their YouTube platform that because they were born in America, and in fact have never seen Africa, this makes them Americans, not "African-Americans." Their logic, based solely on linguistics, is sound.

Related to this is the frequent capitalization of "Black" (designating those of dark or brown skin tone), while "white" (designating those of light tan or whitish skin tone) is never capitalized. Also, people of obvious mixed race—for example, light-skinned blacks who are part Caucasian—always identify as black, but never white. But they are half white. So why do they never say that they are white? In this paradigm of political correctness, whites are being discriminated against.

53. Ibid.

54. Susan Svrluga, "Someone wrote 'Trump 2016' on Emory's campus in chalk. Some students said they no longer feel safe." *The Washington Post*, March 24, 2016. https://www.washingtonpost.com/news/grade-point/wp/2016/03/24/someone-wrote-trump-2016-on-emorys-campus-in-chalk-some-students-said-they-no-longer-feel-safe/ (July 12, 2023).

55. Peter Hart, "Trump Chalk at Emory University." National Coalition Against Censorship, March 24, 2016. https://ncac.org/news/blog/trump-chalk-at-emory-university (July 12, 2023).
56. Ibid.
57. Charlotte Dean, "University bosses order lecturers to stop using capital letters when setting assignments because it might upset snowflake students." *Daily Mail*, November 18, 2018. https://www.dailymail.co.uk/news/article-6402933/University-bosses-order-lecturers-stop-using-capital-letters.html (July 12, 2023).
58. "Educate, don't confiscate: Trainers say Carleton wrong to remove gym scale," CBC News, March 13, 2017. https://www.cbc.ca/news/canada/ottawa/trainer-say-carleton-wrong-remove-gym-scale-1.4023420 (July 12, 2023).
59. Josh Hedtke, "California professors instructed not to say 'America is the land of opportunity.'" *The College Fix*, June 10, 2015. https://www.thecollegefix.com/california-professors-instructed-not-to-say-america-is-the-land-of-opportunity/ (July 13, 2023).
60. Jeannie Suk Gersen, "The Trouble with Teaching Rape Law." *The New Yorker*, December 15, 2014. https://www.newyorker.com/news/news-desk/trouble-teaching-rape-law (July 13, 2023).
61. Gordon Rayner, Eleanor Steafel and Louisa Clarence-Smith, "Schools let children identify as horses, dinosaurs... and a moon." *The Telegraph*, June 19, 2023. https://www.telegraph.co.uk/news/2023/06/19/school-children-identifying-as-animals-furries/ (July 12, 2023).
62. Hunter Stuart, "Hampshire Collete Cancels Afrobeat Band Shokazoba After Concerns Over Mostly White Members." *Huff Post*, October 29, 2013. https://www.huffpost.com/entry/hampshire-college-afrobeat-band-shokazoba-too-white_n_4174231 (July 13, 2023).
63. Adam Steinbaugh and Alex Morey, "Professor Investigated for Discussing Conflicting Viewpoints, 'The Coddling of the American Mind.'" Foundation for Individual Rights and Expression (FIRE), June 20, 2016. https://www.thefire.org/news/professor-investigated-discussing-conflicting-viewpoints-coddling-american-mind (July 12, 2023).
64. Greg Lukianoff and Jonathan Haidt, "The Coddling of the American Mind." *The Atlantic*, September 2015. https://www.theatlantic.com/magazine/archive/2015/09/the-coddling-of-the-american-mind/399356/ (July 13, 2023).
65. Van Jones, discussing safe spaces on college campuses. YouTube video clip, February 24, 2017. www.youtube.com/watch?v=Zms3EqGbFOk (July 18, 2020).
66. Kerri Ann Walsh, "To The Overly-Sensitive College Student." *Odyssey*, March 28, 2016. https://www.theodysseyonline.com/over-sensitive-college-student (July 14, 2023).
67. Mike Adams, "Get Out of My Class and Leave America." *Townhall*, August 28, 2015. https://townhall.com/columnists/mikeadams/2015/08/28/get-out-of-my-class-and-leave-america-n2044785 (July 15, 2020).
68. Chapter 9 discusses in detail the harmful biochemical and physiological changes that occur in someone who's constantly anxious.
   The unusual isolation enforced during the so-called pandemic escalated already high levels of intense depression and anxiety. A Boston University mental health researcher reported that a survey of almost 33,000 college students across the country revealed that half of the students in autumn 2020 "screened positive for depression and/or anxiety." ["Depression, anxiety, loneliness are peaking in college students," *Boston University Science News*, February 19, 2021. https://www.sciencedaily.com/releases/2021/02/210219190939.htm (July 15, 2023).] Two surveys led by the Ohio State University's Office of the Chief Wellness Officer—the first conducted August 2020 and the second, April 2021, found that anxiety rose from 39 percent to 42.6 percent while

depression rose from 24.1 percent to 28.3 percent. The eating of unhealthy food and use of alcohol and tobacco rose, while physical activity decreased. Thirteen percent of students saw a mental health counselor in 2020. Just eight months later that figure rose to 22 percent. ["Survey: Anxiety, depression, burnout rising as college students prepare to return to campus." Ohio State University, Wexner Medical Center, July 26, 2021. https://wexnermedical.osu.edu/mediaroom/pressreleaselisting/survey-anxiety-depression-burnout-rising-among-college-students (July 15, 2023).]

69. Edward Schlosser, "I'm a liberal professor, and my liberal students terrify me." Vox, June 3, 2015. https://www.vox.com/2015/6/3/8706323/college-professor-afraid (July 13, 2023).

70. Arlin Cuncic, "Victim Mentality: Definition, Causes, and Ways to Cope." Very Well Mind, April 4, 2023. https://www.verywellmind.com/what-is-a-victim-mentality-5120615 (July 13, 2023).

71. Scott Barry Kaufman, "Unraveling the Mindset of Victimhood." *Scientific American*, June 29, 2020. https://www.scientificamerican.com/article/unraveling-the-mindset-of-victimhood/ (July 14, 2023).

72. Lisa Marchiano, "What Depth Psychology Can Tell Us About Victimhood Culture." Quillette, December 27, 2017. https://quillette.com/2017/12/27/collision-reality-depth-psychology-can-tell-us-victimhood-culture/ (August 11, 2023).

73. "Parents Lose Custody For Refusing Child Sex-Change." *Pulpit & Pen*, February 16, 2018. https://pulpitandpen.org/2018/02/16/parents-lose-custody-refusing-child-sex-change/ (July 20, 2020).

74. Amanda Prestigiacomo, "Video: James Younger, At Age 3, To Dad: Mommy Tells Me I'm A Girl." *Daily Wire*, October 23, 2019. https://www.dailywire.com/news/video-james-younger-at-age-3-to-dad-mommy-tells-me-im-a-girl (November 20, 2023). The video was removed from YouTube, but the transcript of the clip is in the article. A copy of the clip was captured by a number of viewers before YouTube cancelled the video.

75. James Gordon, "Texas mother trying to transition her seven-year-old son into a girl loses in court as judge orders her to share custody with ex-husband who says boy is just 'confused.'" *Daily Mail*, January 31, 2020. https://www.dailymail.co.uk/news/article-7950655/Mother-trying-transition-son-girl-loses-court-judge-orders-parents-joint-custody.html (July 13, 2023).

76. Juwan J. Holmes, "Texas trans girl's affirming mother gets full custody after father fails to pay child support." LGBTQ Nation, August 10, 2021. https://www.lgbtqnation.com/2021/08/texas-trans-girls-affirming-mother-gets-full-custody-father-fails-pay-child-support/ (July 13, 2023).

77. David Lee, "Father who lost custody of trans child runs for Texas House to outlaw child gender reassignments." Courthouse News Service, December 8, 2021. https://www.courthousenews.com/father-who-lost-custody-of-trans-child-runs-for-texas-house-to-outlaw-child-gender-reassignments/ (July 13, 2023).

78. Snejana Farberov, "Texas dad fears ex-wife plans to 'chemically castrate' 9-year-old son." *New York Post*, January 6, 2023. https://nypost.com/2023/01/06/texas-dad-fears-ex-wife-plans-to-chemically-castrate-9-year-old-son (May 26, 2024).

79. Nicole Russell, "UNT students' reaction to conservative speaker shows how colleges are in deep trouble." *Forth Worth Star-Telegram*, July 13, 2023. https://www.star-telegram.com/opinion/nicole-russell/article259062583.html (July 13, 2023).

80. Ibid.

81. Isabel Brown, "A Girl Was Raped In A Bathroom By A Boy Wearing A Skirt. Her Dad Says The School Is Covering It Up." *Evie*, October 22, 2021. https://www.eviemagazine.com/post/loudoun-county-transgender-policy-sexual-assault-coverup-scott-smith (July 13, 2023).

82. Ibid.

83. Ibid.
84. Luke Rosiak, "Loudoun Schools To Make Bathrooms Co-Ed To Accommodate Trans Students." *Daily Wire*, April 17, 2023. https://www.dailywire.com/news/loudoun-schools-to-make-bathrooms-co-ed-to-accommodate-transgenders (July 14, 2023).
85. Luke Rosiak, "Loudoun Schools To Make Bathrooms Co-Ed To Accommodate Trans Students." *Daily Wire*, April 17, 2023. https://www.dailywire.com/news/loudoun-schools-to-make-bathrooms-co-ed-to-accommodate-transgenders (July 14, 2023).
86. The Virginia Project, April 16, 2023. https://twitter.com/ProjectVirginia/status/1647783451607662592 (July 14, 2023).
87. "Report of the Special Grand Jury on the Investigation of Loudoun County Public Schools, Case No. CL-22-3129," December 2022, pp. 2, 21, 22. https://www.oag.state.va.us/media-center/news-releases/2503-december-5-2022-special-grand-jury-releases-report-on-loudoun-county-public-schools (April 18, 2023).
88. Ibid.
89. Scott Gelman, "Virginia attorney general files to drop remaining charge against former Loudoun Co. schools superintendent." WTOP News, December 22, 2023. https://wtop.com/loudoun-county/2023/12/virginia-attorney-general-drops-remaining-charge-against-former-loudon-co-schools-superintendent/ (March 3, 2024).
90. Charles Homans, "How a Sexual Assault in a School Bathroom Became a Political Weapon." *The New York Times Magazine*, August 5, 2023. https://www.nytimes.com/2023/08/05/magazine/loudoun-county-bathroom-sexual-assault.html (March 2, 2024).
91. Jennifer Smith, "Woke Loudoun County schools $275K-a-year superintendent apologizes for 'failing to protect' female student, 15, from rape by 'boy in a skirt' in the girls' bathroom: He refuses to quit but board member resigns." *Daily Mail*, October 16, 2021. https://www.dailymail.co.uk/news/article-10097271/I-look-forward-simpler-life-Member-woke-Loudoun-School-board-RESIGNS.html (July 13, 2023).

Chapter 9. Making Peace With Your Birth Body

1. Travis Bradberry, "The Most And Least Emotionally Aware Countries." *Forbes*, August 17, 2013. https://www.forbes.com/sites/travisbradberry/2013/08/17/the-most-and-least-emotionally-aware-countries/?sh=605b4c233596 (August 14, 2023).
2. There also can be huge differences in how culture express emotions. For instance, in the U.S., saying "I'm excited" can automatically refer to anything that gives pleasure: an upcoming vacation, the thought of a job well done, or sexual arousal. But in France, if someone utters the same phrase, it's automatically interpreted to mean sexual arousal unless the speaker clarifies otherwise. See Camille Chevalier-Karfis, "French Mistake: Translating I'm Excited In French." French Today, June 7, 2021. https://www.frenchtoday.com/blog/french-vocabulary/excited-in-french/ (August 14, 2023).
   In Japan, it's considered poor taste to publicly display excitement about anything. Etiquette dictates that excitement should be shown only in private. This cultural restraint may force the person to hold back so much energy that it gets stuck.
3. Natalie Terry and Kara Gross Margolis, "Serotonergic Mechanisms Regulating the GI Tract: Experimental Evidence and Therapeutic Relevance." *Handbook of Experimental Pharmacology* 2017; 239: 319–342.
4. Even the bacteria that normally reside in the gut affect our moods as well as digestion. That is why diet plays such a key role in mood. Not only do the nutrients from foods affect one's mood, but different foods encourage the proliferation of different types of bacteria—some beneficial, others not.
5. Alexander Lowen, *Pleasure: A Creative Approach to Life* (Hinesburg, Vermont: The Alexander Lowen Foundation, 2013), p. 22.

6. Contraction of the abdominal muscle also limits peristalsis, the normal wavelike motion of the intestines. A tight abdomen causes the intestinal wall to lose its muscle tone. As a result, the digestive tract becomes sluggish, leading to the putrefaction of food and inflammation of the intestines. Shallow breathing also means that less oxygen reaches the cells. Less oxygen depresses the immune response, thus encouraging harmful anaerobic microbes to thrive. Without sufficient oxygen, the red blood cells also lose some of their electrical charge, which causes them to flatten and clump together—further decreasing the amount of oxygen in the body because the oxygen-carrying ability of the red blood cells has been compromised.

7. Sean Haldane, *Emotional First Aid* (New York: Irvington Publishers, 1984), p. 10.

8. If you notice that you are anxious, or your breathing is irregular, you can try the following breathing exercise standing, sitting, or lying down. Relax the abdomen, place one hand just beneath the ribs or on the upper chest, breathe in slowly and deeply through the nose as you notice the hand rising, and breathe out through either the mouth or nose as you notice the hand falling. To this breathing exercise, you can add exhaling to a count of four, holding the empty lungs to a count of four, inhaling to a count of four, and then holding air in the lungs for a count of four. Do this repeatedly. There are many techniques you can try, but the point is to be mindful of taking relaxed breaths without involving any extraneous muscles.

   For step-by-step exercises to help people become more emotionally aware, see Jack Willis, *Reichian Therapy: A Practical Guide for Home Use* (Los Angeles, California: New Falcon Publications, 2021).

9. Alexander Lowen, *Pleasure: A Creative Approach to Life* (Hinesburg, Vermont: The Alexander Lowen Foundation, 2013), p. 29.

10. Sean Haldane, *Emotional First Aid* (New York: Irvington Publishers, 1984), p. 11.

11. Elizabeth Noble, *Primal Connections* (New York: Simon & Schuster, 1993), p. 97.

12. Michael Nehls, *The Indoctrinated Brain: How to Successfully Fend Off the Global Attack on Your Mental Freedom* (New York, NY: Skyhorse Publishing, 2023), pp. 78, 79.

13. In *The Indoctrinated Brain*, Michael Nehls strongly recommends Vitamin D supplementation for immune function, as most people are highly deficient in it. Fish oil is also vitally important. It not only promotes immune function, but it also helps protect the brain and nervous system. Because most fish are now contaminated with mercury, the best way to ingest fish oil is in the form of a supplement. The product should be molecularly distilled to eliminate mercury and other heavy metals, as well as miscellaneous contaminants. It should also be fresh and not rancid.

14. Lise Van Susteren, "Our Children Face 'Pretraumatic Stress' from Worries about Climate Change." The British Medical Journal (blog), November 19, 2020. Quoted in Michael Nehls, *The Indoctrinated Brain: How to Successfully Fend Off the Global Attack on Your Mental Freedom* (New York, NY: Skyhorse Publishing, 2023), p. 83.

15. Mona Lisa Schulz, *Awakening Intuition* (New York: Harmony Books, 1998), p. 123.

16. There are many ways in which one can "hold back." A former body-mind psychotherapy client of mine, dealing with chronic back problems, one day made a discovery: "I hold back so much in my life. I rarely tell people how I feel, what I think, or what I need. No wonder my back hurts all the time! I am literally 'holding back'—holding my back."

17. Bessel van der Kolk, *The Body Keeps the Score* (New York: Penguin Books, 2014), p. 99.

18. Psychologists use the phrase *inappropriate affect* to describe someone's emotional expression that does not adequately match the reality of what is occurring. This may consist of smiling when receiving upsetting news, or appearing not to care at all. The person's expression can be flat and vacant or excessive and hysterical. Both these states indicate energy that is not moving properly. A vacant or expressionless individual is

contracted, which prevents input from the environment from entering. A hysterical individual is also preventing the reception of accurate environmental input, but is flinging out energy in an exaggerated manner as a barrier. Emotionally stable and mature persons focus on input, whether pleasure or genuine danger, and respond in ways that promote their well-being or protect them against actual threats. Inappropriate affect is a symptom of an underlying issue, which usually cannot be addressed without the help of a qualified mental health professional.

19. Travis Bradberry, "14 Signs You Are Emotionally Intelligent." November 13, 2018. https://www.linkedin.com/pulse/14-signs-you-emotionally-intelligent-dr-travis-bradberry (August 16, 2023).
20. Alexander Lowen, *Pleasure: A Creative Approach to Life* (Hinesburg, Vermont: The Alexander Lowen Foundation, 2013), pp. 1–2.
21. Wilhelm Reich, *Selected Writings* (New York: The Noonday Press/ Farrar, Straus and Giroux, 1961), p. 146.
22. Alexander Lowen, *Pleasure: A Creative Approach to Life* (Hinesburg, Vermont: The Alexander Lowen Foundation, 2013), pp. 29–30.
23. Lily Hayes, "Watch: Trans Child Celebrity Admits They Never Feel Like Themselves Despite Gender-Confirming Surgeries." Louder with Crowder, February 28, 2023. https://www.louderwithcrowder.com/jazz-jennings-themselves (August 11, 2023).
24. Surgery slices through nerves, blood vessels and muscles that were part of the original blueprint of the body. It also ruptures acupuncture meridians through which vital energy is meant to flow. Acupuncture meridians are not an esoteric concept of abstract, intangible or mystical energy. Scientists discovered that meridians are more responsive than other tissue to electric current and ultrasound. The layer of skin is thinner along meridians than non-meridians. And nerves along meridians are connected to mast cells, which are involved in inflammation and allergic responses. Anatomically, meridians appear along the fascia (connective tissue) between muscles, between muscles and bones, and between muscles and tendons. See H. Heine, "Functional Morphology of Acupuncture Points and Meridians," https://icmart.org/icmart99/ab11.htm and Leon Chaitow, "The Amazing Fascial Web, Part I," www.massagetoday.com/mpacms/mt/article.php?id=13204.
25. Miriam Grossman, *Lost in Trans Nation: A Child Psychiatrist's Guide Out of the Madness* (New York, NY: Skyhorse Publishing, 2023), p. xxxi.
26. Bessel van der Kolk, *The Body Keeps the Score* (New York: Penguin Books, 2014), pp. 98–99.
27. Sean Haldane, *Emotional First Aid* (New York: Irvington Publishers, 1984), p. 68.
28. Ibid. pp. 69–70.
29. Miriam Grossman, *Lost in Trans Nation: A Child Psychiatrist's Guide Out of the Madness* (New York, NY: Skyhorse Publishing, 2023), pp. 213, 214.
30. Anna Mason, "'We Don't Even Know What Gender We Are Anymore': Young Mom Calls Women to Get Back to Homemaking, Says Society is Degrading." *The Epoch Times*, September 13, 2023. https://www.theepochtimes.com/bright/we-dont-even-know-what-gender-we-are-anymore-young-mom-calls-women-to-get-back-to-homemaking-says-the-society-is-degrading-5481326?utm_source=morningbriefnoe&src_src=morningbriefnoe&utm_mpaign=mb-2023-09-18&src_cmp=mb-2023-09-18&utm_=O1rpgJbr5kJjGt1bSlorcC%2Fj2ND8NShVjeEFOYvVzfRCC0066dv96dpn24NWlQ%3D%3D (September 18, 2023).
31. See Yang Claire Yang, Courtney Boen, Karen Gerken, et al, "Social relationships and physiological determinants of longevity across the human life span." *Proceedings of the National Academy of Sciences USA*, January 19, 2016, 113(3): 578–583. Also see Julianne Holt-Lunstad, Timothy B. Smith, and J. Bradley Layton, "Social Relationships and Mortality Risk: A Meta-analytic Review." *Plos Medicine*, July 27, 2010.

32. The cost of women's services to their husbands and children—had they been hired for their many and varied skills—was even computed and published in a number of sources, which was considered quite groundbreaking at the time. See Porcshe Moran, "How Much Is A Stay-at-Home Parent Worth?" Investopedia, March 21, 2020, www.investopedia.com/financial-edge/0112/how-much-is-a-homemaker-worth.aspx (July 13, 2020).
33. www.merriam-webster.com/dictionary/feminism (July 15, 2020).
34. https://dictionary.cambridge.org/us/dictionary/english/feminism (July 15, 2020).
35. Ronja Schaber, Marie Kopp, Anna Zähringer, et al, "Paternal Leave and Father-Infant Bonding: Findings From the Population-Based Cohort Study DREAM." *Frontiers in Psychology* 2021; 12:668028.

    Robert Winston and Rebecca Chicot, "The importance of early bonding on the long-term mental health and resilience of children." *London Journal of Primary Care* 2016; 8(1): 12–14.

    Sue Atkins, "The Importance of Father-Child Bonding," June 26, 2023. https://sueatkinsparentingcoach.com/2023/06/the-importance-of-father-child-bonding/ (October 30, 2023).
36. Tony Guerra, "How Much Does Firefighter Gear Weigh?" Career Trend, December 27, 2018. https://careertrend.com/about-4760940-much-does-firefighter-gear-weigh.html (July 15, 2020).
37. "Is A World Beyond Stereotypes Possible?" Wellbeing, April 1, 2020. https://wellbeingmagazine.com/is-a-world-beyond-stereotypes-possible/ (September 21, 2023).
38. Ben Shapiro, Young America's Foundation lecture on June 15, 2022. (No longer available on YouTube.)
39. Jennifer Bilek, "The Billionaire Family Pushing Synthetic Sex identities (SSI)," June 14, 2022. https://www.tabletmag.com/sections/news/articles/billionaire-family-pushing-synthetic-sex-identities-ssi-pritzkers (May 8, 2023).

Appendix A. Highlights of the Gender Wars

1. Estelle B. Freedman, "Women's long battle to define rape." The Daily Item, August 5, 2014. www.dailyitem.com/archives/women-s-long-battle-to-define-rape/article_90666ecb-9430-50a6-a685-ad41c532d18a.html (July 13, 2020).
2. Suzanne Brown, "Feminist History of Rape." *Connections* 9, Spring/Summer 2003, p. 6. www.safeplaceolympia.org/wp-content/uploads/2011/09/A-Feminist-History-of-Rape.pdf (July 13, 2020).
3. Estelle B. Freedman, "Women's long battle to define rape." The Daily Item, August 5, 2014. www.dailyitem.com/archives/women-s-long-battle-to-define-rape/article_90666ecb-9430-50a6-a685-ad41c532d18a.html (July 13, 2020).
4. Alicia Ault reports that Stanton began her activism as an abolitionist, but became disillusioned by that movement when participants at the World's Anti-Slavery Convention (held in London in 1840) debated whether or not women should be allowed to participate. That was a turning point for Stanton, who realized that she needed to focus first on changing women's status—otherwise, women's efforts in any venture would be limited. When Stanton later met with Susan B. Anthony (whose activities had involved temperance and abolition), the two decided to campaign for women's rights, which included the right to vote.

    The Seneca Falls convention was a relatively insignificant event that probably would have been forgotten had not Stanton and Anthony "reprinted the 1848 proceedings and circulated them widely to reinforce their own importance" twenty-five years later. Anthony hadn't even attended the Seneca Falls conference, but because of her association with Stanton she was accepted as one of the suffragist movement founders. Apparently, the tendency toward flagrant self-promotion and aggrandizement is not limited to a particular era or group of people. [Alicia Ault, "How Women Got the Vote Is a Far More Complex Story Than the History Textbooks Reveal." *Smithsonian Magazine*, April 9, 2019. www.smithsonianmag.com/smithsonian-institution/how-women-got-vote-far-more-complex-story-history-textbooks-reveal-180971869/?utm_source=smithsoniandaily&utm_medium=email&utm_campaign=20200818-daily-responsive&spMailingID=43233432&spUserID=NjEyNDI5NjUyMzc0S0&spJobID=1821493361&spReportId=MTgyMTQ5MzM2MQS2 (August 19, 2020).]

5. Ibid.
6. Robin Saks Frankel, "History Of Women And Credit Cards: 1970s To Present." *Forbes Advisor*, https://www.forbes.com/advisor/credit-cards/when-could-women-get-credit-cards/ (September 5, 2022).
7. Nathan Yau, "Most Female and Male Occupations Since 1950." https://flowingdata.com/2017/09/11/most-female-and-male-occupations-since-1950 (July 13, 2020).
8. The article "Men Still Pick 'Blue' Jobs and Women 'Pink' Jobs," in *The Economist*, February 16, 2019, reported that "26 out of the 30 highest-paying jobs in the US are male-dominated. In comparison, 23 out of the 30 lowest-paying jobs in the US are female-dominated." Moreover, when women were employed in male-dominated fields to do the same job, they earn substantially less than the men. This includes the field of journalism, where editors of the nation's 135 most widely distributed newspapers are white males.

    Even acting, a glamorous profession for women, discriminates against them. On average, female stars earn one million dollars less per film than their male counterparts, even if they appear in more scenes and have more speaking lines to memorize. The situation, which has not changed very much since 1980, became so untenable that during her 2015 Oscar acceptance speech, actress Patricia Arquette called for "wage equality once and for all." [Jami Doward and Tali Fraser, "Hollywood's gender pay gap revealed: male stars earn $1M more per film than women." *The Guardian*, September 15, 2019. https://www.theguardian.com/world/2019/sep/15/hollywoods-gender-pay-gap-revealed-male-stars-earn-1m-more-per-film-than-women (Jan 30, 2020).]

    Also, according to WMC Reports, females also accounted for fewer than one-third of speaking characters in 1100 films released from 2006 to 2018. For directing jobs in the highest-grossing films, men comprised 93.4 percent (654 out of 704) while women comprised just 6.6 percent (46 out of 704). ["The Status of Women in U.S. Media 2019." Women's Media Center, February 21, 2019. https://womensmediacenter.com/reports/the-status-of-women-in-u-s-media-2019 (July 15, 2020).]
9. Carolina Aragão, "Gender pay gap in U.S. hasn't changed much in two decades." Pew Research Center, March 1, 2023. https://www.pewresearch.org/short-reads/2023/03/01/gender-pay-gap-facts/ (August 11, 2023).
10. Nicola Davis, "Electroconvulsive therapy mostly used on women and older people, says study." *The Guardian*, October 20, 2017. www.theguardian.com/society/2017/oct/20/electroconvulsive-therapy-ect-mostly-used-women-older-people-nhs (July 14, 2020).
11. Bruce E. Levine, "Electroconvulsive Therapy and Women: Abuse or Treatment?" *Huff Post*, December 24, 2017. https://www.huffpost.com/entry/electroconvulsive-therapy-and-women-abuse-or-treatment_b_5a406a12e4b06cd2bd03dbec (July 14, 2020).
12. Porcshe Moran, "How Much Is A Stay-at-Home Parent Worth?" Investopedia, March 21, 2020, www.investopedia.com/financial-edge/0112/how-much-is-a-homemaker-worth.aspx (July 13, 2020).

    Data from 2019 gives the figure of 178,201 dollars. Adjusted for 1965, the amount would be approximately 22,000 dollars.
13. Veronica Techenor, "Maintaining Men's Dominance: Negotiating Identity and Power When She Earns More." *Sex Roles* 53, August 2005, 191–205.

14. Maya Salam, "What Is Toxic Masculinity?" *The New York Times*, January 22, 2019. www.nytimes.com/2019/01/22/us/toxic-masculinity.html (July 14, 2020).
15. Henry A. Montero, "Depression in Men: The Cycle of Toxic Masculinity." Psycom, June 8, 2022. https://www.psycom.net/depression/depression-in-men/toxic-masculinity (July 28, 2023).
16. Michael Flood, "Toxic masculinity: A primer and commentary." XY, July 7, 2018. https://xyonline.net/content/toxic-masculinity-primer-and-commentary (September 30, 2020).
17. Jaclyn Friedman, "Toxic Masculinity." The American Prospect, March 13, 2013. https://prospect.org/power/toxic-masculinity/ (September 30, 2020).

    Friedman also commented on the globalization of such violence in the name of "culture."

    > The U.N. [United Nations] is in the midst of its 57th Commission on the Status of Women, this year focusing on gendered violence, a global pandemic made all the more urgent by growing evidence that social change leads to increased violence against women. Why? Because destabilizing established social order—even in the interest of what we might agree is progress—can leave people feeling vulnerable. And when men feel vulnerable, toxic masculinity teaches them [that] the way to reassert their power is by dominating women. There's a pall hanging over the proceedings, a real risk that this year's commission may wind up like last year's, failing to come to any policy agreements thanks to the obstructionism of a handful of patriarchal countries who claim that their traditional and religious customs would be infringed upon if they had to take action to end gendered violence in their countries. You can bet that any customs that require impunity for violence against women are built on toxic masculinity. [Jaclyn Friedman, "Toxic Masculinity." The American Prospect, March 13, 2013. https://prospect.org/power/toxic-masculinity/ (September 30, 2020).]

18. Michael Flood, "Toxic masculinity: A primer and commentary." XY, July 7, 2018. https://xyonline.net/content/toxic-masculinity-primer-and-commentary (September 30, 2020).
19. Emily Hopkins, "Wade Davis Has Tough Talk for Men in Tech." w2.0, July 17, 2017. https://women2.com/2017/07/17/wade-davis-has-tough-talk-for-men-in-tech/ (September 30, 2020).
20. Syb, "Purification Rites," April 26, 2022. https://sybmantics.substack.com/p/purification-rites?s=r (August 3, 2023).
21. In the past several years, there has been a great deal of public reference to toxic masculinity. However, to my knowledge there has been no reference, in either literature or pop culture, to its equivalent, "toxic femininity." My conceptualization of the phrase "toxic femininity," along with my decision to write about it, came after talking to some close male friends. These men had been very hurt by cultural expectations to be macho, which primarily affected their ability to be emotionally expressive. But they were also affected by women whose behavior could only be called outright cruel and exploitative.

    Men talk about how belittled they feel from movies, TV, advertisements, politics, and the social arena. One close male friend told me that in most films and television programs, he sees men portrayed as bumbling (though well-meaning) idiots while women are the strong ones, swooping in with their smarts, common sense and wisdom to save the day. Never having been knowledgeable about popular culture to any substantial degree, I never saw it that way. To me, what was most apparent was the denigrating way in which women were portrayed: beautiful ornaments whose sole purpose was to be desirable and pleasing to men. Of course, my friend and I had heightened sensitivity to our own negative experiences, based on our sex. One thing, though, that both of us noticed is that in more recent films and television programs, women have been shown to easily overpower men physically, even if the woman is five-foot-five and the man is a six-foot bodybuilder. One must question the purpose of such highly unrealistic portrayals.

22. Elizabeth Day, "Living dolls: inside the world of child beauty pageants." *The Guardian*, July 10, 2010. https://www.theguardian.com/lifeandstyle/2010/jul/11/child-beauty-queens (October 13, 2023).
23. Laura Goode, "I Was a Child Pageant Star: Six Adult Women Look Back." *New York Magazine*, November 14, 2012. https://www.thecut.com/2012/11/child-pageant-star.html (October 13, 2023).
24. "Female infanticide," BBC, 2014. www.bbc.co.uk/ethics/abortion/medical/infanticide_1.shtml (September 6, 2020).
25. T.A. Smith, "In Study, More Baby Girls Aborted Than Boys." Clinic Quotes, February 23, 2013. https://clinicquotes.com/in-study-more-baby-girls-aborted-than-boys/ (September 6, 2020).
26. Lise Eliot, *Pink Brain Blue Brain* (New York: Houghton Mifflin Harcourt Publishing Company, 2009), pp. 24–25.
27. Emily Davies, "Thousands of girls are aborted due to gender: Study finds couples from cultures in which sons are deemed more desirable are terminating female pregnancies." *Daily Mail*, January 14, 2014. www.dailymail.co.uk/news/article-2539648/Thousands-girls-aborted-gender-Study-finds-couples-cultures-sons-deemed-desirable-terminating-female-pregnancies.html (September 6, 2020).
28. Fengqing Chao, Christophe Z. Guilmoto, Samir K. C., and Hernando Ombao, "Probabilistic projection of the sex ratio at birth and missing female births by State and Union Territory in India." *Plos One*, August 19, 2020, p 1. https://doi.org/10.1371/journal.pone.0236673 (September 6, 2020).
29. Michael Gryboski, "India to have 6.8 million fewer female births by 2030 due to abortion: study." The Christian Post, August 21, 2020. www.christianpost.com/news/india-to-have-68-million-fewer-female-births-by-2030-due-to-abortion-study.html (September 22, 2020).
30. Jonathon Van Maren, "Gendercide: Selection of unborn girls for destruction continues in pro-abortion India." Life Site News, August 28, 2020. www.lifesitenews.com/blogs/gendercide-selection-of-unborn-girls-for-destruction-continues-in-pro-abortion-india (September 22, 2020).
31. "An Updated Definition of Rape." U.S. Department of Justice, Office of the Attorney General, January 6, 2012. www.justice.gov/archives/opa/blog/updated-definition-rape (September 30, 2020).
32. "Victims of Sexual Violence: Statistics." RAINN, www.rainn.org/statistics/victims-sexual-violence (July 2020).
33. Bernice Yeung, "Here are 3 startling new stats on rape." Reveal, November 2, 2017. www.revealnews.org/blog/here-are-three-startling-new-stats-on-rape/ (September 30, 2020).
34. Patrizia Riccardi, "Male Rape" The Silent Victim and the Gender of the Listener." *The Primary Care Companion to the Journal of Clinical Psychiatry*, 2010; 12(6).
35. See "Unhelpful myths about the sexual assault and rape of men," Living Well, February 12, 2019. https://livingwell.org.au/information/unhelpful-myths-about-the-sexual-assault-and-rape-of-men/ (May 9, 2023).
36. Will Storr, "The rape of men: the darkest secret of war." *The Guardian*, July 16, 2011. https://www.theguardian.com/society/2011/jul/17/the-rape-of-men (May 9, 2023).
37. "The global scale of child sexual abuse in the Catholic Church." Aljazeera, October 5, 2021. https://www.aljazeera.com/news/2021/10/5/awful-truth-child-sex-abuse-in-the-catholic-church (October 13, 2023).

38. Will Storr, "The rape of men: the darkest secret of war." *The Guardian*, July 16, 2011. https://www.theguardian.com/society/2011/jul/17/the-rape-of-men (May 9, 2023).
39. Lara Stemple, Andrew Flores, and Ilan Meyer, "Sexual victimization perpetrated by women: Federal data reveal surprising prevalence." *Aggression and Violent Behavior*, May 2017, Volume 34, 302–311; pp. 303–304.
40. Ibid, p. 305.
41. Bryana H. French, Jasmine D. Tilghman, and Dominique A. Maleranche, "Sexual Coercion Context and Psychosocial Correlates Among Diverse Males." *Psychology of Men & Masculinity* 2015, Volume 16, Number 1, 42–53 (November 13, 2020).
42. Ken Armstrong and T. Christian Miller, "Charged With Lying." *The New York Times*, November 24, 2017. https://www.nytimes.com/2017/11/24/opinion/sunday/sexual-assault-victims-lying.html (November 13, 2020).
43. Dean G. Kilpatrick, "The Mental Health Impact of Rape." National Violence Against Women Prevention Research Center Medical University of South Carolina, 2000. https://mainweb-v.musc.edu/vawprevention/research/mentalimpact.shtml (September 30, 2020).
44. "Health Consequences of Sexual Assault," Stop Violence Against Woman, The Advocates for Human Rights, February 1, 2006. www.stopvaw.org/health_consequences_of_sexual_assault (September 30, 2020).
45. Eric Dietrich, "Is the World More Dangerous Now Than Ever?" *Psychology Today*, July 24, 2016. www.psychologytoday.com/us/blog/excellent-beauty/201607/is-the-world-more-dangerous-now-ever (July 16, 2020).
46. Jody Clay-Warner and Mary E. Odem, ed., *Confronting Rape and Sexual Assault* (London: Rowman & Littlefield, 1997).
47. C. Ward, "The Attitudes Toward Rape Victims Scale: Construction, validation, and cross-cultural applicability." *Psychology of Women Quarterly* 12, 1988, 127–146.
48. Shalini Mittal, Tushar Singh, and Sunil Kumar Verma, "Young Adults' Attitudes towards Rape and Rape Victims: Effects of Gender and Social Category." *Journal of Psychology and Clinical Psychiatry* 2017, Volume 7, Issue 4, reprint, p. 5.
49. FBI, Crime Index Offenses Reported, 1996. https://ucr.fbi.gov/crime-in-the.u.s/1996/96sec2.pdf (July 16, 2020).
50. David Lisak, Lori Gardinier, Sarah C, Nicksa, and Ashley M. Cote, "False Allegations of Sexual Assault: An Analysis of Ten Years of Reported Cases," 2010. *Symposium on False Allegations of Rape, Violence Against Women* 16(12) 1318–1334.
51. Cassie Jaye, "Meeting the Enemy: A feminist comes to terms with the Men's Rights movement." TEDx talk, Marin County, California, October 18, 2017. https://www.youtube.com/watch?v=3WMuzhQXJoY (February 12, 2023).

Appendix B. Transgender Athletes in Sports

1. Andrew Langford, "Sex Differences, Gender, and Competitive Sport." Quillette, April 5, 2019. https://quillette.com/2019/04/05/sex-differences-gender-and-competitive-sport (July 14, 2020).
2. Heidi Miller, "Difference Between Male And Female Structures (Mental And Physical)." Steady Health, August 17, 2017. www.steadyhealth.com/articles/difference-between-male-and-female-structures-mental-and-physical (July 16, 2020).
3. J.W. Nieves, C. Formica, J. Ruffing, et al, "Males have larger skeletal size and bone mass than females, despite comparable body size." *Journal of Bone and Mineral Research* 2005, 20(3), 529–535.

4. D.A. Lewis, E. Kamon, and J.L. Hodgson, "Physiological differences between genders. Implications for sports conditioning." *Sports Medicine*, September–October 1986;3(5): 357–369. https://pubmed.ncbi.nlm.nih.gov/3529284/ (July 16, 2020).
5. Thibault, Valérie, Marion Guillaume, Geoffroy Berthelot, et al., "Women and Men in Sport Performance: The Gender Gap has not Evolved since 1983." *Journal of Sports Science and Medicine*, June 2010, 9(2): 214–223.
6. Timothy A. Roberts, Joshua Smalley, and Dale Ahrendt, "Effect of gender affirming hormones on athletic performance in transwomen and transmen: implications for sporting organisations and legislators." *British Journal of Sports Medicine* 2021, No. 55, 577–583.
7. Ibid, p. 581.
8. A. Wiik, T.R. Lundberg, E. Rullman, et al, "Muscle strength, size and composition following 12 months of gender-affirming treatment in transgender individuals: retained advantage for the transwomen." *BioRxiv*, September 26, 2019. https://www.biorxiv.org/content/10.1101/782557v1.full (May 7, 2023).
9. Alison K. Heather, "Transwoman Elite Athletes: Their Extra Percentage Relative to Female Physiology." *International Journal of Environmental Research and Public Health*, August 2022, 19(15). https://www.mdpi.com/1660-4601/19/15/9103 (June 27, 2023).
10. Sumanti Sen, "Who is Mianne Bagger? Transgender golfer calls biological males in women's sports a 'slap in the face.'" MEAWW.COM, April 20, 2022. https://meaww.com/who-is-mianne-bagger-transgender-golfer-opposes-biological-males-in-womens-sports (June 18, 2023).
11. Annamarie Houlis, "The True Story Behind Caitlyn Jenner's Transition." The List, April 15, 2022. https://www.thelist.com/264238/the-true-story-behind-caitlyn-jenners-transition/ (June 18, 2023).
12. Frances Perraudin, "Martina Navratilova criticised over 'cheating' trans women comment." *The Guardian*, February 17, 2019. https://www.theguardian.com/sport/2019/feb/17/martina-navratilova-criticised-over-cheating-trans-women-comments (June 18, 2023).
13. Martina Navratilova, "The rules on trans athletes reward cheats and punish the innocent." *The Sunday Times*, February 17, 2019. https://www.thetimes.co.uk/article/the-rules-on-trans-athletes-reward-cheats-and-punish-the-innocent-klsrq6h3x (June 18 2023).
14. Frances Perraudin, "Martina Navratilova criticised over 'cheating' trans women comment." *The Guardian*, February 17, 2019. https://www.theguardian.com/sport/2019/feb/17/martina-navratilova-criticised-over-cheating-trans-women-comments (June 18, 2023).
15. Richards v. US Tennis Assn, Supreme Court, Special Term, New York County. August 16, 1977. www.leagle.com/decision/197780693misc2d7131654 (July 16, 2020).
16. Emily Bazelon, "Cross-Court Winner." Slate, October 25, 2012. https://slate.com/culture/2012/10/jewish-jocks-and-renee-richards-the-life-of-the-transsexual-tennis-legend.html (July 16, 2020). https://www.ncbi.nlm.nih.gov/pmc/articles/PMC9331831/
17. Karleigh Webb, "Trans cyclist Rachel McKinnon keeps winning championships and her detractors don't like it." *Outsports*, October 23, 2019. https://www.outsports.com/2019/10/23/20928252/rachel-mckinnon-trump-cycling-trans-athletes-transphobia-world-championships (May 7, 2023)
18. Emily Jones, "Transgender Man Who Says He's a Woman Wins Women's World Championship." CBN, December 10, 2022. https://www2.cbn.com/news/us/transgender-man-who-says-hes-woman-wins-womens-world-championship (May 6, 2023).

The headline should have read, "Male Athlete, Mediocre When Competing Against Other Men, Pretends to Be a Woman So He Can Compete Against Female Athletes and Win."

19. Martina Navratilova, "The rules on trans athletes reward cheats and punish the innocent." *The Sunday Times*, February 17, 2019. https://www.thetimes.co.uk/article/the-rules-on-trans-athletes-reward-cheats-and-punish-the-innocent-klsrq6h3x (June 18 2023).

20. "Rachel McKinnon: Transgender athlete sets world best but rules out Tokyo 2020." BBC Sport, October 18, 2019. https://www.bbc.com/sport/cycling/50097423 (June 19, 2023).

21. Warner Todd Huston, "Biological Man Wins Women's Cycling Championship." Breitbart, October 15, 2018. https://www.breitbart.com/sports/2018/10/15/biological-man-wins-womens-cycling-championship/ (June 20, 2023).

22. "Veronica Ivy" [formerly Rachel McKinnon], May 26, 2023. https://en.wikipedia.org/wiki/Veronica_Ivy (June 18, 2023).

23. Karleigh Webb, "Trans cyclist Rachel McKinnon keeps winning championships and her detractors don't like it." *Outsports*, October 23, 2019. https://www.outsports.com/2019/10/23/20928252/rachel-mckinnon-trump-cycling-trans-athletes-transphobia-world-championships (May 7, 2023)

24. Alex Ballinger, "'Preventing trans women from competing is denying their human rights': Transgender athlete Rachel McKinnon returns to defend track world title." *Cycling Weekly*, October 18, 2019. https://www.cyclingweekly.com/news/racing/preventing-trans-women-competing-denying-human-rights-transgender-athlete-rachel-mckinnon-returns-defend-track-world-title-440713 (May 7, 2023).

25. Carolien van Herrikhuyzen, Twitter, October 15, 2018. https://twitter.com/CforCycling/status/1051874220014104576 (June 18, 2023). Also quoted in Emily Jones, "Transgender Man Who Says He's a Woman Wins Women's World Championship." CBN, December 10, 2022. https://www2.cbn.com/news/us/transgender-man-who-says-hes-woman-wins-womens-world-championship (May 6, 2023).

26. Warner Todd Huston, "Trans Cyclist Austin Killips Says Men are 'Underrepresented' in Women's Sports." Breitbart, June 26, 2023. https://www.breitbart.com/sports/2023/06/26/trans-cyclist-austin-killips-says-men-are-underrepresented-in-womens-sports/ (June 27, 2023).

27. Sean Ingle, "UCI hits brakes and will revisit transgender policy after Killips' victory." *The Guardian*, May 4, 2023. https://www.theguardian.com/sport/2023/may/04/uci-recognises-transgender-policy-concerns-reopens-consultation-cycling (June 27, 2023).

28. Ibid.

29. JD Heyes, "16 UPenn swimmers call for transgender Lia Thomas to be banned from women's competition." Natural News, February 9, 2022. https://www.naturalnews.com/2022-02-09-upenn-swimmers-call-for-transgender-to-be-banned-womens-competition.html (February 9, 2022).

30. Yael Halon, "USA Swimming official who resigned over trans swimmer Lia Thomas says athlete is 'destroying women's swimming.'" Fox News, December 27, 2021. https://www.foxnews.com/media/usa-swimming-official-lia-thomas-destroying-womens-swimming (June 18, 2023).

31. *Doping* is the slang term for the illegal consumption of any number of substances to increase muscle mass and strength, endurance, oxygen-carrying capacity, and even imperviousness to pain, in order to gain a competitive edge in an athletic event. Athletes still do this because of the pressure to win and the enormous amounts of money to be made. According to "Doping in Sports, a Never-Ending Story?" there are many ways to improve athletic performance. Testosterone and dihydrotestosterone are commonly utilized. However, other substances include selective androgen receptor

modulators which increase the potency of the steroid hormones that are in the body, peptide hormones and insulin-like growth factors, central nervous system stimulants, narcotics, and even cannabis. Natural ingredients that are not forbidden, but can help with athletic performance, include L-carnitine, an amino acid that's synthesized in the liver and kidneys from two other amino acids, lysine and methionine. (Amino acids are the building blocks of protein.) Arginine, another amino acid, helps improve circulation and hence muscle mass. Yet another amino acid, tyrosine, helps reduce fat. However, it should be used carefully as it's a precursor of adrenaline and noradrenaline and can overstimulate the nervous system. "Other amino acids or derivatives used to increase muscle strength and endurance are: carnosine, citrulline, glutamine, glycine and taurine. Taurine and carnozine have particular effects, being used as energizing substances." [Robert Alexandru Vlad, Gabriel Hancu, Gabriel Cosmin Popescu, and Ioana Andreea Lungu, "Doping in Sports, a Never-Ending Story?" *Advanced Pharmaceutical Bulletin*, November 2018, 8(4): 529–534; 532.] The outstanding benefits of amino acids is why so many athletes drink protein shakes. Whey is especially bio-available for those who can tolerate dairy.

32. John Lohn, "With NCAA Action, the Effects of Lia Thomas Case Are Akin to Doping." *Swimming World*, January 18, 2022. https://www.swimmingworldmagazine.com/news/without-ncaa-action-the-effects-of-lia-thomas-situation-are-akin-to-doping/ (June 18, 2023).
33. Joe Kinsey, "Virginia Swimmers Unite, Speak Out After Biological Male Pulls Lia Thomas, Tries to Join Team." OutKick, October 6, 2023. https://www.outkick.com/virginia-swimmers-unite-biological-male-lia-thomas-team/ (October 7, 2023).
34. Ibid.
35. Shawn Cohen, "We're uncomfortable in our own locker room." Daily Mail, January 27, 2022. https://www.dailymail.co.uk/news/article-10445679/Lia-Thomas-UPenn-teammate-says-trans-swimmer-doesnt-cover-genitals-locker-room.html (June 18, 2023).
36. Samantha Kamman, "Trans swimmer Lia Thomas' former teammate speaks out for the first time: 'Frightening.'" The Christian Post, June 7, 2023. https://www.christianpost.com/news/trans-swimmer-lia-thomas-former-teammate-speaks-out.html (June 18, 2023).
37. "Megyn Kelly blasts Biden's trans health secretary over bizarre gender clinic demand: 'He's a man!'" GB News, August 22, 2023. https://www.youtube.com/watch?v=zRPPBKboXz4 (August 29, 2023).
38. Brady Knox, "Lia Thomas blasts teammates as 'fake' feminists over perceived lack of support." Washington Examiner, April 27, 2023. https://www.washingtonexaminer.com/news/lia-thomas-bashes-teammates-fake-feminists (June 20, 2023).
39. Riley Gaines, "I Was Assaulted by a Transgender Mob and This Is What I Plan To Do Next." OutKick, April 17, 2023. https://www.outkick.com/riley-gaines-i-was-assaulted-by-a-transgender-mob-and-this-is-what-i-plan-to-do-next/ (June 20, 2023).
40. Ibid.
41. Ibid.
42. Victor Nava, "Riley Gains says some 'violated' swimmers 'undressed in the janitor's closet' to avoid Lia Thomas." *New York Post*, June 21, 2023. https://nypost.com/2023/06/21/riley-gaines-says-some-violated-swimmers-undressed-in-the-janitors-closet-to-avoid-lia-thomas/ (June 23, 2023).
43. Sean Ingle, "Transgender women swimmers barred from female competitions by Fina." *The Guardian*, June 19, 2022. https://www.theguardian.com/sport/2022/jun/19/transgender-swimmers-barred-from-female-competitions-after-fina-vote (October 5, 2023).

44. M. Brownstone, "Men Who Identify as Women Banned from Women's USA Powerlifting Competitions." *Gender Identity News for the Mainstream*, February 9, 2019. https://www.womenarehuman.com/men-who-identity-as-women-banned-from-womens-usa-powerlifting-competitions/ (June 27, 2023).

45. Andrew Langford, "Sex Differences, Gender, and Competitive Sport." Quillette, April 5, 2019. https://quillette.com/2019/04/05/sex-differences-gender-and-competitive-sport (July 14, 2020).

46. Kunal Dey, "North Carolina high school female volleyball player injured after trans opponent spikes ball into her face." MEAWW.com/news, October 19, 2022. https://meaww.com/north-carolina-high-school-female-volleyball-player-injured-trans-opponent-spikes-ball-face (June 18, 2023).

47. Luke Gentile, "Transgender rugby player slams female athletes, coach says three injured." *Washington Examiner*, April 14, 2022. https://www.washingtonexaminer.com/news/watch-transgender-rugby-player-slams-female-athletes-coach-says-three-injured (June 18, 2023).

48. "Transgender Guidelines," World Rugby, undated. https://www.world.rugby/the-game/player-welfare/guidelines/transgender (June 18, 2023).

49. Jonathan Kay, "Ignoring Biological Reality Puts Female Hockey Players at Risk." Quillette, December 9, 2022. https://quillette.com/blog/2022/12/09/ignoring-biological-reality-puts-female-hockey-players-at-risk/ (June 18, 2023).

50. Ibid.

51. Ibid.

52. It's no surprise that so little consideration has been given to women with the admission of transgenders into their sports. Women have always been second-class citizens in the sports field. Just one example is women's soccer. Their tournament prize money is only about one-third the amount that men earn. According to one report, "Some players even said that their uniforms were hand-me-downs from the men's teams, and while male players would get to stay at hotels, the women, who were only paid $15 per diem during overseas travel, all bunked in one room at a bed-and-breakfast." [Christopher Parker, "This Summer's Women's World Cup Follows Decades of Challenges On and Off the Field." *Smithsonian Magazine*, July 3, 2023. https://www.smithsonianmag.com/smart-news/womens-world-cup-2023-campaign=editorial&spMailingID=48461467&spUserID=NjEyNDI5NjUyMzc0S0&spJobID=2500295010&spReportId=MjUwMDI5NTAxMAS2 (July 3, 2023).]

53. Timothy A. Roberts, Joshua Smalley, and Dale Ahrendt, "Effect of gender affirming hormones on athletic performance in transwomen and transmen: implications for sporting organisations and legislators." *British Journal of Sports Medicine* 2021, No. 55, 577–583.

54. "Transgender boy wins girls' state wrestling title for second time," *New York Post*, February 25, 2018. https://nypost.com/2018/02/25/transgender-boy-wins-girls-state-wrestling-title-for-second-time/ (June 18, 2023).

55. Isaac Amend, "We need a conversation about transmen in sports." *Washington Blade*, June 2, 2022. https://www.washingtonblade.com/2022/06/02/we-need-a-conversation-about-transmen-in-sports/ (June 26, 2023).

56. Sarah Laframboise, "In the ruling against Caster Semenya, bogus science is being used to stifle the vulnerable." *Massive Science*, May 13, 2019. https://massivesci.com/articles/caster-semenya-track-field-iaaf-olympics-testosterone-hyperandrogenism/ (October 3, 2023).

57. Ariel Levy, "Either/Or." *The New Yorker*, November 19, 2009. https://www.newyorker.com/magazine/2009/11/30/caster-semenya-profile-either-or (October 3, 2023).

58. "Caster Semenya offered to show officials her vagina to prove she is female." *The Guardian*, May 24, 2022. https://www.theguardian.com/sport/2022/may/24/caster-semenya-800m-world-athletics-hbo-interview (October 3, 2023).
59. Melissa Block, "The Sensitive Question of Intersex Athletes." *The Torch*, August 16, 2016. https://www.npr.org/sections/thetorch/2016/08/16/490236620/south-african-star-raises-sensitive-questions-about-intersex-athletes (May 2, 2022).
60. "Caster Semenya offered to show officials her vagina to prove she is female." *The Guardian*, May 24, 2022. https://www.theguardian.com/sport/2022/may/24/caster-semenya-800m-world-athletics-hbo-interview (October 3, 2023).
61. Melissa Block, "The Sensitive Question of Intersex Athletes." *The Torch*, August 16, 2016. https://www.npr.org/sections/thetorch/2016/08/16/490236620/south-african-star-raises-sensitive-questions-about-intersex-athletes (May 2, 2022).
62. Ben Morse, "World Athletics tightens rules on transgender women athletes." CNN, March 24, 2023. https://www.cnn.com/2023/03/23/sport/world-athletics-transgender-ruling-spt-intl/index.html (October 4, 2023).
63. Matthew Brealey, "Caster Semenya—male or female?" September 12, 2020. https://matthewbrealey.medium.com/caster-semenya-male-or-female-c5502364d564 (October 4, 2023).
64. Julian Savulescu, "Ten ethical flaws in the Caster Semenya decision on intersex in sport." *The Conversation*, May 9, 2019. https://theconversation.com/ten-ethical-flaws-in-the-caster-semenya-decision-on-intersex-in-sport-116448 (May 1, 2023).
65. Ibid.
66. Ariel Levy, "Either/Or." *The New Yorker*, November 19, 2009. https://www.newyorker.com/magazine/2009/11/30/caster-semenya-profile-either-or (October 3, 2023).
67. Rebecca Greenfield, "Runner Caster Semenya Looks a Lot More Feminine Than She Did in 2009." *The Atlantic*, June 12, 2012. https://www.theatlantic.com/culture/archive/2012/06/runner-caster-semenya-looks-lot-more-feminine-she-did-2009/327016 (October 3, 2023).
68. Ibid.
69. Ibid.
70. Matthew Brealey, "Caster Semenya—male or female?" September 12, 2020. https://matthewbrealey.medium.com/caster-semenya-male-or-female-c5502364d564 (October 4, 2023).
71. Ibid.
72. Ibid.
73. Ibid.
74. Eddie Pells, "Track bans transgender athletes, tightens rules for Semenya." AP News, March 23, 2023. https://apnews.com/article/transgender-track-semenya-f3499b00b932948f96838adb3b010f11 (May 1, 2023).
75. "Edinanci Silva," Wikipedia, July 29, 2023. https://en.wikipedia.org/wiki/Edinanci_Silva (October 5, 2023).
76. "Teen runners sue to block trans athletes from girls' sports." *The Guardian*, February 13, 2020. https://www.theguardian.com/us-news/2020/feb/13/transgender-athletes-girls-sports-high-school (June 22, 2023).
77. Aaron Katersky, "Female athletes ask to sue over policy allowing transgender athletes to compete in sports." ABC News, June 6, 2023. https://abcnews.go.com/US/female-athletes-sue-policy-allowing-transgender-athletes-compete/story?id=99878569 (June 22, 2023).

78. "Teen runners sue to block trans athletes from girls' sports." *The Guardian*, February 13, 2020. https://www.theguardian.com/us-news/2020/feb/13/transgender-athletes-girls-sports-high-school (June 22, 2023).

79. Rikki Schlott, "'Fastest girl in Connecticut' Chelsea Mitchell suing state after losing to trans athletes." *New York Post*, May 31, 2023. https://nypost.com/2023/05/31/runner-chelsea-mitchell-who-lost-to-trans-athletes-this-is-about-fairness/ (June 22, 2023).

80. Brandon Gillespie, "USA Today blasted as 'garbage' for editing opinion piece opposing trans women in girls' sports." Fox News, May 27, 2021. https://www.foxnews.com/media/usa-today-blasted-censoring-female-track-star-chelsea-mitchell-op-ed-opposing-trans-males-girls-sports (June 22, 2023).

81. Chelsea Mitchell, "I was the fastest girl in Connecticut. But transgender athletes made it an unfair fight." *USA Today*, as revised by editor, May 26, 2021 (originally published on May 22, 2021). https://www.usatoday.com/story/opinion/2021/05/22/transgender-athletes-girls-women-sports-track-connecticut-column/5149532001/?gnt-cfr=1 (June 22, 2023).

82. Ibid.

83. Enrico Trigoso, "Female Athlete Retires After Competing Against Biological Men, Says Girls 'No Longer Have a Fair Chance.'" *The Epoch Times*, May 31, 2023. https://www.theepochtimes.com/sports/female-athlete-retires-after-competing-against-biological-men-says-girls-no-longer-have-a-fair-chance-5301064?utm_source=Aomorningbriefnoe&src_src=Aomorningbriefnoe&utm_campaign=Aomb-2023-06-01&src_ (November 22, 2023).

84. Juliana Kim, "Transgender track and field athletes can't compete in women's international events." National Public Radio, March 24, 2023. https://www.npr.org/2023/03/24/1165795462/transgender-track-and-field-athletes-cant-compete-in-womens-international-events (June 26, 2023).

85. Sean Ingle, "UCI hits brakes and will revisit transgender policy after Killips' victory," May 4, 2023. *The Guardian*, https://www.theguardian.com/sport/2023/may/04/uci-recognises-transgender-policy-concerns-reopens-consultation-cycling (June 27, 2023).

86. USA Powerlifting Transgender Policy, undated. https://www.usapowerlifting.com/transgender-participation-policy/ (June 27, 2023).

87. C. Mandler, "Trans women can compete in USA Powerlifting, ruling says." CBS News, March 7, 2023. https://www.cbsnews.com/news/trans-women-usa-powerlifting-competition-ruling/ (June 27, 2023).

88. Taryn Knox, Lynley C. Anderson, and Alison Heather, "Transwomen in elite sport: scientific and ethical considerations." *Journal of Medical Ethics*, June 2019, 45(6): 395–403.

89. Sean Ingle, "Trans women should not have to reduce testosterone, say new IOC guidelines." *The Guardian*, November 16, 2021. https://www.theguardian.com/sport/2021/nov/16/trans-women-should-not-have-to-reduce-testosterone-say-new-ioc-guidelines (July 29, 2023).

90. International Olympic Committee, *IOC Framework on Fairness, Inclusion and Non-Discrimination on the Basis of Gender identity and Sex Variations*, 2021, p. 2.

91. Ibid, pp. 3–4.

92. Ibid, p. 4.

93. Ibid, p. 5.

94. Ibid, p. 5.

95. Ibid, p. 5.

96. Joe Kinsey, "Birth Gender Should Dictate Sports Participation, 69% of Americans Say in New Poll." *OutKick*, June 12, 2023. https://www.outkick.com/birth-gender-should-dictate-sports-participation-69-of-americans-say-in-new-poll/ (June 20, 2023).
97. Jason Hahn, "Girls High School Basketball Team Forfeits Game Instead of Playing Against Transgender Player." *People*, March 2, 2023. https://people.com/sports/girls-high-school-basketball-team-forfeits-tournament-refuses-face-transgender-player/ (March 13, 2024).
98. Yaron Steinbuch, "Girls' high school basketball coach banned for forfeiting game over transgender player has no regrets: 'Asking for injury.'" *New York Post*, February 27, 2024.

Selected References

Complete references for each chapter can be found in the Notes section.

Abbruzzese, E., Stephen B. Levine and Julia W. Mason. "The Myth of 'Reliable Research' in Pediatric Gender Medicine: A critical evaluation of the Dutch Studies—and research that has followed," *Journal of Sex and Marital Therapy*, January 2, 2023. Online: January 2, 2023. https://www.tandfonline.com/doi/full/10.1080/0092623X.2022.2150346 (July 10, 2023).

Aboli, Laura. "Transhumanism: The End Game," November 14, 2023. https://twitter.com/Yolo304741/status/1724556707097932054 (November 15, 2023). A longer version can be found on YouTube, June 20, 2023. https://www.youtube.com/watch?v=FCh6auCKYS0&t=5s (November 15, 2023).

"A Gender Variance Who's Who: Christiane Völling," May 30, 2008. https://zagria.blogspot.com/2008/05/christiane-vlling-1960-nurse.html (June 22, 2023).

Alzahrani, T., T. Nguyen, A. Ryan, et al. "Cardiovascular Disease Risk Factors and Myocardial Infarction in the Transgender Population," *Circulation: Cardiovascular Quality and Outcomes*, April 5, 2019; Vol.12, No. 4.

Angell, Marcia. "Drug Companies and Doctors: A Story of Corruption," *The New York Review of Books*, January 15, 2009. nybooks.com/articles/archives/2009/jan/15 (July 2, 2015).

Aragão, Carolina. "Gender pay gap in U.S. hasn't changed much in two decades." Pew Research Center, March 1, 2023. https://www.pewresearch.org/short-reads/2023/03/01/gender-pay-gap-facts/ (August 11, 2023).

Asscheman, h., L.J.G. Gooren, and P.L.E. Eklund. "Mortality and morbidity in transsexual patients with cross-gender hormone treatment," *Metabolism* 1989, Number 38 (9): 867–873.

Barnes, James. "I'm a Trans Man. I Didn't Realize How Broken Men Are," *Newsweek*, August 6, 2023. https://www.newsweek.com/trans-man-broken-men-1817169 (January 7, 2024).

Barres, Ben A. "Does gender matter?" *Nature*, July 13, 2006, Volume 442.

Barres, Ben A. *The Autobiography of a Transgender Scientist* (Cambridge, Massachusetts: The MIT Press, 2018).

Bateman, Ashley. "The Whole Transgender Industry Is Founded On Two Faulty Studies," The Federalist, February 1, 2023. https://thefederalist.com/2023/02/01/the-whole-transgender-industry-is-founded-on-two-faulty-studies/ (July 10, 2023).

Bear, Julia B. and Peter Glick. "Breadwinner Bonus and Caregiver Penalty in Workplace Rewards for Men and Women," *Social Psychological and Personality Science*, December 14, 2016.

Bem, Sandra. *An Unconventional Family* (New Haven, Connecticut: Yale University Press, 1998).

Bian, Lin, Sarah-Jane Leslie, and Andrei Cimpian. "Gender stereotypes about intellectual ability emerge early and influence children's interests," *Science*,

Volume 244, Number 6323, 389–391, January 27, 2017. https://www.science.org/doi/10.1126/science.aah6524 (July 28, 2023).

Biggs, Michael. "Puberty Blockers and Suicidality in Adolescents Suffering from Gender Dysphoria," *Archives of Sexual Behavior* 2020, 49(7): 2227–2229. https://www.ncbi.nlm.nih.gov/pmc/articles/PMC8169497/ (July 26, 2023).

Biggs, Michael. "The Dutch Protocol for Juvenile Transsexuals: Origins and Evidence," *Journal of Sex and Marital Therapy* 2023, Volume 49, Issue 4: 348–368.

Biggs, Michael. "The Open Society Foundations and the transgender movement," 4th Wave Now, May 25, 2018. https://4thwavenow.com/2018/05/25/the-open-society-foundations-the-transgender-movement/ (September 22, 2023).

Bilek, Jennifer. "The Billionaire Family Pushing Synthetic Sex identities (SSI)," Tablet, June 14, 2022. https://www.tabletmag.com/sections/news/articles/billionaire-family-pushing-synthetic-sex-identities-ssi-pritzkers (May 8, 2023).

Blanchard, Ray. "The concept of autogynephilia and the typology of male gender dysphoria," *The Journal of Nervous and Mental Disease* 1989, Number 177, 616–623. Quoted from "Autognephilia," LGBT Project Wiki. https://lgbt.wikia.org/wiki/Autogynephilia (August 21, 2020).

Blum, Brian. "Would you give up on orgasm?" *Jerusalem Post*, June 2, 2022. https://www.jpost.com/opinion/article-708397 (May 16, 2023)

Bradbard, Marilyn R., Carol Lynn Martin, Richard C. Endsley, et al. "Influence of Sex Stereotypes on Children's Exploration and Memory. A Competence Versus Performance Distinction," *Developmental Psychology*, July 1, 1986, 481–486.

Bradberry, Travis. "14 Signs You Are Emotionally Intelligent," November 13, 2018. https://www.linkedin.com/pulse/14-signs-you-emotionally-intelligent-dr-travis-bradberry (August 16, 2023).

Brealey, Matthew. "Caster Semenya—male or female?" September 12, 2020. https://matthewbrealey.medium.com/caster-semenya-male-or-female-c5502364d564 (October 4, 2023).

Brownlow, Sheila, Amanda J. Janas, Kathleen A. Blake, et al. "Getting by with a Little Help from My Friends: Mental Rotation Ability after Tacit Peer Encouragement," *Psychology*, Volume 2, Number 4, July 2011, 363–370.

Canadian Paediatric Society, "Concerns for the use of soy-based formulas in infant nutrition." *Paediatrics Child Health*, February 2009, 14(2): 109–113.

Caprino, Kathy. "Gender Bias Is Real: Women's Perceived Competency Drops Significantly When Judged As Being Forceful," *Forbes*, August 25, 2015. https://www.forbes.com/sites/kathycaprino/2015/08/25/gender-bias-is-real-womens-perceived-competency-drops-significantly-when-judged-as-being-forceful/?sh=7f68601e2d85 (August 1, 2023).

Casey, Kennedy, Kylee Novick, and Stella F. Lourenco. "Sixty years of gender representation in children's books: Conditions associated with overrepresentation of male versus female protagonists," *Plos One* 16(12), December 15, 2021.

Cass, Hilary. Letter to National Health Service England, July 19, 2022. https://cass.independent-review.uk/wp-content/uploads/2022/07/Cass-Review-Letter-to-NHSE_19-July-2022.pdf (September 2, 2023).

Chao, Fengqing, Christophe Z. Guilmoto, Samir K. C., and Hernando Ombao. "Probabilistic projection of the sex ratio at birth and missing female births by State and Union Territory in India." *Plos One*, August 19, 2020.

Chapman, Benjamin P., Kevin Fiscella, Ichiro Kawachi, et al. "Emotion Suppression and Mortality Risk Over a 12-Year Follow-up," *Journal for Psychosomatic Research*, October 2013, 75(4): 381–385.

Chase, Cheryl. "Genital Surgery On Intersexed Children," letter to a judge in Columbia, South America, February 7, 1998. https://www.healthyplace.com/gender/inside-intersexuality/genital-surgery-on-intersexed-children (August 10, 2023).

Chatard, Armand, Serge Guimond, and Leila Selimbegovic. "'How good are you in math?' The effect of gender stereotypes on students' recollection of their school marks," *Journal of Experimental Social Psychology* 2007, Number 43, 1017–1024.

Chemaly, Soraya. "All Teachers Should Be Trained To Overcome Their Hidden Biases," *Time*, February 12, 2015. https://time.com/3705454/teachers-biases-girls-education (July 15, 2020).

Clark, Malcolm. "The tragedy of Jazz Jennings," Spiked, August 20, 2023. https://www.spiked-online.com/2023/08/20/the-tragedy-of-jazz-jennings (September 18, 2023).

Cohen, Elizabeth. "Study shows convalescent plasma works for immune-compromised Covid-19 patients, but it can be hard to find," CNN, January 12, 2023. https://www.cnn.com/2023/01/12/health/convalescent-plasma-immune-compromised-covid/index.html (July 11, 2023).

Colapinto, John. *As Nature Made Him: The Boy Who Was Raised as a Girl* (HarperCollins, 2001).

Cole, Chloe. "Detransitioner Chloe Cole's full testimony to Congress is a 'final warming' to stop gender surgery," *New York Post*, August 9, 2023. https://nypost.com/2023/07/28/detransitioner-chloe-coles-full-testimony-to-congress-is-a-final-warning-to-stop-gender-surgery/ (August 9, 2023).

Cooper, Brett. "My Biology Is Not Your Costume," The Comments Section with Brett Cooper, YouTube, January 31, 2023. https://www.youtube.com/watch?v=iq_1PWEEzOs&t=7s (March 21, 2023).

Correll, Shelley J. "Gender and the Career Choice Process: The Role of Biased Self-Assessments," *American Journal of Sociology*, May 2001, Volume 106, Number 6.

Cortes, Laura R., Carla D. Cisternas, and Nancy G. Forger. "Does Gender Leave an Epigenetic Imprint on the Brain?" *Frontiers in Neuroscience*, Volume 13, Article 173, February 26, 2019.

Dallas, Kai, Paige Kuhlman, Karyn Eilber, Victoria Scott, et al. "Rates of Psychiatric Emergencies Before and After Gender Affirming Surgery." *The Journal of Urology*, Volume 206, Issue Supplement 3, September 1, 2021.

D'Angelo, Roberto, Ema Syrulnik, Sasha Ayad, et al. "One Size Does Not Fit All: In Support of Psychotherapy for Gender Dysphoria," *Archives of Sexual Behavior* 2021, Number 50, 7–16.

Davies, Paul, Steven Spencer, and Claude Steele. "Clearing the Air: Identity Safety Moderates the Effects of Stereotype Threat on Women's Leadership Aspirations," *Journal of Personality and Social Psychology*, 88(2), 276–287.

Davies, Paul, Steven Spencer, Diane M. Quinn, and Rebecca Gerhardstein Nader. "Consuming Images: How Television Commercials That Elicit Stereotype Threat Can Restrain Women Academically and Professionally," *Journal of Personality and Social Psychology*, December 2002. 28(12): 1615–1628.

"Depression, anxiety, loneliness are peaking in college students," Boston University Science News, February 19, 2021. https://www.sciencedaily.com/releases/2021/02/210219190939.htm (July 15, 2023).

"Detransition Facts and Statistics 2022: Exploding the Myths Around Detransitioning," June 21, 2021. https://www.gendergp.com/detransition-facts/ (August 4, 2023).

Dhejne, Cecilia, Paul Lichtenstein, Marcus Boman, et al. "Long-Term Follow-Up of Transsexual Persons Undergoing Sex Reassignment Surgery: Cohort Study in Sweden," *Plos One*, February 2011, Volume 6, Issue 2. https://journals.plos.org/plosone/article?id=10.1371/journal.pone.0016885 (July 13, 2023).

Diaz, Suzanna and J. Michael Bailey. "Rapid Onset Gender Dysphoria: Parent Reports on 1655 Possible Cases," *Archives of Sexual Behavior* (March 29, 2023) 52:1031–1043. https://link.springer.com/article/10.1007/s10508-023-02576-9#change-history (July 9, 2023).

Dion, Jacinthe, Marie-Eve Blackburn, Julie Auclair, et al. "Development and aetiology of body dissatisfaction in adolescent boys and girls," *International Journal of Adolescence and Youth*, April 3, 2015, 20(2): 151–166.

Duty, Susan M., Narendra P. Singh, Manori J. Silva, et. al. "The relationship between environmental exposures to phthalates and DNA damage in human sperm using the neutral comet assay," *Environmental Health Perspectives* July 2003; 111(9):1164–1169.

Eisenberg, Albert. "The Plight of the Detransitioners," *National Review Magazine*, May 29, 2023. https://www.nationalreview.com/magazine/2023/05/29/the-plight-of-the-detransitioners/ (August 4, 2023).

Eisenberg, Nancy and Randy Lennon. "Sex Differences in Empathy and Related Capacities," *Psychological Bulletin* 1983, Volume 94, No. 1.

Erhardt, Virginia Editor. *Head Over Heels: Wives Who Stay With Cross-Dressers and Transsexuals* (New York: Routledge, 2007).

Eliot, Lise. *Pink Brain Blue Brain* (New York: Houghton Mifflin Harcourt Publishing Company, 2009).

Fausto-Sterling, Anne. *Sexing the Body: Gender Politics and the Construction of Sexuality* (New York: Basic Books, 2020).

"Female infanticide." BBC, 2014. www.bbc.co.uk/ethics/abortion/medical/infanticide_1.shtml (September 6, 2020).

Fine, Cordelia. *Delusions of Gender: how our minds, society, and neurosexism create difference* (New York: W.W. Norton & Company, 2010).

Fine, Cordelia. *Testosterone Rex: Myths of Sex, Science, and Society* (New York: W.W. Norton & Company, 2017).

Fisher, Helen. *Why Him? Why Her?* (New York: Henry Holt and Company, 2009).

Flood, Michael. "Toxic masculinity: A primer and commentary," XY, July 7, 2018. https://xyonline.net/content/toxic-masculinity-primer-and-commentary (September 30, 2020).

Formuzis, Alex. "Landmark BPA Study Finds Troubling Health Effects at FDA's 'Safe' Levels," Environmental Working Group, September 14, 2018. www.ewg.org/release/first-us-bpa-lab-study-humans-finds-troubling-health-effects-levels-deemed-safe-fda-epa (July 23, 2020).

Futterweit, Walter. "Endocrine therapy of transsexualism and potential complications of long-term treatment," *Archives of Sexual Behavior*, March 31, 1998, 27(2), 209–226.

Gaines, Riley. "I Was Assaulted by a Transgender Mob and This Is What I Plan To Do Next," OutKick, April 17, 2023. https://www.outkick.com/riley-gaines-i-was-assaulted-by-a-transgender-mob-and-this-is-what-i-plan-to-do-next/ (June 20, 2023).

Gays Against Groomers. https://www.gaysagainstgroomers.com/faq and https://www.gaysagainstgroomers.com/about (July 8, 2023).

Gharibyan, Hasmik. "Gender Gap in Computer Science: Studying Its Absence in One Former Soviet Republic," *2007 American Society for Engineering Education Conference Proceedings*, Honolulu, Hawaii. https://peer.asee.org/gender-gap-in-computer-science-studying-its-absence-in-one-former-soviet-republic (October 5, 2022).

Gluck, Genevieve. "'Cis' Coined by 'Pedosexual' Physician," 4W Feminist News, January 5, 2022. https://4w.pub/cis-coined-by-pedosexual-researcher/ (June 21, 2023).

Good, Catherine, Joshua Aronson and Jayne Ann Harder. "Problems in the pipeline: Stereotype threat and women's achievement in high-level math courses," *Journal of Applied and Developmental Psychology*, Volume 29, Number 1, January 2008, 17–28.

Greenfield, Rebecca. "Runner Caster Semenya Looks a Lot More Feminine Than She Did in 2009," *The Atlantic*, June 12, 2012. https://www.theatlantic.com/culture/archive/2012/06/runner-caster-semenya-looks-lot-more-feminine-she-did-2009/327016 (October 3, 2023).

Grossman, Miriam. *Lost in Trans Nation: A Child Psychiatrist's Guide Out of the Madness* (New York, NY: Skyhorse Publishing, 2023).

Grossman-Scott, Amanda. "8 Ways A Predator Might Groom Your Child," undated. https://educateempowerkids.org/8-ways-predator-might-groom-child/ (July 8, 2023).

Gunderson, Elizabeth A., Sarah J. Gripshover, Carissa Romero, et a. "Parent Praise to 1-3 Year-Olds Predicts Children's Motivational Frameworks 5 Years Later," *Child Development*, September 2913, 84(5): 1526–1541. www.ncbi.nlm.nih.gov/pmc/articles/PMC3655123/ (September 29, 2020).

Gustafsson, Erik, Florence Levréro, et al. "Fathers are just as good as mothers at recognizing the cries of their baby," *Nature Communications* 2013, Volume 4, Article number 1698.

Hafezi, Shirin A. and Wael M. Abdel-Rahman. "The Endocrine Disruptor Bisphenol A (BPA) Exerts a Wide Range of Effects in Carcinogenesis and Response to Therapy," *Current Molecular Pharmacology*, August 2019; 12(3): 230–238.

Haldane, Sean. *Emotional First Aid* (New York: Irvington Publishers, 1984).

Heather, Alison K. "Transwoman Elite Athletes: Their Extra Percentage Relative to Female Physiology." *International Journal of Environmental Research and Public Health*, August 2022, 19(15). https://www.mdpi.com/1660-4601/19/15/9103 (June 27, 2023).

Hedtke, Josh. "California professors instructed not to say 'America is the land of opportunity,'" The College Fix, June 10, 2015. https://www.thecollegefix.com/california-professors-instructed-not-to-say-america-is-the-land-of-opportunity/ (July 13, 2023).

Heyer, Walt. "62.7% of Transgenders Have Untreated Mental Disorders," December 15, 2016. https://waltheyer.com/62-7-of-transgenders-have-untreated-mental-disorders (July 14, 2020).

Heyer, Walt. "Gender dysphoria diagnoses are too general, and they're destroying people," Life Site News, August 19, 2019. https://www.lifesitenews.com/opinion/gender-dysphoria-diagnoses-are-too-general-and-theyre-destroying-people/ (August 9, 2023).

Heyer, Walt. "Hormones, surgery, regret: I was a transgender woman for 8 years—time I can't get back." *USA Today*, February 11, 2019. https://www.usatoday.com/story/opinion/voices/2019/02/11/transgender-debate-transitioning-sex-gender-column/1894076002/ (August 4, 2023).

Holland, Brynn. "Human Computers: The Early Women of NASA," History, September 28, 2023. https://www.history.com/news/human-computers-women-at-nasa (October 29, 2023).

Hruz, Paul, Lawrence Mayer, and Paul McHugh. "Growing Pains: Problems with Puberty Suppression in Treating Gender Dysphoria," *The New Atlantis*, Spring 2017.

Ibrahim, Eyal and Ruth Feldman, "Oxytocin and Fathering," The Good Men Project, June 7, 2018. https://goodmenproject.com/featured-content/oxytocin-and-fathering-sjbn/ (September 26, 2020).

Imai, Hideyuki, Hiroto Nishikawa, Asai Suzuki, et al. "Secondary Hypogonadism due to Excessive Ingestion of Isoflavone in a Man," *Internal Medicine*, October 1, 2022; 61(19), 2899-2903.

"I'm Transgender, and I Oppose the Medical Transition of Children." The Center for Bioethics and Culture Network, April 2, 2020. https://cbc-network.org/2020/04/im-transgender-and-i-oppose-the-medical-transition-of-children/ (October 2, 2023).

Ingle, Sean. "Trans women should not have to reduce testosterone, say new IOC guidelines." *The Guardian*, November 16, 2021. https://www.theguardian.com/sport/2021/nov/16/trans-women-should-not-have-to-reduce-testosterone-say-new-ioc-guidelines (July 29, 2023).

International Olympic Committee, *IOC Framework on Fairness, Inclusion and Non-Discrimination on the Basis of Gender identity and Sex Variations*, 2021.

"Interview: Scott Newgent," Gender Dysphoria Alliance, December 18, 2021. https://www.genderdysphoriaalliance.com/post/meet-scott-newgent (August 9, 2023).

Ioannidis, John P.A. "Why Most Published Research Findings Are False," *Plos Medicine*, August 30, 2005. journals.plos.org/plosmedicine/article?id=10.1371/journal.pmed.0020124 (July 2, 2015).

Irwig, Michael S. "Detransition Among Transgender and Gender-Diverse People—An Increasing and Increasingly Complex Phenomenon," *Journal of Clinical Endocrinology & Metabolism*, Volume 107, Issue 10, October 2022, e4261–e4262.

"Is A World Beyond Stereotypes Possible?" Wellbeing, April 1, 2020. https://wellbeingmagazine.com/is-a-world-beyond-stereotypes-possible/ (September 21, 2023).

Jakupcak, Matthew, Matthew T. Tull, and Lizabeth Roemer. "Masculinity, Shame, and Fear of Emotions as predictors of Men's Expressions of Anger and Hostility," *Psychology of Men and Masculinity*, October 2005.

James, Matt. "React vs. Respond: What's the Difference?" *Psychology Today*, September 1, 2016. www.psychologytoday.com/us/blog/focus-forgiveness/201609/react-vs-respond (July 14, 2020).

Jeffreys, Sheila. *Gender Hurts* (London and New York: Routledge, 2014).

Jeffreys, Sheila. "The politics of the toilet: A feminist response to the campaign to 'degender' a women's space," *Women's Studies International Forum* 45 (2014), 42–51.

Joel, Daphna Ariel Persico, Moshe Salhov, et al. "Analysis of Human Brain Structure Reveals that the Brain 'Types' Typical of Males Are Also Typical of Females, and Vice Versa," *Frontiers in Human Neuroscience*, Volume 12, Article 399, October 18, 2018.

Joel, Daphna, Zohar Berman, Ido Tavor, et al. "Sex beyond the genitalia: The human brain mosaic," *Proceedings of the National Academy of Sciences*, December 2015, 112(50): 15468–15473.

Kaufman, Scott Barry. "Unraveling the Mindset of Victimhood," *Scientific American*, June 29, 2020. https://www.scientificamerican.com/article/unraveling-the-mindset-of-victimhood/ (July 14, 2023).

Kay, Jonathan. "An Interview With Lisa Littman, Who Coined the Term 'Rapid Onset Gender Dysphoria,'" Quillette, March 19, 2019. https://quillette.com/2019/03/19/an-interview-with-lisa-littman-who-coined-the-term-rapid-onset-gender-dysphoria/ (August 9, 2023).

Kay, Jonathan. "Ignoring Biological Reality Puts Female Hockey Players at Risk," Quillette, December 9, 2022. https://quillette.com/blog/2022/12/09/ignoring-biological-reality-puts-female-hockey-players-at-risk/ (June 18, 2023).

Kearns, Madeleine. "California's Transgender Prison Policy Is a Disaster for Women," *National Review*, June 26, 2019. www.nationalreview.com/2019/06/californias-transgender-prison-policy-is-a-disaster-for-women/ (August 4, 2020).

Kearns, Madeleine. "Women-Only Rape-Relief Shelter Defunded, Then Vandalized," *National Review*, August 28, 2019. www.nationalreview.com/2019/08/women-only-rape-relief-shelter-defunded-then-vandalized/ (August 25, 2020).

Kerschner, Helena, Interview with Ben Shapiro. "Former Transgender Teenager Shares Powerful Story About Going In and Out of Transition," YouTube, April 28, 2022. https://www.youtube.com/watch?v=HwVyozpWWAU&t=872s (August 11, 2023).

Kilgore, Billy Doidge. "The key to letting boys actually be boys? See them as the emotional beings they are," *The Washington Post*, November 12, 2019. https://www.washingtonpost.com/lifestyle/2019/11/12/key-letting-boys-be-boys-see-them-emotional-beings-they-are/ (July 28, 2023).

Koenig, Anne M. "Comparing Prescriptive and Descriptive Gender Stereotypes About Children, Adults, and the Elderly," *Frontiers in Psychology*, June 2018, Volume 9, Article 1086.

Kohlhepp, Jacob. "California students now given six 'gender identity' choices on college admissions applications, *The College Fix*, July 27, 2015. www.thecollegefix.com/calif-students-now-given-six-gender-identity-choices-on-college-admissions-applications (July 17, 2020).

Kyan, Mahreen, Amirali Minbashian, and Carolyn MacCann. "College students in the western world are becoming less emotionally intelligent: A cross-temporal meta-analysis of trait emotional intelligence," *Journal of Personality*, December 2021, Volume 89, Issue 6, 1176–1190.

Laidlaw, Michael K., Quentin L. Van Meter, Paul W. Hruz, et al. Letter to the Editor: "Endocrine Treatment of Gender-Dysphoric/Gender-Incongruent Persons: An Endocrine Society Clinical Practice Guideline," *Journal of Clinical Endocrinology & Metabolism*, March 2019, 104(3):686–687. https://academic.oup.com/jcem/article/104/3/686/5198654.

Langford, Andrew. "Sex Differences, Gender, and Competitive Sport," Quillette, April 5, 2019. https://quillette.com/2019/04/05/sex-differences-gender-and-competitive-sport (July 14, 2020).

Leaper, Campbell and Melanie M. Ayres. "A meta-analytic review of gender variations in adults' language use: talkativeness, affiliative speech, and assertive speech." *Personality and Social Psychology Review*, November 2007, 11(4): 328–363.

Lewis, D.A., E. Kamon, and J.L. Hodgson. "Physiological differences between genders. Implications for sports conditioning," *Sports Medicine*, September-October 1986;3(5): 357–369. https://pubmed.ncbi.nlm.nih.gov/3529284/ (July 16, 2020).

Liberman, Mark. Language Log, "Blinding Us With Science," June 19, 2007. itre.cis.upenn.edu/~myl/languagelog/archives/004 (November 2, 2023).

Lindahl, Hans and Stephani Lohman. "Congenital Adrenal Hyperplasia Surgery: A Mom and Nurse Busts 5 Myths," *InterAct*, July 8, 2020. https://interactadvocates.org/genital-surgery-and-congenital-adrenal-hyperplasia/ (September 4, 2020).

Lidinsky-Smith, Grace. "There's No Standard for Care When it Comes to Trans Medicine," *Newsweek*, June 25, 2021. https://www.newsweek.com/theres-no-standard-care-when-it-comes-trans-medicine-opinion-1603450 (August 4, 2023).

Lipton, Bruce. *The Biology of Belief* (Carlsbad, California: Hay House Inc: 2015).

Little, Becky. "When Computer Coding Was a 'Woman's' Job," History, February 9, 2021. https://www.history.com/news/coding-used-to-be-a-womans-job-so-it-was-paid-less-and-undervalued (October 29, 2023).

Littman, Lisa. "Individuals Treated for Gender Dysphoria with Medical and/or Surgical Transition Who Subsequently Detransitioned: A Survey of 100 Detransitioners," *Archives of Sexual Behavior* 2021, Number 50, 3353–3369.

Littman, Lisa. "Parent reports of adolescents and young adults perceived to show signs of a rapid onset of gender dysphoria," *Plos One*, August 16, 2018, 1–44. https://journals.plos.org/plosone/article/file?id=10.1371/journal.pone.0202330&type=printable (August 9, 2023).

Lohn, John. "With NCAA Action, the Effects of Lia Thomas Case Are Akin to Doping," *Swimming World*, January 18, 2022. https://www.swimmingworldmagazine.com/news/without-ncaa-action-the-effects-of-lia-thomas-situation-are-akin-to-doping/ (June 18, 2023).

Lowen, Alexander. *Pleasure: A Creative Approach to Life* (Hinesburg, Vermont: The Alexander Lowen Foundation, 2013).

Lukianoff, Greg and Jonathan Haidt, "The Coddling of the American Mind," *The Atlantic*, September 2015. https://www.theatlantic.com/magazine/archive/2015/09/the-coddling-of-the-american-mind/399356/ (July 13, 2023).

Marchiano, Lisa. "Misunderstanding a New Kind of Gender Dysphoria," Quillette, October 6, 2017. https://quillette.com/2017/10/06/misunderstanding-new-kind-gender-dysphoria/ (August 10, 2023).

Marchiano, Lisa. "The Ranks of Gender Detransitioners Are Growing. We Need to Understand Why," Quillette, January 2, 2020. https://quillette.com/2020/01/02/the-ranks-of-gender-detransitioners-are-growing-we-need-to-understand-why/ (August 9, 2023).

Marchiano, Lisa. "Trans Activism's Dangerous Myth of Parental Rejection," Quillette, July 20, 2018. https://quillette.com/2018/07/20/trans-activisms-dangerous-myth-of-parental-rejection/ (August 11, 2023).

Marchiano, Lisa. "Transgenderism and the Social Construction of Diagnosis," Quillettee, March 1, 2018. https://quillette.com/2018/03/01/transgenderism-social-construction-diagnosis/ (August 10, 2023).

Marchiano, Lisa. "What Depth Psychology Can Tell Us About Victimhood Culture," Quillette, December 27, 2017. https://quillette.com/2017/12/27/collision-reality-depth-psychology-can-tell-us-victimhood-culture/ (August 11, 2023).

Marwha, Dhruv, Meha Halari, and Lise Eliot. "Meta-analysis reveals a lack of sexual dimorphism in human amygdala volume," *NeuroImage*, Volume 147, February 15, 2017, 282–294.

Marx, David M. and Jasmin S. Roman. "Female Role Models: Protecting Women's Math Test Performance," *Personality and Social Psychology Bulletin*, Volume 28, Number 9, September 2002, 1183–1193.

Mascaro, Jennifer S., Kelly E. Rentscher, Patrick D. Hackett, et al. "Child gender influences paternal behavior, language, and brain function," *Behavioral Neuroscience*, June 2017, Volume 131(3), 262–273.

Matuszczak, Ewa, Marta Diana Komarowska, Wojciech Debek, and Adam Hermanowicz. "The Impact of Bisphenol A on Fertility, Reproductive System, and Development: A Review of the Literature," *International Journal of Endocrinology*, Volume 2019, Article ID 4068717. https://doi.org/10.1155/2019/4068717.

"Mayo Clinic Disciplinary Letter to Michael J. Joyner, March 5, 2023," FIRE (Foundation for Individual Rights and Expression). https://www.thefire.org/research-learn/mayo-clinic-disciplinary-letter-michael-j-joyner-march-5-2023 (July 11, 2023).

McCall, Becky. "75% of Transgender Women Fail to Suppress Testosterone," Medscape, March 1, 2018. https://www.medscape.com/viewarticle/893280?form=fpf (August 22, 2023).

McComb, Carly A., Eric J. Vanman, and Stephanie J. Tobin, "A Meta-Analysis of the Effects of Social Media Exposure to Upward Comparison Targets on Self-Evaluations and Emotions," *Media Psychology*, February 23, 2023.

McHugh, Paul. "Psychiatric misadventures," *American Scholar* 61 (7):497–510. Also at https://www.transgendermap.com/politics/psychiatry/paul-mchugh/ (November 15, 2023).

McHugh, Paul. "Surgical Sex: Why We Stopped Doing Sex Change Operations," First Things, November 2004. www.firstthings.com/article/2004/11/surgical-sex (July 23, 2020).

McHugh, Paul. "Transgenderism: A Pathogenic Meme," *Public Discourse*, June 10, 2015. www.thepublicdiscourse.com/2015/06/15145 (July 20, 2020).

McLean, Dorothy Cummings. "At world's first gender 'detransition' conference, women express regret over drugs, mutilation," Life Site News, December 2, 2019. www.lifesitenews.com/news/at-worlds-first-gender-detransition-conference-women-express-regret-over-drugs-mutilation (August 25, 2020).

McLean, Siân, Rachel F. Rodgers, Amy Slater, et al. "Clinically significant body dissatisfaction: prevalence and association with depressive symptoms in adolescent boys and girls," *European Child & Adolescent Psychiatry*, December 2022; 31(12): 1921–1932.

"Men Still Pick 'Blue' Jobs and Women 'Pink' Jobs," *The Economist*, February 16, 2019. www.economist.com/finance-and-economics/2019/02/16/men-still-pick-blue-jobs-and-women-pink-jobs (July 13, 2020).

Meybodi, Azadeh Mazaheri, Ahmad Hajebi, and Atefeh Ghanbari Jolfaei. "Psychiatric Axis I Comorbidities among Patients with Gender Dysphoria," *Psychiatry Journal* 2014: 971–814.\

Diane Woods Middlebrook. *Suits Me: The Double Life of Billy Tipton* (Boston & New York: Houghton Mifflin Company, 1998).

Mitchell, Chelsea. "I was the fastest girl in Connecticut. But transgender athletes made it an unfair fight," *USA Today*, as revised by editor, May 26, 2021 (original published on May 22, 2021). https://www.usatoday.com/story/opinion/2021/05/22/transgender-athletes-girls-women-sports-track-connecticut-column/5149532001/?gnt-cfr=1 (June 22, 2023).

Mondschein, Emily R. Karen Adolph, and Catherine S. Tamis-LeMonda. "Gender Bias in Mothers' Expectations about Infant Crawling," *Journal of Experimental Child Psychology*, December 2000, 77(4).

Mones, Paul. "What Is Grooming?" 2023. https://www.paulmones.com/what-is-grooming/ (July 8, 2023).

Montero, Henry A. "Depression in Men: The Cycle of Toxic Masculinity," Psycom, June 8, 2022. https://www.psycom.net/depression/depression-in-men/toxic-masculinity (July 28, 2023).

Moorhead, Joanna. "Boys will be boys? How schools can be guilty of gender bias," *The Guardian*, April 23, 2019. www.theguardian.com/education/2019/apr/23/school-guilty-bias-against-boys-gender-gap-education (July 15, 2020).

Mordowanec, Nick. "Biden Official Praising Clinic Calling Moms 'Egg Producers' Sparks Outrage," *Newsweek*, August 17, 2023. https://www.newsweek.com/biden-official-praising-clinic-calling-moms-egg-producers-sparks-outrage-1820629 (October 8, 2023).

Muižnieks, Nils. *Human Rights and Intersex People*, April 1, 2015. Available at https://intersexrights.org/coe/issue-paper-human-rights-and-intersex-people/ (June 22, 2023).

National Sex Education Standards Core Content and Skills, K-12, Second Edition (Future of Sex Education Initiative: 2020). https://advocatesforyouth.org/wp-content/uploads/2020/03/NSES-2020-web.pdf.

Navratilova, Martina. "The rules on trans athletes reward cheats and punish the innocent," *The Sunday Times*, February 17, 2019. https://www.thetimes.co.uk/article/the-rules-on-trans-athletes-reward-cheats-and-punish-the-innocent-klsrq6h3x (June 18 2023).

Nehls, Michael. *The Indoctrinated Brain: How to Successfully Fend Off the Global Attack on Your Mental Freedom* (New York, NY: Skyhorse Publishing, 2023).

Newgent, Scott. "We Need Balance When It Comes To Gender Dysphoric Kids. I Would Know," *Newsweek*, February 9, 2021. https://www.newsweek.com/we-need-balance-when-it-comes-gender-dysphoric-kids-i-would-know-opinion-1567277 (August 9, 2021).

Newman, Kurt, Judson Randolph, and Kathryn Anderson. "The Surgical Management of Infants and Children With Ambiguous Genitalia," *Annals of Surgery*, June 1992, 215(6): 644–653.

Newman, Sandra. "Man, weeping," Aeon, September 9, 2015. https://aeon.co/essays/whatever-happened-to-the-noble-art-of-the-manly-weep (July 28, 2023).

Nieves, J.W., C. Formica, J. Ruffing, et al, "Males have larger skeletal size and bone mass than females, despite comparable body size," *Journal of Bone and Mineral Research* 2005, 20(3), 529-535.

"Ninety Day Notice of Intent to Sue Pursuant to C.C.P. § 364," November 9, 2022, Limandri & Jonna LLP. https://www.dhillonlaw.com/wp-content/uploads/2022/11/Letter-of-Intent-Chloe-Cole.pdf

Noble, Elizabeth. *Primal Connections* (New York: Simon & Schuster, 1993).

Ann Oakley, *Sex, Gender, and Society* (U.S. and UK: Routledge, 2015).

Oransky, Matthew and Jeanne Marecek. "'I'm Not Going to Be a Girl': Masculinity and Emotions in Boys' Friendships and Peer Groups," *Journal of Adolescent Research*, January 2009, 24(2): 218–241.

Paoletti, Jo. *Pink and Blue: Telling the Girls From the Boys in America* (Bloomington and Indianapolis: Indiana University Press, 2012).

"Parents Lose Custody For Refusing Child Sex-Change." Pulpit & Pen, February 16, 2018. https://pulpitandpen.org/2018/02/16/parents-lose-custody-refusing-child-sex-change/ (July 20, 2020).

Parents with Inconvenient Truths about Trans (PITT). "Learning from the Detransitioners," April 29, 2022. https://pitt.substack.com/p/learning-from-the-detransitioners (August 3, 2023).

Pasha-Robinson, Lucy. "Children feel they are treated differently because of their gender, finds survey," *Independent*, January 18, 2018. www.independent.co.uk/news/uk/home-news/gender-difference-children-education-teachers-parents-family-survey-a8164321.html (September 29, 2020).

Patel, Jainish and Prittesh Patel. "Consequences of Repression of Emotion: Physical Health, Mental Health and General Well Being," *International Journal of Psychotherapy Practice and Research*, Volume 1, Issue 3, February 12, 2019, 16–21.

Patterson, Meagan M. and Rebecca S. Bigler. "Preschool Children's Attention to Environmental Messages About Groups: Social Categorization and the Origins of Intergroup Bias," *Child Development*, Volume 77, Issue 4, July 25, 2006, 847–860.

Payne, Daniel. "The Transgender Suicide Rate Isn't Due To Discrimination," *The Federalist*, July 7, 2016. https://thefederalist.com/2016/07/07/evidence-the-transgender-suicide-rate-isnt-due-to-discrimination (July 17, 2020).

Perry, Louise. "What Is Autogynephilia? An Interview with Dr Ray Blanchard," Quillette, November 6, 2019. https://quillette.com/2019/11/06/what-is-autogynephilia-an-interview-with-dr-ray-blanchard/ (May 1, 2023).

Pong, Yuan-Hung, Yu-Chuan Lu, Vinscent F.S. Tsai, et al. "Acute manic and psychotic symptoms following subcutaneous leuprolide acetate in a male patient without prior psychiatric history: A case report and literature review," *Urological Science* 25, 2014, 22–24.

Radke, Elizabeth G., Audrey Galizia, Kristina A.Thayer, and Glinda S.Cooper. "Phthalate exposure and metabolic effects: a systematic review of the human epidemiological evidence," *Environmental International* Volume 132, November 2019.

"Report of the Special Grand Jury on the Investigation of Loudoun County Public Schools, Case No. CL-22-3129," December 2022. https://www.oag.state.va.us/media-center/news-releases/2503-december-5-2022-special-grand-jury-releases-report-on-loudoun-county-public-schools (April 18, 2023).

Ridgeway, Cecilia L. and Shelley J. Correll. "Unpacking the Gender System: A Theoretical Perspective on Gender Beliefs and Social Relations," *Gender & Society*, Volume 18, Number 4, August 2004, 510–531.

Rigbgy, Sara. "22 pioneering women in science history you really should know about," Science Focus, March 8, 2023. https://www.sciencefocus.com/science/10-amazing-women-in-science-history-you-really-should-know-about/ (May 11, 2023).

Roberts, Timothy A., Joshua Smalley, and Dale Ahrendt. "Effect of gender affirming hormones on athletic performance in transwomen and transmen: implications for sporting organisations and legislators," *British Journal of Sports Medicine* 2021, No. 55, 577–583.

Rostad, Whitney, Daniel Gittins-Stone, Charlie Huntington, et al. "The Association Between Exposure to Violent Pornography and Teen Dating Violence in Grade 10 High School Students," *Archives of Sexual Behavior* 48, July 15, 2019, 2137–2147.

Rudman, Laurie A. and Peter Glick. "Feminized Management and Backlash Toward Agentic Women: The Hidden Costs to Women of a Kinder, Gentler Image of Middle Managers," *Journal of Personality and Social Psychology* 1999, Volume 77, Number 5.

Rufo, Christopher F. "The Real Story Behind Drag Queen Story Hour," *City Journal*, Autumn 2022. https://www.city-journal.org/article/the-real-story-behind-drag-queen-story-hour (July 11, 2023).

Saiphoo, Alyssa N., Lilach Dahoah Halevi, and Zahra Vahedi. "Social networking site use and self-esteem: A meta-analytic review," *Personality and Individual Differences* Volume 153, January 15, 2020.

Salam, Maya. "What Is Toxic Masculinity?" *The New York Times*, January 22, 2019. www.nytimes.com/2019/01/22/us/toxic-masculinity.html (July 14, 2020).

Samuel, Sigal. "Elon Musk reveals his plan to link your brain to your smartphone, Vox, July 17, 2019. https://www.vox.com/future-perfect/2019/7/17/20697812/elon-musk-neuralink-ai-brain-implant-thread-robot (October 16, 2023).

Schaber, Ronja, Marie Kopp, Anna Zähringer, et al. "Paternal Leave and Father-Infant Bonding: Findings From the Population-Based Cohort Study DREAM," *Frontiers in Psychology* 2021; 12:668028.

Schemmel, Alec. "FDA warns puberty blocker may cause brain swelling, vision loss in children," ABC National Desk, July 26, 2022. https://katv.com/news/nation-world/fda-warns-puberty-blocker-may-cause-brain-swelling-vision-loss-in-children-rachel-levine (September 4, 2022).

Schilt, Kristen. "Just One of the Guys?: How Transmen Make Gender Visible at Work," *Gender and Society* 2006, 20 (4):465–490.

Schlosser, Edward. "I'm a liberal professor, and my liberal students terrify me," Vox, June 3, 2015. https://www.vox.com/2015/6/3/8706323/college-professor-afraid (July 13, 2023).

Schulz, Mona Lisa. *Awakening Intuition* (New York: Harmony Books, 1998).

Scott Newgent website, https://www.scottnewgent.com/ (August 9, 2023).

"Scott Newgent Unboxing | Becoming Trans Ruined My Life," undated. https://thestoryboxpodcast.com/podcast/scott-newgent-unboxing-becoming-trans-ruined-my-life/ (August 10, 2023).

Senefeld, Jonathon W., Massimo Franchini, Carlo Mengoli, et al. "COVID-19 Convalescent Plasma for the Treatment of Immunocompromised Patients: A Systematic Review and Meta-analysis," *JAMA Network Open*, January 12, 2023. https://jamanetwork.com/journals/jamanetworkopen/fullarticle/2800275?utm_source=For_The_Media&utm_medium=referral&utm_campaign=ftm_links&utm_term=011223 (July 11, 2023).

Servin, A., G. Bohlin, and L. Berlin. "Sex differences in 1-, 3-, and 5-year-olds' toy-choice in a structured play-session," *Scandinavian Journal of Psychology* March 1999; 40(1):43–48.

"Sex Reassignment Surgery Market to hit USD 1.5 Bn by 2026: Global Market Insights, Inc.," March 31, 2020. https://www.globenewswire.com/news-release/2020/03/31/2009112/0/en/Sex-Reassignment-Surgery-Market-to-hit-USD-1-5-Bn-by-2026-Global-Market-Insights-Inc.html (July 30, 2023).

Shaffi, Sarah. "Four times more male characters in literature than female, research suggests," *The Guardian*, April 12, 2022. https://www.theguardian.com/books/2022/apr/27/four-times-more-male-characters-in-literature-than-female-research-suggests (July 24, 2023).

Sharkey, Colleen. "New study first to define link between testosterone and father' social roles outside the family," Medical Xpress, September 24, 2020. https://medicalxpress.com/news/2020-09-link-testosterone-fathers-social-roles.html (September 26, 2020).

Shrier, Abigail. *Irreversible Damage: The Transgender Craze Seducing Our Daughters* (Washington, DC: Regnery Publishing, 2020).

Shumer, Daniel, Aser Abrha, Henry A. Feldman, and Jeremi Carswell. "Overrepresentation of Adopted Adolescents at a Hospital-Based Gender Dysphoria Clinic," *Transgender Health* 2017, 2(1): 76–79.

Smith, David, Judith Rosenstein, Margaret C. Nikolov, and Darby A. Chaney. "The Power of Language: Gender, Status, and Agency in Performance Evaluations," *Sex Roles* 2019, 80: 159–171.

Soares Filho, L.C., R.F.L. Batista, V.C. Cardoso, et al. "Body image dissatisfaction and symptoms of depression disorder in adolescents," *Brazilian Journal of Medical and Biological Research*, 2021, Volume 54 (1).

St. James, James. "25 (More) Examples of Male Privilege as Experienced By a Trans Man," Everyday Feminism, June 21, 2015. https://everydayfeminism.com/2015/06/more-male-privilege-trans-man/ (April 25, 2022).

St. James, James. "These 25 Examples of Male Privilege from a Trans Guy's Perspective Really Prove the Point," Everyday Feminism, May 30, 2015. https://everydayfeminism.com/2015/05/male-privilege-trans-men/ (January 14, 2021).

Storr, Will. "The rape of men: the darkest secret of war." *The Guardian*, July 16, 2011. https://www.theguardian.com/society/2011/jul/17/the-rape-of-men (May 9, 2023).

"Suicide Facts and Myths," Transgender Trend, undated. www.transgendertrend.com/the-suicide-myth/ (July 18, 2020).

Syb. "Purification Rites," April 26, 2022. https://sybmantics.substack.com/p/purification-rites?s=r (August 3, 2023).

Tabassum, Naznin and Bhabani Shankar Nayak. "Gender stereotyping is considered to be a significant issue obstructing the career progressions of women in management," *IIM Kozhikode Society & Management Review*, February 10, 2021, Volume 10, Issue 2, 192–208.

"Teacher Bias: The Elephant in the Classroom," Marco Learning, August 27, 2018. www.thegraidenetwork.com/blog-all/2018/8/1/teacher-bias-the-elephant-in-the-classroom/#download-teacher-bias (July 15, 2020).

Techenor, Veronica. "Maintaining Men's Dominance: Negotiating Identity and Power When She Earns More," *Sex Roles* 53, August 2005, 191–205.

"The global scale of child sexual abuse in the Catholic Church." Aljazeera, October 5, 2021. https://www.aljazeera.com/news/2021/10/5/awful-truth-child-sex-abuse-in-the-catholic-church (October 13, 2023).

Therapy or Torture? The Truth About Electroshock: A Supplement to the Documentary. Citizens Commission on Human Rights, 2019. https://www.cchr.org/ban-ect/?utm_campaign=redirecttherapy-or-torture-the-truth-about-electroshock.html&utm_medium=direct&utm_source=watch (October 10, 2023).

"The Status of Women in U.S. Media 2019." Women's Media Center, February 21, 2019. https://womensmediacenter.com/reports/the-status-of-women-in-u-s-media-2019 (July 15, 2020).

Thibault, Valérie, Marion Guillaume, Geoffroy Berthelot, et al. "Women and Men in Sport Performance: The Gender Gap has not Evolved since 1983," *Journal of Sports Science and Medicine*, June 2010, 9(2): 214–223. Also at https://www.ncbi.nlm.nih.gov/pmc/articles/PMC3761733/

Thoman, Dustin B., Paul H. White, Niwako Yamawaki, and Hirofumi Koishi. "Variations of Gender-math Stereotype Content Affect Women's Vulnerability to Stereotype Threat," *Sex Roles* 58, February 14, 2008, 702–712.

Tinari, Paul D. "Circumcision Permanently Alters the Brain," undated. https://circumcision.org/circumcision-permanently-alters-the-brain/ (May 8, 2018).

Todd, Erica V., Oscar Ortega-Recalde, Hui Liu, et al. "Stress, novel sex genes, and epigenetic reprogramming orchestrate socially controlled sex change," *Science Advances* 2019; Vol 5, No 7. https://www.science.org/doi/10.1126/sciadv.aaw7006 (June 15, 2023).

Tomey, Ramon. "Former trans teens express regret over gender reassignment procedures," Transhumanism.News, July 15, 2022. https://transhumanism.news/2022-07-15-former-trans-teens-express-regret-gender-reassignment.html# (August 9, 2023).

Transgender Regret, 2018 Dutch documentary. https://www.youtube.com/watch?v=1bV8AaeYKjQ (October 1, 2023).

Trigoso, Enrico. "Female Athlete Retires After Competing Against Biological Men, Says Girls 'No Longer Have a Fair Chance,'" *The Epoch Times*, May 31, 2023. https://www.theepochtimes.com/sports/female-athlete-retires-after-competing-against-biological-men-says-girls-no-longer-have-a-fair-chance-5301064?utm_source=Aomorningbriefnoe&src_src=Aomorningbriefnoe&utm_campaign=Aomb-2023-06-01&src_ (November 22, 2023).

Twenge, Jean M. "Have Smartphones Destroyed a Generation?" *The Atlantic*, September 2017.

Vandenbussche, Elie. "Detransition-Related Needs and Support: A Cross-Sectional Online Survey," *Journal of Homosexuality* 2022, Volume 69, Number 9, 1602–1620.

van der Kolk, Bessel. *The Body Keeps the Score* (New York: Penguin Books, 2014).

Van Loo, Katie J. and Robert J. Rydell. "On the experience of feeling powerful: perceived power moderates the effect of stereotype threat on women's math performance," *Personality and Social Psychology Bulletin*, March 2013; 39(3): 387–400.

Varela, Anna. "Society's Gender Expectations Alter Brain Cells," April 17, 2019, Futurity, www.futurity.org/gender-identity-brains-2037992 (July 15, 2020).

Welner, Michael. "Child Sexual Abuse: 6 Stages of Grooming," October 18, 2010. https://www.oprah.com/oprahshow/child-sexual-abuse-6-stages-of-grooming/all (July 8, 2023).

Wiik, A., T.R. Lundberg, E. Rullman, et al. "Muscle strength, size and composition following 12 months of gender-affirming treatment in transgender individuals: retained advantage for the transwomen," *BioRxiv*, September 26, 2019. https://www.biorxiv.org/content/10.1101/782557v1.full (May 7, 2023)

Winston, Robert and Rebecca Chicot. "The importance of early bonding on the long-term mental health and resilience of children." *London Journal of Primary Care* 2016; 8(1): 12–14.

Witmer, Denise. "The Media and Your Teen's Body Image," Very Well Mind, April 4, 2020. https://www.verywellmind.com/body-image-issues-teens-and-the-media-2609236#citation-1 (August 2, 2023).

"Women are beautiful, men rational," *Neuroscience News*, August 27, 2019. https://neurosciencenews.com/male-female-adjectives-14804/ (August 1, 2023).

"WPATH Gender Affirming Doctor Shows Concern For Mental Health of Minors After Transition Surgeries." Project Veritas, October 6, 2022. https://www.youtube.com/watch?v=9EYdzTPaguU (July 30, 2023).

Wright, Colin. "Intersex Is Not as Common as Red Hair," Reality's Last Stand, December 7, 2020. https://www.realityslaststand.com/p/intersex-is-not-as-common-as-red (August 18, 2023).

Wright, Colin. "Sex Chromosome Variants Are Not Their Own Unique Sexes," Reality's Last Stand, December 1, 2020. https://www.realityslaststand.com/p/sex-chromosome-variants-are-not-their (August 18, 2023).

Wright, Colin. "What is a Woman? Debunking Myths About the Biology of Sex," ICONS [Independent Council on Women's Sports] Conference, June 27, 2022, Las Vegas, Nevada. https://www.youtube.com/watch?v=5-rhLH5lYi4&t=805s (July 3, 2023).

Index

46,XY, 31, 293, 296
Aboli, Laura, 188–189
Abortion, 264–266
Acronyms, 193–194
Activity/energy levels of boys versus girls, 16
Academy of Breastfeeding Medicine, 196
Acupuncture meridians, effects of surgery on, 350
ADD / ADHD as a factor in transgendering, 114, 239
Adrenal glands
    diseases of, 28–29
    physiology of, 4–5
    stress symptoms of, 226–227
Affirmative action, 245
American Psychiatric Association, 109–110
American Psychological Association, 111
Amygdala, 47, 66–67
Androgen hormones, 5, 27–28, 29, 31, 32, 103, 290, 293, 296, 300
Androgen Insensitivity Syndrome (AIS), 27–28
Atrazine as endocrine disruptor, 135–136. *See also* Puberty blockers for children
Athletes. *See* Sports
Autism as a factor in transgendering, 91, 114, 133, 165, 239, 261
Autogynephilia, 146–147
Autonomic nervous system, 52, 225–226, 229
Barres, Ben, 56, 71, 153–156
Bathrooms
    segregated (racially), 72
    shared ("gender-neutral"), 110, 118–119, 216–218
Bailey, J. Michael, 125, 146
Beauty
    pageants, 199, 263
    standards of, 80–81, 141, 199–200, 305
Biggs, Michael, 126–127, 184
Bilek, Jennifer, 177, 184–186, 187, 247–248
Bisexuality. *See* Homosexuality
Blanchard, Ray, 88–89, 146
Body image in girls and women, 141, 199–200, 305
Body-oriented expressions, 223–224
Bono, Chaz, 98
Bottom surgeries, 105–108
Bowers, Marci, 104
BPA (Bisphenol A) as endocrine disruptor, 134–135, 333. *See also* Puberty blockers

Brain. *See also* Neurotransmitters
    effects of stress on, 227–228
    hormonal influences on, 12–14
    myths of male versus female brains, 11–21
    neuroplasticity (malleability) of, 7–9, 51–80, 318
    protective supplements for, 349
Breasts
    binding of breasts, 107
    breastfeeding, 196
    removal of, including complications, 107, 167
Breathing
    exercise, 349
    physiology and function of, 224–225
    sexual sensation and, 234
    shallow, effects of, 349
Budweiser ad campaign, 183
Categorizing versus assigning (sex), 38–39
Chemical castration. *See* Puberty blockers
Chromosomes, 3-4, 24
Circumcision, 312
"Cis" terminology, 194–195
Clothing, 80–82, 317
"Coddling of the American Mind," 208, 211
Cole, Chloe, 166–168
Colleges. *See* Schools
Colors, gender-specific, 317
Competitiveness, 19–20, 307
Congenital Adrenal Hyperplasia, (CAH) 28–29
Convalescent plasma therapy, 202–205, 344
Cooper, Brett, 121
Corpus callosum, 9–11
Cross-dressing, 145, 147
Crying,
    ease of, comparing males and females, 67, 68, 69
    and estrogen, 96
    father's sensitivity to in infant, 77
    history of, 65–66
Cult, characteristics of, 200–201
De la Chapelle Syndrome, 30–31
Detransitioner accounts, 162–173
Detransitioning
    percentage of detransitioners, 158–160
    roadblocks to, 157–162
Diagnostic and Statistical Manual of Mental Disorders (*DSM*), 132, 143
Divergences (or Differences) of Sexual Development (DSD)
    surgery for, 32–38, 144–145
    social treatment of, 156
    types of, 24–32
DNA, 3, 51–52, 72, 77, 134
Dopamine and the brain, 21–22, 207
Doping, 284, 290, 291, 294

Doping alternatives, 357–358
Doxing, 117
Drag
    history of, 179–180
    performances for children, 180–181
Drag Story Hour (DSH). *See* Drag
Drug "side" effects, 99–104, 103, 126, 127, 166–167, 308–309. *Also see* individual drugs
Electroshock, 201–202, 255
Eliot, Lise, 4, 9, 10, 11, 14, 16, 18, 20, 45, 55, 62, 63, 66–67, 68, 69, 80, 306
Emotional awareness
    in boys, 65–70
    in college students, 206, 207–214
    in the general population, 222–223
    in girls, 69–70
Emotions. *See also* Trauma
    and breathing, 224
    cultural differences in, 348
    and pleasure 231–235
    stifling, effects of, 68–70, 223–235
Empathy, 76–80
Endocrine disrupters, 134–136, 333. *See also* Puberty blockers
Epigenetics, 51–55, 63–65, 77, 318. *See also* Brain, neuroplasticity (malleability) of
Eskridge, Ash, 178
Estrogen
    and the brain, 12–14, 22, 23, 77
    emotions and, 154
    nonsexual effects of, 6
    sex-linked physical effects of during normal development, 5–6
    transgendering effects of, 95–96
Equality between the sexes, 242–249
Eye contact, 225
Fatherhood, 52–53, 76–80
Fausto-Sterling, Anne, 10, 26, 34, 72–73, 82, 315
Female genital mutilation (FGM), 311–312
Femininity. *See also* Masculinity
    definition of, 48–51
    toxic, 262–264, 353–354
Feminism
    definitions of, 244–246
    first wave feminist movement, 251–254, 351–352
    phony feminists, 258
    second wave feminist movement, 254–258
    third wave feminist movement, 258–274
Fine, Cordelia, 4, 12–14, 19–20, 21, 46–47, 51, 58, 59, 64, 75, 77, 79–80
Finch, Alan, 123, 199
Fisher, Helen, on four brain types, 21–23
Friedan, Betty, 255
GABA (gamma-aminobutyric acid), 22, 226, 228, 308–309
Gaines, Riley, 286–287
Gays. *See* Homosexuality

Gays Against Groomers, 182, 184, 193, 275
Gender
    "affirmation" 88, 192–193
    cross-cultural differences, 324
    meaning of, 43–45
    "reassignment," 87–108
    roles. *See* Sex role stereotypes
    versus biological sex, 43–45
Gender dysphoria 87–93, 109–111
Genitals. *See also* Intersexuals and Surgery
    ambiguous, 24–25
    destruction of (female genital mutilation or FGM), 311–312
    destruction of (male circumcision), 311
Grooming (sexual), 181–182
Grossman, Miriam, 45, 94–95, 105, 139, 176, 235, 238–239
Gynecomastia, 100, 136
Haldane, Sean, 67, 68–69, 224, 225, 237–238
Heyer, Walt 111–112, 147–148, 162–163
Homosexuality
    acceptance of children by parents, 93–95
    as different from transgenderism, 193
    fear of, 18, 49, 67–68, 143, 151–152
    sex role nonconformity and, 82–84
Hormones. *See also* Estrogen, Testosterone, and other individual hormones
    costs, 175–176
    cross-sex hormone treatments, 87, 95–98. *See also* Puberty blockers
    functions of, 4–6
    and sex differentiation, 4
Hormone Replacement Therapy (HRT), 92, 95–98, 176. *See also* Hormones
Housework, value of, 243, 255–256
Internet algorithms favoring transgenders, 115–116. *See also* Social media
Intersexuals
    chromosomal and hormonal differences in, 24–38
    conditions ascribed to, 27–32
    incidence of, 25–27, 308
    in sports, 292–298
    surgery performed on, 32–38
Jane, Layla, 168–169
Jaye, Cassie, 274
Jeffreys, Sheila, 83, 105–106, 119, 122, 174, 195, 196, 198, 203
Jennings, Jazz, 105, 137–139, 235
Job satisfaction, 242–244
Jones, Van, 211–212
Jorgensen, Christine, 83
Joyner, Michael, 203–204
Kelly, Megyn, 198–199, 286
Kerschner, Helena, 169–170
Krolczyk, Olivia, 197–198
Labiaplasty, 314–315
Language as propaganda and indoctrination, 191–200, 296
Lawsuits, 36, 120, 121, 166, 168, 216–218, 298–299

Leadership, 49–50, 51, 74–75
Lesbianism. *See* Homosexuality
Liberman, Mark, 47, 62
Littman, Lisa, 90, 140, 159–160, 203
Loudoun County rape case, 216–218
Lowen, Alexander, 224, 225, 231–232, 234
Lupron, 100, 103, 126, 127, 166–167
Male bashing, 264
Marchiano, Lisa, 90–91, 93–94, 98, 129, 143–144, 162, 213
Masculinity. *See also* Femininity
    definition of, 48–51
    toxic, 258–261, 353
Mathematics ability, 58–61
McHugh, Paul, 96–97, 102, 109, 122, 200
Medication costs for transgenders, 175–176
Mental illness, 109–130, 346
Metoidioplasty, 108
Microaggressions, 208, 345
Military
    and drag queens, 182
    and rape, 267–268
Mind-body connection, 221–231
Money, John 312–313
Montero, Henry, 68, 259
Motherhood, 52–53, 76–80
Neuroplasticity. *See* Brain, neuroplasticity (malleability) of
Neurotransmitters, 21–23, 221, 223, 226, 227–228, 308–309
Newgent, Scott, 123–124, 156, 158, 171–173, 175
"Niceness" syndrome, 74–76
North Face drag advertising, 183
Oakley, Ann, 43–44
OCD (obsessive-compulsive disorder) as a factor in transgendering, 133, 165, 239
Orgasm. *See also* Pleasure
    benefits of, 77, 104, 234
    breathing and, 234
    emotional repression and, 256
    interference via hormones and surgery, 33, 34, 104, 139, 157, 163–164
Owens, Candace, in *The Greatest Lie Ever Sold*, 184
Oxytocin, 5, 76–77, 104, 226, 228
Pain threshold, 15
Parasympathetic nervous system, 52, 225, 230
Parents
    custody battles, 215–216
    support of their children, 93–95
    schools against, 114–115
Parents with Inconvenient Truths about Trans (PITT), 133
Pedophilia, 180, 181–82, 342. *See also* Grooming
Penis, fake
    construction of, 107–108
    problems with after surgery, 107–108
Phalloplasty, 107–108

Pinkett, Matt, 56–57
Plastics. *See* Endocrine disrupters
Play, 16. *See also* Toys
Political correctness, 210, 211, 345
Polycystic Ovary Syndrome (PCOS), 29, 103, 296
Pornography, 142
Praise, person versus process, 53–54, 60
Progesterone, 5
Promiscuity, 307–308
Pronouns, 198–199
Propaganda. *See* Language as propaganda and indoctrination
Psychotherapy
    choosing a therapist, 238–240
    questions to ask would-be transitioners, 240–241
    mistreatment of transitioners during, 90–91, 117
    versus drugs and surgeries for trans-identified clients, 128–130
Puberty blockers for children, 98–104, 139
Quotas, 245
Raab, Michaela, 36–37
Rape (of both females and males), 266–274
Rapid-onset gender dysphoria (ROGD), 90–91, 125
Reassignment. *See* Gender "reassigment"
Reimer, David, 312–314
Reproductive organs, simultaneous male and female, 33
Research, scientific
    Dutch studies known for being fraudulent, 112–114
    fraudulent or misleading, general, 45–47
Richards, Renée, 279–280
Rufo, Christopher, 179–180
Schools
    anti-parent agendas, 114–115
    learning issues for boys and girls, 55–58. *See also* individual subjects
Science
    and female participation in, 70–74
    studies falsified, 45–47, 112–113
Semenya, Caster, 292–297
Serotonin, 21, 22, 223, 308–309
Sex
    act, as pleasure, 266
    assignment, 38–39
    change in animals, 315–316
    development in humans, 3–7
    versus gender, 43–45
Sexism
    in books, 50, 57–58
    in business, 74–76, 153–154
    general, 148-151
    social, 67–69

Sex role stereotypes
    causing changes in the brain, 51–55
    effects of, 48–80
    and sexual orientation, 82–84
Sexual
    abuse. *See* Grooming
    dimorphism, 26, 67, 154
    orientation. *See* Homosexuality
Shapiro, Ben, 169, 246–247
Shrier, Abigail, 89–90, 114, 139–140, 142, 143, 144, 178, 197, 199
Social contagion, 91, 140, 169
Social media
    effects of, 206–208
    as weapon of trans agenda, 140, 157–158, 168, 170, 178, 188
Soy as endocrine disruptor, 136
Spatial skill, 61–62, 63–65
Sports
    biological and physiological differences between males and females, 275–279
    injuries to women by male-bodied athletes, 288–290
    International Olympic Committee (IOC), 301–303
    intersexuals in sports, 292–298
    men and MtF transgenders in women's sports, 280–290
    wage disparity between male and female pro athletes, 359
    women and FtM transgenders in men's sports, 290–292
Standard of care, 92, 176
Steroids. *See* Hormones and Doping
Students. *See also* School
    anxiety in, 346–347
    infantilizing of, 206–214
Suicide, 96, 100, 103, 111–113, 122-127, 172, 202, 229, 239, 247, 264
Surgery
    costs, transgender-related, 114, 175–176
    FtM, 107–108
    MtF, 105–106
Syb (a detransitioner), 165
Sympathetic nervous system, 52, 225–230
Target "pride" displays, 1183
Teacher biases, 55–58, 61, 70–71
Testosterone
    and the brain, 12–14, 22, 23
    and dominance / aggression, 321
    gestational effects of, 4
    nonsexual effects of, 6–7
    sex-linked physical effects of during normal development, 5
    transgendering effects of, 97–98, 144, 169–170, 171–172
Tipton, Billy, 307
Toxic femininity, 262–264, 353–354
Toxic masculinity, 258–261

Toys, 16–19, 60 (Barbie), 306–307, 318
Transgendering. *See also* Hormones and Surgery
    costs of hormones and surgeries, 114, 175–176
    definition of, xiv–xv
Transgender movement
    as a cult, 200–201
    funding of, 175–177
    retaliation and violence from, 117, 118–122, 160–162, 202–203
Transgender Regret (Dutch documentary), 116–117
Transhumanism, 186–189
Transition
    how to help those considering, 238–242
    protocols, 87–108
Transitioning, reasons for
    boys, 114, 133–139
    girls, 114, 139–144
    men, 145–148
    women, 148–153
    adults with Divergences of Sexual Development, 153–156
Trauma. *See also* Detransitioner accounts and Psychotherapy
    biochemistry of, 237–238
    contributing to desire to transition, 90–91, 111–112, 140–141, 143, 145, 147–148, 151, 157–158, 159–160
Tullip (a detransitioner), 163–164
Twiggy, 199–200
Universities. *See* Schools
U.S. Transgender Survey, 106, 107, 108, 142, 158, 159
Vaccines, 344
Vagina, biological
    appearance, 314–315
    function, 105–106
Vagina, fake
    construction of, 105–106
    problems with after surgery, 33–36, 105–106, 138–139, 163–164, 165, 171–172
van der Kolk, Bessel, 230, 237
Verbal fluency, 61–63
Victimhood, 206–214
Voice changes for FtM transgenders, 107, 144, 151, 172
Violence against females. *See* Bathrooms, shared ("gender-neutral") and Rape
Violence against males. *See* Rape
Visual orientation of boys, 15
Völling, Christiane, 36
Wage disparity, 75–76, 351, 352
Women, derogatory terms pertaining to and negating, 196–200
WPATH (World Professional Association for Transgender Health), 113, 176, 185, 188
Wright, Colin, 24, 26–27, 37
XY with 5-α-Reductase Deficiency, 30
Younger, Jeffrey, 215–216

About the Author

Carla Curtis participated in the second wave feminist movement, later becoming active in the gay and bisexual liberation movements as well. For twenty years she worked as a body-mind psychotherapist, incorporating numerous holistic healing modalities into her practice. Her writing on sexuality, feminism, and psychology (under a different name) has appeared in many magazines, journals and anthologies, as well as books published by Simon & Schuster and Skyhorse Publishing. This is her first book with Gays Against Groomers.

About Gays Against Groomers

www.GaysAgainstGroomers.com

Gays Against Groomers is a nonprofit organization of gays, lesbians, and others in the community who oppose the sexualization, indoctrination, and mutilation of children under the guise of radical "LGBTQIA+" activism. We are moms and dads, couples, siblings, husbands and wives, families and friends, typical gay American men and women who live our lives just like everyone else. Our mission is twofold: to end the war on children being carried out in our name, and to reclaim the community we once called our own, which at this point has become unrecognizable.

What we are witnessing is mass-scale child abuse being perpetuated on an entire generation, and we will no longer sit by and watch it happen. From its inception in 2022, Gays Against Groomers has shut down "family-friendly" drag shows aimed at children, lobbied for bills preventing child abuse and mutilation, given speeches at school board meetings, organized rallies and protests, spoken out from within the community, and endorsed candidates who unequivocally condemn the current state of the gender movement as much as we do.

Gender ideology isn't just a neo-religious cult; it is biotechnological warfare in drag. The propaganda machine is relentless, like a multi-headed hydra with claws in every corporate sector. The fervent disciples of this ideology—who endorse it in mainstream media—fail to represent the interests and concerns of gay people. Trans agenda proponents have sold their souls to a belief system that is wreaking havoc in our schools, in our government and legal sector, and in the medical establishment, at the expense of millions like us who disagree with prioritizing so-called "gender identity" over material reality. We of Gays Against Groomers are determined to put a stop to this insanity once and for all. All like-minded individuals are welcome to join us in our goal to protect children.

—*Michael Costa, head of Gays Against Groomers Publishing*

Helpful Resources:
gaysagainstgroomers.com/resources

Helpful Studies:
radar.gaysagainstgroomers.com/posts/categories/studies

Support Gays Against Groomers:
gaysagainstgroomers.com/donate

Get official Gays Against Groomers merchandise:
shop.gaysagainstgroomers.com

Listen to The Dark Side of the Rainbow podcast:
gaysagainstgroomers.com/podcast

Join Gays Against Groomers
gaysagainstgroomers.com/join